W9-BXM-719

POLIO AND ITS AFTERMATH

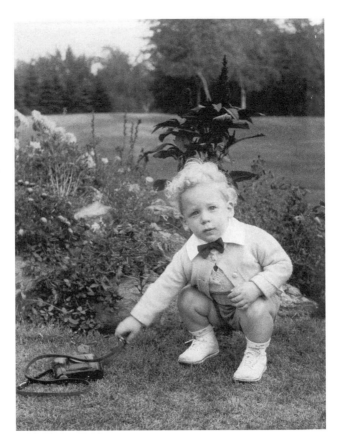

Picking up where he left off.

POLIO AND ITS AFTERMATH

THE PARALYSIS OF CULTURE

MARC SHELL

HARVARD UNIVERSITY PRESS
Cambridge, Massachusetts
London, England
2005

Library of Congress Cataloging-in-Publication Data

Shell, Marc.
    Polio and its aftermath : the paralysis of culture / Marc Shell.
      p. cm.
    Includes bibliographical references and index.
    ISBN 0-674-01315-8
    1. Poliomyelitis—Social aspects—United States.   2. Poliomyelitis—Biography.
    3. People with disabilities in motion pictures.   I. Title.

RC181.U5S53 2005
616.8′35—dc22   2004060562

Aftermath: Second or later mowing; the crop of grass which springs up after the mowing in early summer.

—*A New English Dictionary on Historical Principles*, 1884–1928

Contents

POLIO AND ITS AFTERMATH

PROLOGUE

It isn't the war that matters, it's the after-war. The world we're going down into.

—George Orwell, *Coming Up for Air* (1939)

For seventy years, polio traumatized the world. The epidemic closed down New York City during the two-month quarantine of Manhattan Island. An American president suffered from its paralyzing effects. So did sixty million other people worldwide. Even when polio did not kill its victims outright, it often crippled them for life. The survivors were the visible reminder of polio's ever-increasing power to slay, maim, and deform. The children of the relatively affluent middle class were affected as much as other people. No one knew what caused the disease, and there was no cure. All therapeutic and rehabilitative methods failed. During the seventy years in which polio epidemics were widespread, the various electronic media— cinema, radio, and television—were also coming into their own: polio influenced the formation of these media as much as they influenced the perception of polio on the part of terrified people and nation-states. The polio epidemics crystallized human uncertainties at the time of the two world wars, and the celebrated vaccine itself came on the scene a few years into the Cold War.

After all, it is no wonder that "the conquest of polio" in the mid-1950s was raised to genuinely iconic status in the West. The Salk vaccine was heralded as the beginning of a brave new world of universal health and safety. From now on, the world would be safe from polio and its ilk—perhaps, indeed, from all epidemic diseases. So great was the euphoria about the end of polio that, within a few years, the scientific hunt—the search to understand what polio had been and the research into what were the ongoing effects of polio on individual bodies and on bodies politic—was abruptly ended. A "total victory" was declared on polio—along the lines of Truman's declaration of total military victory against the Axis powers and of Cold War rhetoric.

The success of the polio prophylaxis made it easier, if not also politically inevitable, for researchers to put off medical investigation into what caused polio and what was still causing diseases like it. Areas of ignorance certainly remained, and problems just beneath the surface of celebration, but at that time we set aside searching for what therapeutic cures or rehabilitative treatments might be available for polio sufferers and others like them. We still do not know for sure even how the polio enterovirus enters the spinal column. There is still no cure for polio or even an effective treatment; the hundreds of thousands of cases of polio that the unvaccinated part of the world has seen since the 1950s bear testimony to the public health issues. Moreover, the purely prophylactic approach to polio put off important investigations in the social sciences. In the area of public health, for example, "the victory over polio" allowed us to take for "granted" the historically idiosyncratic combination of public and private philanthropy that had supported American polio research and treatment and to apply the private model to other medical issues, sometimes thoughtlessly. And even as the new vaccine made people supremely confident that the age of world epidemics was ended forever, it made it apparently unnecessary to deal with the various sociopathological approaches—military, pedagogical, cultural, familial, and medical—relevant to this disease and its tens of millions of crippled survivors. In the same way, belief in the victory over polio obscured just how polio was still affecting key aspects of our culture—literature, cinema, music, and the media and health businesses.

The conceptual misprision of polio in the twentieth century is already an old complaint: our raising the polio vaccine to the status of factotum helped erase awareness of the continuing presence of polio during the latter part of the twentieth century. Just that kind of erasure is, of course, a common trait of traumatic incidents in the development of individual human beings as well as of bodies politic. Reactions to the great influenza pandemic provide an example—its twenty million dead are all but forgotten. And yet, as we shall see, there is something peculiarly gripping about the case of polio, informing not only the reaction to the influenza pandemic at the beginning of the twentieth century but also the reaction to AIDS (acquired immuno-deficiency syndrome) at the end of that century.

Illness Narrative

> Men and germs are not widely different from each other.
>
> —Mark Twain, *Three Thousand Years among the Microbes* (1905)

Polio and Its Aftermath is a study of polio—its still evolving cultural, political, and medical history as well as its longstanding place in traumatic memory and suppressed memory. This study is pursued simultaneously on several methodological fronts. One of these fronts involves what is sometimes called the illness narrative. Dr. Roland Berg, in his midcentury medical book *Polio and Its Problems*, says half-tragically that his study is "the biography of a disease. Would that it were its obituary!"[1] Berg wished for something like the vaccine that Salk would discover just a few years later. As it turned out, however, the Salk vaccine was not enough to put polio to rest—as Salk himself knew.[2] That is *one* reason we still need an apt "biography" of polio.

Bentz Plagemann, in his first-person polio narrative *My Place to Stand*, reports that his wife half-comedically called his book about his polio years "the biography of an illness."[3] Mrs. Plagemann's gallows humor derives partly from the fact that a biography is "a written record of the life an individual"; it is not usually a history of a pandemic malady that affects the lives of millions of individuals.[4] Yet the disease polio lends itself well—at least in aesthetic terms—to being the subject of a biography. That is because polio was often thought of as being like an individual: first, in the particular way that the paralyzed person, "a polio," *becomes* his disease, polio—or vice versa (as in the boxed dialogue); and second, in that the lifespan of polio as a major worldwide epidemic (about seventy years) was close to that of an individual person.

Consider this nominal confusion between the name of the disease *(polio)* and the label attached to a person who has had that disease *(a polio)*, which stays with him, after the period of infection, throughout his life.[5] In this regard, the disease and its survivor are unique. Many people with some

A *Polio:* Dialogue

Moi: I don't much like the term *polio* when it means "a person who has had polio."

Lui: Well, *polio* is the usual dictionary term for "person who has had polio"—or "PWHHP." The term *polio* as such was much used in both medical and popular literature. A well-known, nationally syndicated series of newspaper articles was "I Am a Polio." And . . .

Moi: I don't like it. Polio suggests that the disease leaves its stamp on entire persons—even on their personalities. A person who has sickle-cell anemia would dislike being called a *sickler;* a person with leprosy ought to dislike being called *leper.*

Lui: I see what you mean. But no matter what the social stigma of having had polio (or lack of stigma), and no matter what the individual denial of having had polio (or acceptance of having had it), the PWHHP remains marked, if not also informed, by his disease.

Moi: Maybe. But mightn't we get along with some such term as *cripple?*

Lui: Not all cripples are polios. And not all polios are cripples. The same problem obtains for using the recently fashionable term *crip.* . . .

Moi: Why not use the term *polio survivor?* Those who have had polio have lived on past the initial event, whether damaged or not.

Lui: But the event, as you call it, is not over and done with. It has its sequelae. The event is ongoing—for some people or for many, perhaps even for all. The term *polio* manages to combine the period of initial contagion, as it were, with its lifelong consequences.

Moi: But is it the initial onslaught of polio that they never survive? Or is it, as you say, polio's sequelae that they fail to survive?

Lui: Again, the disease polio and its sequelae are, in this context, the same. One lives in the present. The sequelae and second coming, if they are not now, are to come. One does not live on—after them. Between a terminal condition and a comorbid one, it's only a matter of timing.

(continued)

> *Moi:* So no one has "survived" until he is dead?
>
> *Lui:* Yes. I suppose so *[He laughs, bitterly]*—as when Euripides enjoins us, in *The Trojan Women,* "Call no one happy until he is dead."
>
> *Moi:* It is an odd problem. *[Wonderingly]* Is the problem unique?
>
> *Lui:* Not . . . for Euripides.
>
> *Note:* Turnley Walker, *Rise Up and Walk* (New York: Dutton, 1950), refers to the series of magazine and newspaper articles entitled "I Am a Polio," syndicated by the North American Newspaper Alliance.

other illness or medical condition come to identify psychologically with their diseases, or their family members and compatriots may come to identify them sociologically with the disease affecting them.[6] Other illnesses than polio sometimes entail names for the disease and the diseased person that are merely similar.[7] However, polio and polios are different from most others. To begin with, polio is often personified as the Crippler, for example, as a shadowy, almost human sculptor who leaves his handiwork behind for all to see (photograph in Chapter 3).

More significantly, precise nomenclature for polio suggests that not only did his one-time encounter with polio, now "over," shape the polio's body; that momentous encounter with paralysis also shaped, and continues to shape, his mind. In her "Prologue" to *Small Steps,* the polio Peg Kehret writes about her encounter at the age of twelve with the disease: "When I began to write about my polio days, long forgotten memories bubbled to the surface. I was astonished by the intense emotions these memories brought with them. . . . Those months, more than any other time of my life, molded my personality."[8]

Leonard Kriegel, in his *Falling into Life,* writes, "I came to understand that my war with the virus would never be over. For the virus had created me."[9] Mark Twain's *Three Thousand Years among the Microbes* (1905), whose narrator pretends to have translated "the original manuscript" into English from "the original Microbic" language, is the fantastic autobiography of a germ which, through an accident of scientific experiment, has been transformed into a human being.[10]

The second way that polio was conceived as being like an individual person—the usual subject of biography—is that polio, as understood and historicized during the 1950s, had the same active life *(bios)* in chronological terms as does an individual human being: seventy years or so. The epidemics in North America were also believed to have begun around 1885, with the Vermont epidemic of 1893–1894 standing out as a key originating event; they mostly ended around 1955.[11] Hence, polio had a rhetorically reassuring "beginning," "middle" and, as we have stressed, "end," relatively easy to pinpoint.

The congruence of disease and person has affected polio's historiography considerably in the past half-century, and the rhetoric surrounding the disease made it too easy for the very few historians of medicine who have attempted to write the history of polio to organize those histories as if they were biographies.

Even so, biographies of polios lend themselves peculiarly well to access certain cultural problems. Part 1 of *Polio and Its Aftermath,* by including the story of my polio in relation to tens of others, demonstrates why this is the case, even as it offers more a focused comparative "metapathography" in the sociopathology of twentieth-century culture than an autobiography.[12]

Any account of what it means to live on *after* (survive) polio and simultaneously to live *with* (convive) its familial, social, and medical consequences has two methodological purposes that exist in productive tension with each other.[13] In telling a single person's story, with its all idiosyncrasies, I seek to close the differentiating gap between the individual and the general. While telling my own polio story, I provide citations from and references to hundreds of other accounts. Hence, by virtue of its strongly comparatist perspective, my illness narrative, however idiosyncratic, is not merely clinical, in the sometimes pejorative sense of "coldly detached and dispassionate, like a medical report or examination."[14]

Most autobiographies written by polios and many biographies written about polios depend on triumphant survival as an organizational structure, one that we usually also encounter in the post-Salk histories of polio.[15] Authors of such autobiographical and biographical works usually seem unaware of one another; yet they often offer the same wise counsel—about lifestyle, religion, love, and medical knowledge and the lack thereof.[16] They further record sage advice about how the reader too might survive in similar circumstances to those faced by a polio. Several books addressed by doctors to polio patients do the same.[17]

Polio and Its Aftermath makes reference to hundreds of book-length first-person polio narratives, not only in order to present certain aesthetic, literary, and occasionally eccentric aspects of other illness histories and stories (and in this way suggest how one might resolve their sometimes informing narratological difficulties) but also in order to demonstrate to what extent polio has been forgotten in the history of literature and medicine and to help recuperate the loss as far as possible. Dozens of these polio narratives are referenced here for the first time anywhere. (Four dozen are not listed in a single library catalogue *anywhere* in the world. I found most of them at secondhand bookstores in Canada, the United States, Tasmania, Australia, South Africa, Zimbabwe, Singapore, Mexico, France, and Germany.) Recently, a few reunion books have been put together containing various short polio testimonials, heavily edited into third-person stories or interviews. Among these would be Aitken, Caron, and Fournier's collection for Quebec, Ochoksla's for Poland, North's for Great Britain, and Sass's for the United States.[18] Such books movingly commemorate hospital-school reunions, but still more immediate and valuable are the original accounts written closer to the time of the events they describe—letters, scrapbooks, diaries, self-published work, and much else.

Library materials about polios from outside the usual commercial publishers' arena were especially difficult for me to find. Unpublished book manuscripts, self-published books, and even so-called children's books have been strangely "disappeared."[19] Their absence from the libraries, as well as from the general histories of childhood and the sociology of childhood disease, mirrors not merely the commercial publishing practices of the past but also the general reception of polio literature and the general repression of the memory of polio.[20]

Demography

Polio was a crisis not only for the individual but also for the group—both the family and the polis. *Polio and Its Aftermath* thus considers the various jurisdictions and administrative spaces in which the polio lives and is publicly defined and militarily controlled. The illness narrative of Part 1, for example, starts in Quebec and moves to the United States. This move across borders provides a cross-cultural viewpoint, politically as well as economically heterogeneous.

Beyond that, the chapters present a panoply of demographically and politically diverse viewpoints. As is true for most pandemics, the study of polio is usually sorted out by temporal and geographic category; for example, Whysall's essay "The 20 Who Can't Forget the 1953 Polio Epidemic" (1978) and Taylor's book *Polio '53* both focus on the single year 1953—a form of myopia that serves *faute de mieux* to define their subject.[21] Similarly myopic with regard to political space, Whysall discusses only Winnipeg (one city), and Taylor discusses only Alberta (one province).

No study yet written attempts in any way to take in the whole world of the polio pandemics or allows us to see the universal in the particular in the sense that a painting, say, might. Certainly, studies by the inclusively named World Health Organization do not comprehensively cover the world. All previous studies look instead for their defining limits to intraglobal units. Some use nation-state boundaries—as is the case of Chungkuo's study of China, Rutty's of Canada, and Schanke's of Norway.[22] Other studies examine smaller intranational or provincial units—Killalea's book on Tasmania or Lovett and Emerson's early work on Massachusetts.[23] Several studies are broken down by county.[24] Dozens of monographs are devoted to individual cities—as is Goodale's study of Buffalo and Emerson's of New York City.[25] Several works discuss smaller administrative units of a different sort—for instance, studies of polio hospital-schools, like Rancho los Amigos, Hope Haven, Santa Monica Rehabilitation, Warm Springs in Georgia, and Warm Springs in Texas.

All such works are defined by administrative, political, financial, or institutional limits. This focus has the artificial advantage of making narratology relatively easy and, in many ways, thorough. Such studies can even serve to guard against complicating matters by trying to account for differences of economic class, race, religion, or language within the same region or time. Thus, the distinction within the United States between the experiences of the black and the white populations is rarely addressed in such works as Lovett's. Likewise, the distinction within North America between the public health and research institutions in publicly funded Canada and the privately funded United States is rarely pursued, or even that between anglophone and francophone institutions in Quebec. Only recently has the field of medical geography begun to deal directly with this problem, an example being newer class-based studies of polio in Germany and Sweden.[26]

In the past, institutional funding organizations concerned with public health usually provided support according to certain political and administrative boundaries. That is why a proper historiography of polio must now include the study of the sociopathology—or at least the biases—of the public health, medical, and disability rights systems in a political jurisdiction.

In *Polio and Its Aftermath,* I am particularly interested in the American medical profession's approaches to polio, especially in the mid-twentieth century. Our main exemplary study in this area concerns hydrotherapy, whose widespread practice during the first five decades of the twentieth century and relative disappearance in the latter five unfortunately mimics the historical fate of polio studies. Among other medical responses to polio at this time are such treatments as the movement-arresting corset treatment (a subject in cinematographic—literally, "movement-writing" —works like *Rear Window* and paintings by the polio Frida Kahlo), the Sister Kenny method (which made its Australian inventor "the most popular woman in America"), and the injections of cobra venom and cod liver oil. Customary psychological treatments of polio at the time included play therapy, various psychoanalytic approaches, instruction in passing as a nonpolio, and deflection of concern with treating the patient toward concern with treating the caretakers. Our representative study here concerns tough love. Institutionally endorsed sociological treatments for dealing with polios include founding hospital rehabilitation schools for polios, orphanage hospitals for polio children unwanted by their parents, and various forms of programs aimed at reintegrating polios back into mainstream society or at allowing them to live on their own.

Similarly, we discuss various theories about the causes of polio in the first place. Flies? White bread? Pasteurization of milk? Poor diet in general? Lack of religious faith? Filthy Italian immigrants? Did dirty water cause polio? Alternatively, did clean water cause polio?[27] William McNeill, in his *Plagues and Peoples,* caught the irony that cleanliness was the culprit.[28] Had we dealt better in the first instance with the motivations behind all such false etiologies, it would have enabled us to confront the AIDS epidemic more intelligently.

Other ways in which the polio epidemic affected the culture in North

America as a whole touch on such matters as the flight to the suburbs and a remarkable institution of "handi-capitalism" supported by celebrity culture and the entertainment business: the art industry.

The Arts of Paralysis

In some ways, the relevant cultural effects of polio were overplayed in the first half of the century and then underplayed in the second half. Those effects range from literature to cinematography, from changing ideas about the image of the child to transforming notions about public health, and from a philosophy of static disability to one of kinetic ability.

In the literary realm, polio is a subject of much fiction and poetry. But literature about polio has been largely overlooked in all histories of the disease and most histories of literature. Here too the research for writing *Polio and Its Aftermath* involved working with secondhand bookstores at home and overseas. One of the best quasi-fictional books about polio is J. G. Farrell's novel *The Lung* (1965). Not one library or secondhand bookstore in the United States seemed then to have it. Eventually I found a copy in a secondhand bookstore in Cambridge, England.

Polio and Its Aftermath helps bring to the fore a school of literature—the Polio School—and offers examples of both narrative and poetic art. It is the mindfully understood link between body and mind that helps to characterize this literature. Leonard Kriegel, in his autobiographical novel, *The Long Walk Home*, writes, concerning the poliomyelitic scission of mind from body: "The knife of the virus severed legs from will and I found myself flat on my back, paralyzed with polio."[29] More than one psychiatrist has it that the patient who has had "paralytic polio" is differently aware than others—or than other paralyzed persons—are of being "trapped" inside a body. (*Trapped* is a common title of polio narratives.)[30] This is what the playwright Charles Mee says in his memoir, *A Nearly Normal Life*:

My sense of who I am . . . would never reside in a body that let me down; it moved instead into a mind that promised to be more trustworthy, more devious and elusive, that can escape when it needs to; that still, today, lives in a realm where it can take flight; that cannot be pinned down; that refuses to place its faith or trust in the *material* world. . . . I'm not crazy; I don't have multiple personalities; but I do know that the body I drag around and put here and there in the world is something separate from *my self.* In addition, sometimes I still want to hurt it for what it did to me, to take revenge against it, to let its aches and pains go unnoticed and untreated.[31]

This "sense" is far more than mental alienation as understood by physiotherapeutic and medical theorists. Such theorists often confused polio with the hysterical paralysis of shell shock and argued that alienation of mind from body was ultimately psychological in origin—a matter of "will."[32] The term *mental alienation* was used as a technical expression in the polio therapy of Elizabeth Kenny, which helped many thousands of polios come to uncertain terms with their paralysis—as Noreen Linduska reminds us in *My Polio Past.* As we shall see, however, the Kenny theory falls short.[33]

In the art of painting, too, we discover a Polio School, even as we consider the same in such arts of human movement as dance, puppetry, and ventriloquism. Along with music, opera, and theater, these are expressive forms involving self-conscious and willed bodily manipulation.

One of *the* central cultural developments of the twentieth century is cinematography. Cinematography was concerned, from its beginning, with defining the problem of stasis (paralysis) in still photography and then making it kinetic in some way; and, as it happens, the historical origin of cinematography coincided with that of the polio epidemics. Cinematography was part of an attempt—one that included early medical photography—to cure people stilled by still photography. As polio still-photographers like Dorothea Lange knew, cinematography cures by means of kinesis. The dozens of movies dealing with paralysis that are referenced in *Polio and Its Aftermath* would, if taken together, constitute a reinterpretation of the history of cinema.

I test and illustrate my propositions about cinematography in several ways. First, *Polio and Its Aftermath* refers explicitly to dozens of movies about polios or about persons with poliolike disabilities or illnesses as well as to television shows. Especially interesting archival cinematographic material exists from around the time of the earliest movies, when polio was just beginning to show its true colors. Second, *Polio and Its Aftermath* refers to some hundred and fifty movies that by their subject matter seem not to have to do with polio and yet are essentially concerned with paralysis and stasis. Third, I consider the cinematographic style and general themes of several movie directors paralyzed by polio. Finally, I have chosen for close analysis a particular text to test our main thesis. That text is the mid-twentieth-century movie *Rear Window* (1954), with its curiously corseted hero, a Hitchcock movie that came out halfway through the historical chronology of the cinema, as seen from the perspective of our own time. *Rear Window* provides our case study for kinesis and stasis of the body per se. The movie concerns paralysis—paresis and vertigo being common themes in Hitchcock—and *Rear Window*'s success derives from a careful balance between two apparent extremes: it is about polio, which was a concern central to its time, but it appears not to be about polio, an avoidance that was also central to its time.

Besides literature, painting, and cinema, another object of cultural study considered in *Polio and Its Aftermath* is the notion of childhood—an expected subject when one is considering the disease polio, often called infantile paralysis. Here, too, I encountered severe archival problems. Literature written *for* child polios had not been collected—except as a sort of accidental byproduct. Nor had writing *by* polio children, either published or not, been collected. Moreover, historians had made almost no attempt to consult the tens of thousands of letters written by children. The historian Naomi Rogers, in her *Dirt and Disease: Polio before FDR,* bemoans the absence of such material from the polio historiography; yet Rogers's book, which is excellent in its own right, repeats the same omission. When it comes to the disabled community, children in the twentieth century were hardly "the unexpected minority" (a phrase that forms the title of the 1982 book by Gliedman and Roth).[34] *Polio and Its Aftermath* thus helps bring to light a twentieth-century "history of childhood and disability." At the same time, it sheds light on the literary treatment of variably paralytic diseases in the case of such literary figures as the young Roman emperor Claudius (as described by Suetonius) and the lame prince Dolor (the main character in Craik's Victorian children's novella).[35]

One important stylistic aspect of this book about polio is its attention to specifically formal linguistic and photographic aspects of the representation of paralysis. That is what the polio Walter Scott, in contemplating his own way of fashioning sentences, viewed as the "paralytic custom of stuttering with my pen."[36]

A Face-Off

Many first-person narratives about illness attempt to heal, or at least to control the situation, by means of narrative reinterpretation of the self after an account of some moment of transformation.[37] Numerous other narratives train on the subject a certain professional acumen, or at least an intellectualizing coercion, that seems to transcend aesthetic and political perspectives in a different way. In recent decades, for example, two New York writers brought their "professional" experience to bear on the diseases they had just recently contracted: Robert Murphy and Susan Sontag. Both had relatively late-onset diseases (late, that is, compared with the onset of polio in childhood); and both have written meta-autobiographies relating to their profession.

The anthropologist Murphy's *Silent Body* concerns a case of adult-onset paralysis that leads to death. Murphy, who is dying, writes that his book "was conceived in the realization that my long illness with a disease of the spinal cord has been a kind of extended anthropological field trip, for through it I have sojourned in a social world no less strange to me at first than those of the Amazon forests. And since it is the duty of all anthropologists to report on their travels . . . this is my accounting."[38]

Murphy says that *The Silent Body* is "not my autobiography."[39] And claiming qua professional anthropologist that "disability is defined by society and given meaning by culture; it is a social malady," Murphy attempts to get at the "logic and meaning of his paralysis" in cross-cultural context.[40] Whereas the adult Murphy interprets his life before illness as a preparation for dealing with spinal paralysis, the childhood-onset polio sufferer sees his disease as a preparation for the life that follows polio—or as the preparation for what is now his whole life. Murphy remains ignorant even of the existence of such paralyzed colleagues at his own Columbia University as the polio Edward Le Comte, who published *Long Road Back* (1958) after an onset of polio in adulthood.

A more influential example of the omission of polio from a purportedly general account of disease in the twentieth century would be Susan Sontag's work. Sontag, who wrote in the wake of the Frankfurt School of social criticism, had cancer in 1976, when she wrote *Illness as Metaphor*. Written in lieu of a memoir, the book claims to consider tuberculosis and

cancer (her own illness) as problematic metaphors.[41] Having beaten cancer
("I . . . was cured of my own cancer, confounding my doctors' pessimism,"
she writes in *Illness as Metaphor*), Sontag went on to write a sequel, *AIDS
and Its Metaphors*.[42]

Sontag's general argument is that tuberculosis, cancer, and AIDS were
and are received metaphorically but that diseases should be received un-
metaphorically. Such an argument seems to rely on the notion that there is
such a thing as a "relatively appropriate, unmetaphorical reaction" to a disease.[43] Curiously, Sontag claims to find that reaction only in relation to polio. For our present purpose, the most telling aspect of Sontag's two books
concerns the author's otherwise near silence about polio—remarkable,
given the important place it has in her thinking about disease and metaphor; her outright errors about polio on the two occasions when she
breaks that silence; and the significance of that near silence, given the importance Sontag assigns to polio in her argument about the cultural sociology of twentieth-century diseases and given the concomitant silence
about polio in the twentieth century as whole.

Here is the first of the two passages that have to do explicitly with polio:
"Polio's effects could be horrific—it withered the body—but it did not
mark or rot the flesh: it was not repulsive. Further, polio affected the body
only, though that may seem ruin enough, not the face. The relatively appropriate, unmetaphorical reaction to polio owes much to the privileged
status of the face, so determining of our evaluation of physical beauty and
of physical ruin." Sontag here says that polio does not affect the face. This
claim matters to her argument, insofar as it allows her to argue that the reaction to polio was relatively "appropriate" and unmetaphorical. In fact,
however, polios are sometimes affected in their faces. Take, for example,
the case of Jean Chrétien, the former prime minister of Canada, part of
whose face is "frozen." Tens of first-person polio narratives carefully describe the relevant moments when their authors first see their own reflections in the mirror. Enid Foster of Southern Rhodesia, for example, reports in her autobiography, *It Can't Happen to Me*, how she first learns that
her mouth has been frozen into an unflinching grimace and her eyes paralyzed into an unblinking stare.[44] Such facially deforming cases as those of
Chrétien and Foster bear comparison, in this regard, with the sort of polio
that a curiously closeted Sontag seems to have had in mind: namely that of
President Franklin Delano Roosevelt. Roosevelt's paralysis, which seemed

to affect only his lower body, tends too much to define the understanding of polio by American intellectuals in the twentieth century.

In the passage quoted earlier, Sontag says that the effect of polio was not repulsive. Yet, polio did commonly result in something many people found distressing or off-putting. Polio's asymmetrical freezing of various muscles made for deformities so visually disturbing that the science or art of orthopedics partly owes its development to "making the crooked straight" in the age of the polio epidemics. (The name of this branch of medicine comes from the Greek terms *orthos,* "straight," and *paidos,* "child.") Orthopedists explicitly promised parents that their surgeries would make their polio children more attractive. Tens of thousands of untreated polios were called deformed, misshapen, or hunchbacked. Even the "fixed grimace" face of bulbar polios came up for consideration. Polios who could not afford surgeries often earned their living in the freak shows alongside the "repulsive slime woman" or "serpent boy." The polio Frog-Boy performed at circuses in New York in the 1940s—while Sontag was growing up there.[45] Many a magazine article from the 1950s had some such title as "I Married a Polio Victim" (1956).[46]

In the other passage where she mentions polio, Sontag also makes telling statements about the disease:

Cholera was perhaps the last major epidemic disease to fully qualify for plague status for almost a century. (I mean cholera as a European and American, therefore a nineteenth-century disease; until 1817 there had never been a cholera epidemic outside the Far East.) Influenza, which would seem more plague-like than any other epidemic in this century if loss of life were the main criterion, and which struck as suddenly as cholera and killed as quickly, usually in a few days, was never viewed metaphorically as a plague. Nor was a more recent epidemic, polio. One reason why plague notions were not involved is that these epidemics did not have enough of the attributes perennially ascribed to plagues. (For instance, polio was construed as typically a disease of children—of the innocent.)

Sontag is right that polio was generally seen in the United States as a disease of children. Yet polio was also sometimes a disease of adults. When, in Quebec, polio wiped out half the population of a town, most cases involved older adolescents and adults; and adults had the more severe cases.[47] And if, in the typical view in the United States, polio was misconstrued as a disease of childhood, one cannot conclude, as Sontag does, that the American reception of the disease was quintessentially without the usual fiction and metaphor that surround the social construction of disease. Equally telling is Sontag's claim here that "polio was construed as typically a disease . . . of the innocent." In fact, polio was often construed to be, like syphilis, a sort of punishment for sexual activity. The medical profession itself sometimes confused syphilitic paresis with poliomyelitic paralysis. Moreover, many polios recall the doctrine of sin inculcated into them by the nursing and medical professions alike. If one did not get better ("rise up and walk"), then it was because one was guilty (in other words, *not* innocent) of not *trying* hard enough. Otherwise, it was because one was guilty of not *wanting* to get better. Both these sins led the polio to the priest or psychiatrist. Freud too confused "hysterical paralysis" with poliomyelitis.

Sontag writes that polio was "never viewed metaphorically as a plague." In fact, polio was viewed as plague almost throughout its short history.[48] There are three ways to consider this matter: First, polio is *called* a plague. In Quebec, houses with polio quarantine signs were called plague-houses or *maisons de fléau*. Where polio still exists in the world today, as it does in Angola, it is still called a *fléau*.[49] In so famous a speech as his first inaugural address, Franklin Roosevelt himself alludes to polio as plague.[50] Second, the kill rate of polio is quite high. Sontag suggests that loss of life ought to be a "main criterion" in determining whether or not a disease is to be considered a plague. She asserts that the kill rate for polio was low—but any kill rate needs to be measured in terms of time and space. If we consider the relevant space for measurement to be the world taken as a whole for a single year, as Sontag seems to do, then the loss of life occasioned by the great flu epidemic would be something like 20 million out of a total world population in 1916 of 1.8 billion people.[51] *Viewed as such, the Great Influenza killed .01 percent of the total population at that time.* However, if we consider the relevant space to be Chesterfield Inlet—a township in the Northwest Territories of Canada, 150 miles north of Churchill Falls—then, during the winter of 1948–49, polio paralyzed 57 out of a total population of 275, and it killed 14 people. *Viewed as such, polio killed 5 percent of the total population at that time.*[52] What is more, polio in Chesterfield Inlet left 20 percent of the population behind as visibly crippled reminders of the event. For those who lived in the isolated township of Chesterfield Inlet, that *was* the entire world. Third, Sontag suggests that because polio was usually viewed (as she would have it) as a childhood disease and the plague was not, polio could not be a plague. In fact, though, polio was also known as a disease of adults (as we have already seen). And, what is more important, discussions of the plague often do include children, sometimes preeminently. Plagues *did* affect children—and people knew it precisely from the stories and metaphors of the period. The ten plagues of Egypt, for example, included the death of the first-born children, and that plague was usually popularly construed, especially in first half of the twentieth century, as affecting children.[53] Consider Cecil B. DeMille's blockbuster movie *The Ten Commandments* (1956), made at precisely the moment of "conquest" over polio. In this movie, the pharaoh Ramses II is tormented by the death of his young son at the hands of a shadowy Angel of Death. (DeMille's Angel is markedly similar to the shadowy personification of Polio in the movie *The Crippler* of the 1940s, in which Polio wanders the land seeking out child victims—Figure 8).[54]

Why did Sontag make all these errors about polio? For Sontag to have known nothing of polio would be almost impossible, for someone who grew up in New York. New York history included the New York epidemic of 1916, with a quarantine that was the largest in world history. In that year there were more than twenty-seven thousand reported cases of polio in the United States—and more than seven thousand deaths.[55] New York City had a similar outbreak of polio in 1931, just a couple of years before Sontag's birth. Throughout the period 1942–1952—when Sontag was between nine and nineteen years of age—polio continued to appear in the headlines of the *New York Times*. In 1949, when Sontag was sixteen years old, New York State had more than five thousand reported cases of polio out of a total for the United States of about thirty-eight thousand.[56] In 1952, there were sixty thousand reported cases in the United States. One of the best-known photographs of 1952, *The Face of Polio*, was displayed prominently in Sontag's hometown of New York City when Sontag was nineteen years old. It was printed and reprinted myriad times in all New York newspapers and was pasted onto buses, subway cards, and billboards.

It is more likely that Sontag "forgot" what she once knew about polio in much the fashion that twentieth-century America, traumatized by this epidemic, all but forgot it. On the one hand, Sontag is probably correct in assigning to polio a central role in the twentieth-century "dialectic" between illness and metaphor, although, as we shall see, that dialectic was quite different from the one she has in mind. On the other hand, Sontag's hypostatization of polio as unmetaphorical, though it gets her to the point where she can make the politically simple statement that "it is highly desirable for an especially dreaded disease to come to seem ordinary," misrepresents polio.[57] More important, that hypostatization also reiterates the problem in the historiography of disease that Sontag pretends to solve and calls into question a good part of her thesis in *Illness and Metaphor*. The unstated and unexamined irony is that Sontag's calling the treatment of polio unmetaphorical is itself a *merely* metaphorical move. Far from original, Sontag's argument is yet another typical reflection of the long-standing cultural denial and—even oblivion—about disease and epidemic that still affect much of the historiography of disease.

Comparative Diseases

> *Dr. Emma Brookner (a polio):* There's always a plague. Of one kind or another. I've had it since I was a kid.
>
> —Larry Kramer, *The Normal Heart* (1985)

Some diseases appear frequently in literary history and others rarely. For example, tuberculosis, called the French disease, was often thematized in nineteenth-century novels, and many writers of the period had tuberculosis; influenza, though it killed tens of millions of people at the end of World War I, gave rise to very little literature.[58] Similarly, different diseases seem to give rise to different sorts of literary writers and literary production.

If indeed "different diseases or conditions of physical disability give rise to different sorts of first-person writing"—which hypothesis commonly informs writing in the academic field known as literature and medicine—then what might explain the difference? Do different diseases differently affect the brain, in such a way that the victim of one disease will narrate or metaphorize differently from the victim of another? Do different diseases variously change the victim's understanding of his body and its relation to the spirit? Do sociological reactions toward one disease, or toward its physical and psychological symptoms, vary from those toward another disease in such a way as to result in predictably varying kinds and qualities of first-person narratives? When such questions involve polio, ancillary queries arise. Do diseases that strike in childhood—as polio often does—differ, in the eventual literary production they inspire, from those which usually strike in adulthood?[59] Do diseases that strike with sudden intensity—as polio usually does—differ from those which work up to a gradual intensity? Do diseases that usually result in "comorbid" conditions—as polio does—differ from mortal diseases, which we believe no one outlives?

With regard to the last two questions, consider the terminal diseases—like cancer, tuberculosis, and AIDS—that give the ill person a chance to aestheticize the experience of the disease and to write about it before dying. Thus, in Robert Dessaix's novel *Night Letters,* the narrator is diagnosed with an evidently incurable disease, probably AIDS; then he writes a series of letters home to a friend that intertwine reflections on his mortality with accounts of his real and imagined journeys.[60] Polio is usually too traumatic, both physically and psychologically, for that. Many polios died from that trauma. (The number of deaths is far greater than most people expect.[61] One historian of polio reports that in some decades "something like 25 percent of people who caught polio [in the United States] died of it within the first two weeks."[62] In the polio wards that I remember, the older children hardly dared to ask the attending nurse the question that Scrooge, in Charles Dickens's *A Christmas Carol,* asks the Ghost about the paralyzed boy: "Spirit, . . . tell me if Tiny Tim will live.")[63] After all, first-person polio literature is written only by survivors of polio—that is, those who live in the aftermath of polio. Where there seem to be day-by-day accounts, or journals, written by polios that take us through the critical days of the disease itself, it is always participant-observers who write them. Thus, Charles Schwab's *Man in a Wheelchair* (1961), which includes a foreword by its polio-publisher, Edward Uhlan, consists of "journal entries" written over a five-year period beginning the day Schwab attended his friend Bill Blake in the polio hospital: "July 5, 1952: Bill Blake is hopeless paralyzed."[64]

Some first-person polio-narrators feel that they have triumphed by virtue of religion—as does Richard Chaput in *Not to Doubt* (1964). They may feel that their polio experience has charmed the rest of their lives.[65] A few narrators believe that they have overcome, or passed through, death, or a deadly stillness, in something like the way Jesus did. In the novel *Crossing to Safety,* by Wallace Stegner—who also wrote about the influenza epidemic—one of the main characters, Sally, pauses before a painting by Piero della Francesca.[66] Piero's painting shows the recently resurrected Jesus, half in and half out of the grave. Sally's husband Larry (the novel's narrator) then tells us how Sally reacted to the work: "But I noticed that Sally stood a long time on her crutches in front of that painting propped temporarily against a frame of raw two-by-fours. She studied it soberly, with something like 'recognition' or acknowledgement in her eyes, as if those who have been dead understand things that will never be understood by those who have only lived." It is as if life after polio (survival) were, for this polio, the same as afterlife (death); the material importance of the artificial distinction between life and death affects the distinction between literary works involving diseases one survives and works about those to which one succumbs.

Does the kind of isolation that a disease or social condition foists upon a person matter to the literary output of the diseased person? Do diseases whose sufferers are totally quarantined result in different literary production than do diseases whose sufferers had experiences that are more communal? What difference might it make if such patients were gathered together for a limited period in hospital wards or rehabilitation spas—as at the spa for tuberculars in Thomas Mann's novel *The Magic Mountain* (1924)? What happens to patients when they are permanently quarantined—as they were in the leper colonies that still operated in the United States during the period of the polio epidemics?[67] How is the production of literature, both oral and written, affected when healthy but fearful people isolate themselves in time of plague—as they did in Giovanni Boccaccio's *Decameron*?

If, as some say, sexual desire and death are key and motivating themes, then the subject of venereal disease leading to death—which, like the subject of AIDS, might allow for expression of various connections between sexuality and death—would seem to have the aesthetic advantage, when it comes to making great literature, over a presumably nonvenereal, nonmorbid disease like polio. In fact, the etiology of polio at many periods in its historical reception was believed to be nonvenereal—unrelated to sexual activity. (That was partly because polio paralyzed and killed infants and children—creatures whom the popular imagination often understood as creatures without sexual desire.) There are, however, at least three countervailing factors to consider.

1. During the 1880s, poliomyelitic paralysis was considered a condition with a definite sexual etiology. The paralytic effects of what we now know as polio were confused with paresis of the sort transmitted venereally by syphilis. Sir Thomas Clouston, in an 1877 medical case study of a sixteen-year-old, was probably the first to recognize the connection between paresis and congenitally transmitted syphilis.[68] Henrik Ibsen's portrayal of the lame Oswald Alving's paresis in his play *Ghosts* (1881) owes much to Clouston. *General paresis* was the "term used by some for progressive paralysis of the insane,"[69] a designation that helps explain the claim of some political literature of the 1930s that polio had made the paralyzed FDR crazy.

2. An extraordinary belief prevailed in twentieth-century popular culture that polio could not be a disease of concupiscence, because it usually affected children, and children do not experience sexual desire. The long-known (and long-ignored) fact that children do have sexual desires came to scandalous prominence in North American life only during the heyday of polio—just around the time Nabokov's *Lolita* was published (1955) and Freudian theory was being popularized.

3. Popular prejudice often applies to adult polios the sexlessness already falsely attributed to all children. As we shall see, a public myth had it that when polio strikes after an adult has reached sexual maturity, polio "neutralizes" sexual feelings. Polio was further believed to dull all sensation and to make childbirth impossible. Countless novels, movies, and plays assume wrongly that adult polios are sexless beings—among these artworks being Kramer's *Normal Heart* (1985), written about the polio who first brought AIDS to the light of day.

Consider, then, the irony that in earlier times, going as far back at least as Greek antiquity, being "oversexed" was considered a consequence of—or compensation for—being crippled. Thus, we read in Montaigne's essay *On Cripples* (1575): "'Tis a common proverb in Italy, that he knows not Venus in her perfect sweetness who has never lain with a lame mistress. Fortune, or some particular incident, long ago put this saying into the mouths of the people; and the same is said of men as well as of women; for the queen of the Amazons answered the Scythian who courted her to love,

'Lame men perform best.'"[70] Amazon women purposely crippled their infant male children ("elles les stropioient dès l'enfance"). So too Jocasta sees to it that Oedipus is lamed and eventually grows up oversexed.

After Afterness

> Pain—expands the Time—
> Ages coil within
> The minute Circumference
> Of a single Brain—
>
> Pain contracts—the Time—
> Occupied with Shot
> Gamuts of Eternities
> Are as they were not—
>
> —Emily Dickinson, "Pain—Expands the Time"

Child-onset polio authors write in the wake of a disease that changes definitions of time and recovery afterward, that affects understanding of the mind-body relationship, and that drastically alters the relationships between the polio and his or her immediate family.[71] Not surprisingly, their narratives emphasize the moment of contracting polio as a genesis. (Most other biographies begin conceptually with the moment of birth in the context of familial genealogy.)[72] A few polio-authors present themselves as having two lives, BP and AP—before polio and after polio. For others, the moment of poliomyelitic "rebirth" is marked off as if the polio had graduated from something like a university or school. Such common monikers as "Polio Class of 1953, Warms," recall graduation, or rebirth, from an alma mater like Warm Springs.[73]

My title, *Polio and Its Aftermath,* suggests "post-polio (syndrome)"— contemporary medical science's name for the late effects of polio or the sequelae of polio.[74] The usual view is that a person contracts polio, then has the virus "active and destructive" and has "classic" polio symptoms for a couple of weeks. Then follow "obviously discernible" effects—like paralysis. Then it is over—except for the lifelong debilitation and injuries that result from that initial bout with polio. However, this view of polio is wrong. Decades after polio mows down its victim the first time, it can return, boomerang-style, to make a second mowing. This is, literally, the aftermath—meaning "after mowing"—of polio. Many people have longer-term aftereffects, or sequelae, of polio—that is to say, they have post-polio syndrome (PPS).[75] This "condition" affects the skeletal, neurological, and muscular functions, and comes to most polios within four or five decades. Despite claims to the contrary, post-polio syndrome is not a recently discovered or freshly invented condition; as we shall see, it was known at least as far back as 1879.[76] In each generation, people want to forget that PPS exists—and they do. The history of polio is the history of forgetting polio.

Some individuals who had polio will not develop overt symptoms of PPS. On the other hand, some who thought they did not have polio actually did have polio (though without knowing it).[77] That is because in most cases—probably 99 percent—the disease presented as a mild case of "influenza." One contemporary researcher has it that six million North Americans had this sort of "nonparalytic" polio.[78] Many of these people—some researchers suggest as many as 65 percent—will develop symptoms of PPS, usually without ever receiving proper diagnosis of their condition.[79] Helen Henderson thus writes that "some people who never even realized that they had polio as children are now struggling with the crippling after-effects of post-polio syndrome." Oftentimes they struggle alone: medical advisers attribute such patients' symptoms—incorrectly—to old age or to some such condition as chronic fatigue syndrome or fibromyalgia. That is one reason the media today like to call PPS a time bomb for the twenty-first century, and what shattering results it will have—in addition to those other half-forgotten cultural and political implications of polio and its aftermath—time alone will tell.[80]

AUTOBIOGRAPHIES OF A DISEASE

I'll be your staff, for I am one that hath
Lived long and gathered in Life's aftermath—

—*A Masque of Poets* (1878)

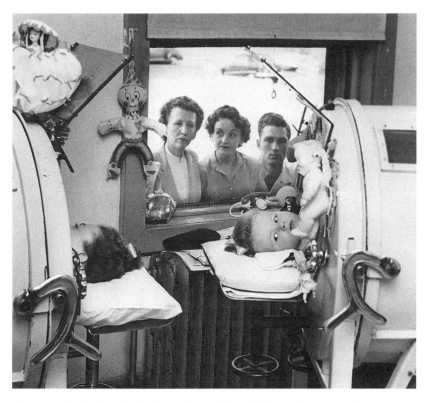

The face of polio. Linda Gunther, eight (left), and Mary Jo Moss, two, lie in iron lungs equipped with rearview mirrors and puppets. Their parents watch at an observation window. Memphis Isolation Hospital, Tennessee, 1952.

1 ONE POLIO STORY

Ball one, low and outside
Paralyzed, I lay on my bed
—Mark O'Brien, "How I Survived Childhood," in *Love and Baseball*

1953. What was that year like for poliomyelitis research? *July:* the hostilities of the Korean War, which had kept many American polio workers occupied with trying to keep the troops relatively safe from polio, ended. *September:* the World Health Organization's Expert Committee on Poliomyelitis was holding its principal meeting.[1] *October:* the Immunization Committee of the National Foundation for Infantile Paralysis sided with Jonas Salk on how to further test the inactive vaccine that he had developed in 1952. *December:* the Foundation proposed that the evaluation team be headquartered at the University of Michigan.

February 1954. D. T. Francis presented his plan to inject placebo or vaccine into 650,000 school children. Eventually 1,800,000 children participated. For these children in 1954, February really was a great moment in the history of medicine. Anyhow—that is what we were told. My peers who took the first vaccine were certified as heroic "pioneers."[2] And by 1955, teachers across North America were writing this message on classroom blackboards: "April 19, 1955. Making History. We are among the first children ever to be given Polio shots. So we are really making History today. We are lucky."[3] Popular histories of the twentieth century still mark the introduction of the Salk vaccine as one of that century's real highlights. It was not so good for some of the children who received placebos instead of vaccine.

This polio's eye view of 1953 and 1954 pushes out of mind other events of relevance for medical progress, such as the discovery of the double-helix structure of DNA by Francis Crick and James Watson or the establishment of the U.S. Department of Health, Education and Welfare. In addition, it leaves out other events of 1953 that we shall have occasion to discuss in *Polio and Its Aftermath.* On the music charts were songs like "How Much Is That Doggie in the Window?" and "O My Papa!" In the movie houses were such films as *Caddy, Lili, Road to Bali,* and *Call Me Madam,* as well as two Marilyn Monroe hits, *How to Marry a Millionaire* and *Gentlemen Prefer Blondes.* Marilyn Monroe appeared on the cover of the first issue of *Playboy Magazine.* John Michael Hayes completed the script for Alfred Hitchcock's movie *Rear Window.* Sir Edmund Hillary and Tenzing Norgay reached the summit of Mount Everest. Ethel and Julius Rosenberg were executed. Longtime polio sufferers like Frida "Peg-leg" Kahlo, who had polio at the age of six, were painting and writing about their experiences.[4]

As for me—I move away now from the big picture, back to the narrow world of my childhood experience—Salk's polio vaccine came too late. *September 1953:* I was beginning first grade at Van Horne School in Montreal. *October 14:* I contracted polio. It was the same day that the foundation backed Jonas Salk's proposal to test his vaccine.

Our movie direction now requires us to focus a wider-angle lens on the times. Most North Americans, then and now, mistakenly consider polio "a summer plague." Tony Gould, who got polio in 1959, makes this error, and the belief that polio is a summer plague was already an adage when *Canadian Magazine* published Davies's "Death Walks in the Summer" in 1932.[5] Even so, people had plenty of experience, especially in northern Canada, of polio epidemics occurring also in the fall and winter seasons, as Dr. Joseph Moody describes in his first-person narrative *Arctic Doctor.*[6] Quebecers knew from the terrible polio epidemic in Saint-Augustine near the Labrador border that it did not strike only in summer.[7] In Vermont, moreover, Dr. Charles Caverly—who greatly influenced the fields of epidemiology, disease quarantine, public health, and treatment—had already warned in 1893 about the prevalence of polio in the fall season.[8]

A close-up explanation of the strange game of epidemiological roulette that sidelined me on that October day would take us too soon into the metaphysical realm of theodicy—which we will consider below. For now, a brief rundown on the statistics of place, disease, and time will serve to locate how things fell out for me, an individual, in terms of demographic variables and may point to the larger statistical surveys that one might still

Places, Diseases, Times

Place: Manitoba had 286.4 reported cases of polio per 100,000 persons in 1953. So the chance of getting polio was far less in Quebec than in Manitoba. *Disease:* Tuberculosis was reported that year, for all Canada, at a rate of 65.7 cases per 100,000 persons. In the same year, polio was reported, for all Canada, at 59.8 cases per 100,000. My risk of getting polio in Canada that year was less than my chance of getting tuberculosis.

1931. The polio rate in Quebec was 37.5 reported cases per 100,000 persons.

1932. The polio rate in Quebec was 24.2 reported cases per 100,000 persons. The 1932 outbreak of poliomyelitis was much discussed in the medical literature. The recollection of the outbreak shaped the memory of my parent's generation.

1946. The polio rate in Quebec was 44.4 reported cases per 100,000 persons.

1959. The polio rate in Quebec was 23.2 reported cases per 100,000 persons. In 1959, there were 1,886 reported cases in all Canada, of which 1,171 were from Quebec. Of the 182 all-Canadian deaths from polio that year, 106 were from Quebec. (The polio vaccine might have prevented most such deaths. In Quebec, however, there was resistance to the vaccine, coming mostly from the Catholic Church. Likewise, a more widespread use of the smallpox vaccine would have prevented the terrible smallpox outbreak in Montreal in 1885—according to Drs. Hingston and Osler.)

Sources: On 1953, see R. Kohn, "Some Figures on Poliomyelitis in Canada," *Canadian Journal of Public Health* 45 (June 1954): 225–235; Christopher J. Rutty, "'Do Something! . . . Do Anything!' Poliomyelitis in Canada, 1927–1962," Ph.D. diss., University of Toronto, 1995, 396. On tuberculosis, see Rutty, "'Do Something!'" 402. On 1932, see A. R. Foley, "The Present Outbreak of Poliomyelitis in Quebec," *Canadian Public Health Journal* 23 (October 1932): 494–497. More relevantly, see also A. R. Foley, "The 1932 Outbreak of Poliomyelitis in Quebec," *Canadian Public Health Journal* 25 (June 1934): 260–274. On 1959, see Rutty, "'Do Something!'" 395.

conduct. In 1953, Quebec had 488 reported cases of polio. (Canada as a whole that year had 8,878 reported cases.)[9] To put it another way, Quebec in 1953 had 11.4 reported cases of polio per 100,000 people. How are we to understand these figures with respect to different places, diseases, and times?

Many statistics involving other places, diseases, and times suggest that, "all other things being equal" (a condition whose doubtful groundwork we will reexamine), my chances of getting polio in Quebec in 1953 were relatively small. However, two extenuating circumstances—not untypical for the polio epidemics of the twentieth century—militate against this conclusion. First, the reported mortality figures for polio in Quebec for 1953 are extraordinarily high compared with the figures reported for other Canadian provinces (and most other parts of the world). Of the 494 deaths from polio that year in Canada, fully 333 were from Quebec.[10] One would need to conclude that, for that year in Quebec, either polio was being underreported or the polio strain was particularly virulent.

In fact, polio was underreported. But not reporting is also part of the stories of many other Quebecers, anglophone and francophone. Even the most renowned cases of polio in Canadian history, including Franklin Delano Roosevelt's—he contracted the disease on Campobello Island, New Brunswick, in August 1921—went officially unreported.[11]

If children did not lose their lives in the roulette of polio that year, then, at the least, they lost their childhood. Mia Farrow, who got polio in 1954 when she was nine years old, begins her memoir *What Falls Away* with the dramatic statement "I was nine years old my when childhood ended."[12] If, like Farrow, one was already old enough to know something of what was going on when one got polio, and if, after having had polio, one could remember what had gone before, the advent of the disease could indeed affect one in that way. I was six years old in 1953—old enough. For me, too, polio was the pioneer—the old mole—who undermined the then current notion of my childhood.[13]

Several polios recall in the first sentences of their memoirs that premature ending of childhood—or that new rebirth as a polio (the person) or existence after polio (the disease)—as an awakening from a dream or nightmare. In his memoir *Closer to the Sun,* for example, Garth Drabinsky writes: "I wakened into the air-conditioned nightmare. It was September 1953."[14] These narrators frequently begin with a description of their becoming ill in the first place—as if the advent of disease were, to all intents and purposes, the real beginning of the life they are about to tell. Many polios, concomitantly, forget their lives before polio, in a way that is often psychologically needful. Among such authors are Earl Bailly in *His Trials and Triumphs* and Vivienne Overheu in her *It Helps to Be Stubborn*. Bailly asks: "How far back can I remember? Can I remember before I was stricken with polio? I am afraid I cannot recall very vividly much that happened in my life before that period." Overheu starts her memoir as follows: "The year was 1954. The twelfth of March. I was twenty-two years of age. On this day I had to begin my life all over again, as someone I did not understand, know, or wish to be."[15] Scores of polio accounts, autobiographical or not, offer some such sentence as this one in the semifictional novel *Joyride,* by the polio Betty Cavanna: "Actually, Susan couldn't remember a time when she hadn't been lame."[16] Some persons, like Jenny Danielson—who had polio at fourteen in 1955—remember nothing of their lives before the advent of the physical and psychological trauma of the disease itself.[17] In some polio narratives—including Judith Rossner's novel *Looking for Mr. Goodbar*—this loss of the memory of a previous existence is attributed to a change of personality, which the poliomyelitis and associated physical or social situations somehow trigger.[18] In other narratives—including Owen Dixson's memoir *My Way with Polio*—the polio's loss of memory before the appearance of the disease is simply attributed to the early age at which polio usually strikes.[19]

One might recall certain notions about the relation between trauma and narrative theory. Peter Brooks promulgates the view in "Freud's Masterplot," for example, that "plot starts . . . from the moment at which the story, or 'life,' is stimulated from quiescence into a state of narratability, into a tension, a kind of irritation which demands narration."[20] Here we understand trauma as "being possessed by an image or event," hence needing to begin over again repeatedly, boomerang-style.[21] It is that way in Martha Ramsey's rape memoir, *Where I Stopped: Remembering Rape at Thirteen.* Writes Susan Brison in her essay "Trauma Narratives and the Making of the Self," "Narrative memory is not passively endured; rather, it is an act on the part of the narrator, a speech act that defuses traumatic memory, giving shape and a temporal order to the events recalled, establishing more control over their recalling, and helping the survivor to remake a self."[22]

So trauma ends childhood, even as it provides the motive spring or narratological strategy for writing. Writes Leonard Kriegel, in his memoir *Falling into Life*, of the "meeting"—the bout with poliomyelitis that paralyzed him at age eleven: "Almost everything prior to our meeting could be dismissed. Life for the writer began with the death of legs. Passion was rooted in the absence and the desires absence evoked."[23]

If polio helps destroy—or encourages the destruction of—(the memory of) a childhood *before* polio, it also makes all but impossible a regular childhood *after* polio. This is not just to say that the child, now a polio, can no longer play on the monkey bars, although it is true that most such children could not. It is to say that the polio's relationship to his family and to his body has changed, prematurely, at once toward greater dependence and toward greater independence, with all the inner spiritual conflict and sometimes inconsistency that change can bring with it.

The book of Genesis says about the adult man: "Therefore shall a man leave his father and his mother."[24] The requirement to leave one's own family is felt by the child polio earlier than the usual moment of manly adulthood. Polio narratives almost always involve children being separated physically from their parents because of the legal need for quarantine or the medical need for treatment.[25] The polio is away from "healthy" people; or, he is together with "unhealthy" people. Quarantines were already standard practice by 1910.[26] American culture knew them well from the New York City typhus and cholera epidemics of 1882. And by the time of the great polio epidemic of 1916, quarantines had begun to affect the sociopathology of the disease in definite ways. In fact, attempts to quarantine polios mark a significant moment in the history of public health and, indeed, in the history of moving or isolating large groups of people.[27] Dr. John R. Paul, in his *History of Poliomyelitis*—still the only standard history of the disease—writes that the New York City polio epidemic of 1916 "will go down in history as the high-water mark in attempts at enforcement of isolation and quarantine measures."[28] Elsewhere, too, families could not even visit their loved ones. The military aspects of the enforced sequestration in New York City—of the sick population (concentrated in guard camps) from the healthy—was not lost on the people of the United States.

Social scientists have not pursued the similarity and differences between the quarantines and such other militarily enforced American wartime experiments in population control as the displacement of the Cherokee Na-

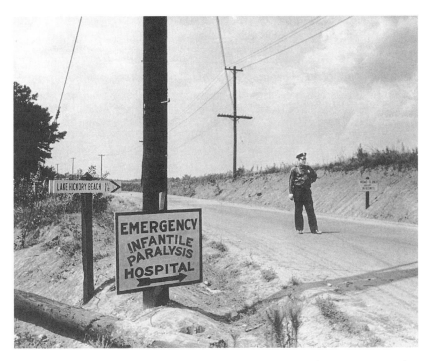

Military quarantine at Hickory: armed serviceman ensuring the quarantine at the Emergency Infantile Paralysis Hospital.

tion, compelled to take the Trail of Tears (1831–1833), and the relocation of Japanese-Americans into internment camps (1942–1946). The latter was an important subject for the photographer Dorothea Lange—as a polio, especially wary of such situations.[29] From the viewpoint of the child polio, however, there was at least one important difference between the internment camps and the polio wards. The Cherokee and Japanese-American children were isolated together with their parents and extended families; child polios, on the other hand, were separated from their families. This separation from family and home could last weeks, months, or years. Tom Atkins's first-person account *One Door Closes, Another Opens: Personal Experiences of Polio,* describes how he was entirely isolated from his family from the age of three to the age of seven.[30] In many cases, the end of the quarantine period meant legal orphanhood or permanent institutionalization by the state. In some cases, even after returning home, patients *felt* separated from family and society by a never-voiced yet all-pervasive anxiety. Nancy Frick, in her presentation on "the development of the polio personality," writes, "Polio survivors were the AIDS people of their generation. Nobody wanted to have anything to do with [them]. Everybody was terrified of polio survivors, and even their families, for years."[31] This separation usually affects a person quite as much as the lasting physical disabilities that polio imposes.

Some earlier works by polios, like my own, privilege the cultural over the medical implications of polio. The ethnographer Fred Davis focuses on family crises and the like in the case of polio; his book *Passage through Crisis* is among the first studies in American sociology to take into more than incidental account the patient's perspective and its implications for the illness experiences of people.[32] There are also sociological-autobiographical works by polios—for example, Robert Lovering, *Out of the Ordinary,* and Irving Kenneth Zola, *Missing Pieces.*[33] But *Polio and Its Aftermath* differs from these, not least by virtue of its formal recognition of the afterness that dogs the lives of polios before and after post-polio and that both motivates and inhabits their lives and work.

The Hour of Lead

A markedly memorable paralysis inhabits the hardly leaden poetry of Emily Dickinson:

> This is the Hour of Lead—
> Remembered, if outlived,
> As Freezing persons, recollect the Snow—
> First—Chill—then Stupor—then the letting go—[34]

The feeling of despair can be not merely recollected but relived, resumed, as Camille Savard expresses: "I take note of how terrible it is to have suffered so much, with so much effort and work, only to find myself, today, back at the departure point."[35] One unique quality of polio is the way, if one outlives it and lives long enough, it comes back or returns one, post-polio, to the beginning. Peg Kehret can write, forty years after she succumbed to polio in 1949, "After all these years, I have drawn inner strength from my victory over polio, feeling that if I could beat polio, I could handle anything. It was painful to discover that the enemy was not vanquished, as I had thought, but had merely gone under cover, waiting to strike once more. My battle with polio is not yet over."[36] This peculiar ability of polio to strike again and to shape the lives of the survivors (the ones who live on and out) whom it visits affects my narrating voice now, some fifty years after polio first struck me down in 1953.

To explain this boomerang effect that polio can have, let me contrast polio and polios with certain other disabling diseases and the people who suffer from them. Many polios believed for forty years that polio had finished its work with them, however well or badly off it had left them. But years afterward, as post-polio patients, they are compelled in some fashion to relive certain aspects of their childhood experiences with paralysis and "recovery" and to face up to the fact that the disease is a continuing process that will not finish with them until death. (The word *comorbidity* comes up in conversations with medical professionals discussing such conditions—as if life itself were not always comorbid. Another term that comes up is *remission*.) After four decades or so, the polio sufferer becomes aware of a new yet also familiar neuromuscular degeneration. Consider how the polio Robert Mauro looks at the second coming of polio—or the appearance of PPS—in his poem "My Iron Lung et Cetera":

> When I was but a boy of five,
> an iron lung did breathe for me.
> It pumped and pumped around the clock,
> a yellow tank with pressure lock.
> And while inside the only touch
> was through a rubber gasket just.
> And then when I was only seven,
> they pulled me out and turned to heaven.
> For eighteen years I had a ball.
> Then PPS did take its toll.
> A rocking bed they laid me on;
> no lady fair would come upon.
> At forty-three they took the bed
> and ventilated me instead.
> and now when lovers with me lay,
> I hap'ly take their breath away![37]

So Mauro moves from iron lung only to ventilator. It is useful here to consider two kinds of survivors of diseases. On the one hand are those victims of chronic diseases who know that their condition will not finish with them until they are dead. Such terminal or comorbid diseases include multiple sclerosis and AIDS. On the other hand are those victims of disease and accident who, no matter how painful or misshapen their body has become, believe that their problem has at least finished with them—many people who are left quadriplegic after an automobile accident, for example.

Where does the polio survivor fit in? During the first years after he has contracted the disease, the polio generally believes that he falls into this second category. He is "a survivor," no matter how scarred by polio. The terrible suffering and the temperately triumphant sense of survivorship may be one reason that young polios so often seemed more grown up than others their age. It is as if they had already passed through that *midlife crisis*—a favorite term of the 1950s—which confers mature wisdom and tolerance. Many polios, and almost all of the 1.6 million polios who are still alive in the United States, were praised for "getting on" with their lives— and in some ways also getting along, smilingly, with other people—almost as if nothing had happened.

Most polios survived. They outlived the disease. "This is the Hour of Lead," writes Emily Dickinson in "After great pain a formal feeling comes," "Remembered, *if* outlived." Quite a few polio survivors claimed to have had, or were told that they had had, something like gracious "spontaneous recoveries"—a common tale about a "triumph over adversity" in the pleasant Horatio Alger tradition.[38] Canadian magazines in the 1950s published upbeat articles with such bizarre titles as "I'm Glad I Had Polio" about people who were supposedly 98 percent cured.[39] In 1953, doctors in Canada were claiming (falsely) in the newspapers that three-fourths of the "victims recover fully from polio."[40]

In fact, several researchers—among them, Butterfield and Ross in their New Zealand study *Mind over Muscle*—still like to say (fallaciously) that people adopted one of three social and psychological strategies of coping with having had polio and surviving the experience.[41] Polios in the first group pass as if they had never had polio—as if they were fully recovered. Those in the second group minimize their having had polio. Those in the third group identify as being polios.

Polios who believed in tales of complete recovery—many are described in Sass's *Polio's Oral Legacy*—became passers of an extreme sort.[42] These passers keep their having had polio—or, if you prefer, their being polios—a secret from other people. In most cases, they also kept it a secret from themselves. Nancy Carter Baldwin thus writes in her *Myths and Chicken Feet*:

> For most of us, resolving physical problems was the first order of business after we had polio. We wanted to get on with it. We worked out ways to do what needed to be done and charged into life. Before long these ingenious substitutions for the way "normies" do things became routine, and we began to think of ourselves as one of the gang.
>
> In fact, many of us got so good at the charade that we fooled ourselves.[43]

In some other cases, in fact, passer-polios did not know themselves that they had had polio. Some were too young or too traumatized to remember. (A few were still too traumatized decades later to "recover" memories of having had polio. In the realm between *un*covering and *dis*covering the past lies confusion about what "really" happened to body and spirit.) Others were never told the name of the disease they had had. In some cases, no one knew. In other cases, the hope was to protect them from acting too uncomfortably like polios. I was an all-but-unwitting passer.

No matter which of these three types he may be, the childhood-onset polio, if he lives long enough, has a good chance of developing post-polio syndrome, and if that condition is properly recognized or diagnosed, he will eventually discover that he did not, after all, conquer the disease. If he is a passer who was too young, and hence ignorant, he may not ever have known that he had polio. He is not who, or what, he thought he was. Much as Oedipus grown up eventually discovers that the problem with his Achilles tendon is worse than—as well as both etiologically and teleologically different than—he had thought, so the polio confronting post-polio syndrome needs to confront again his past injury and its story. However much this polio has been praised by others for having conquered or learned to live with the disability—and likewise however much he may have accommodated himself, Oedipuslike, to his crutch(es)—the lame man comes to learn that, all along, he was really an unwitting member of the group of passers. He learns that, in some ways, at least, his life until now has been counterfeit.

The diagnosis of post-polio syndrome is, in this narrow sense, like the argument, or *mythos,* of the plot of Sophocles' *Oedipus the Tyrant* in the fifth century BC. If the polio's mind, forty years later, will not remember that he is a polio, then his body will do the remembering—the memoir—for the mind. After all, in post-polio syndrome, body trumps mind![44] That order of precedence gives old urgency and new meaning to the Jesuit dictum "Give me a child until he is seven and he will be mine for the rest of his life." In that powerful medley of fear and pity that is Sophocles' *Oedipus the Tyrant,* the three-legged tragic hero—with his mysteriously hobbled swollen feet and his cripple's walking stick—is forced to relive his childhood and to recognize the reality of his present.[45]

The riddle of the Sphinx was "Who walks on four legs in the morning, two at noon, and three in the evening?"[46] Oedipus of Thebes, as a normal four-legged infant (crawling on all fours), was thus already sufficiently handicapped in relation to his two-legged parents. Nevertheless, they maimed him (further) by driving stakes through his ankle(s): hobbled Oedipus' very name means "swollen foot."[47] Then the adults abandoned him to die on Mount Cithaeron. It was not enough for the gods to make Oedipus a pain-ridden physical cripple able now to know better than others the answer to the riddle of the Sphinx. More than that, during the course of Sophocles' drama Oedipus, with all his impediments, has to relive the riddle of his origins at another more terrible—because now witting—level. The hero now has to learn how he got his scars and what they really mean for him. Far from being marks of an old wound that now merely hobble him, the scars are actually living wounds that go right through him.[48]

What is it like to be a polio abandoned by one's parents? Many polios have scars whose original "purpose," if any, they do not know, except to say that it had something to do with their having had polio and someone's having treated them.[49] Countless polios have those scars from having had a leg bone surgically shortened or lengthened, or tendons cut or unwrapped, in order to avoid, by means of medically induced deformity, further disease-induced deformity. Not a few polio survivors have had their heel cords "repaired" in infancy, in order to avoid "foot drop." Myriad such operations were deemed medically necessary. In the present context, it does not matter why the surgeons did these operations on polios. Was the conscious intention to improve the physical well-being of the patient? Was the purpose to boost the psychological well-being of parents and doctors who did not want to feel powerless and who were driven, in a culture where orthopedic deformity was taboo, to do something—anything at all?[50] Was the purpose merely to enrich the surgeons? What does matter, in the present context, is that many of those who had surgery when they were very young children were never told about that surgery when they were older. For these children grown up, their scars are a bodily mystery. Such grown-up polios are like Oedipus in Corinth—before the drunkard in Sophocles' play tells him, "You are a counterfeit *[plastos]*."[51] That statement is what spurs three-legged Oedipus—with his two hobbled legs and his one walking stick—to visit the oracle; for Oedipus has been told nothing of what was deliberately done to hobble him during his infancy. For all he knows, the cripple's scars might almost be the remnants of all-but-forgotten tortures.[52]

Seen in this light, the regularly misunderstood trauma or terror that some people experience when they confront their post-polio condition as a return to polio—when they remember the parts of a body once whole— is spiritual as well as physical.[53] Not without reason does Kenny Fries make the title of his disability memoir *Body, Remember* (1997). Fries, whose deformities are congenital, has had unexplained physical and psychological scars for as long as he can remember; his book documents the long-forgotten surgeries and other interventions that were meant to re-member his body and hence make him whole. Fries takes his title from Constantine Cavafy's poem of the same name, "Body, Remember."[54]

Here I am speaking, then, of the psychological scars that are inflicted to make physical deformity tolerable. If surgeries do not make things directly tolerable for the patient (they rarely do), they do make them tolerable for others. Since the attitudes of those around the young polio—often the family at home—help determine what is tolerable for the patient, surgeries help the patient indirectly.

At Home

When I had polio, I was kept at home, instead of being hospitalized.[55] Historians are still a little puzzled by my experience. Legal regulations in Quebec required that polios be hospitalized—or, at the very least, quarantined in a space clearly marked with official posters; and elsewhere parents of polios were accused of criminal acts and even military violations for keeping an occurrence of polio secret (as Miner and Kimball describe in their *Camilla*).[56] Despite such regulations, however, many hospitals in North America feared to accept polio cases "because of the attitude of the public and because of their own ignorance on the subject."[57] And regardless of what the regulations said or what hospitals wanted, parents might have good private—if not public health–oriented—reasons for keeping their children at home. Thus, some parents in Quebec absolutely refused to allow their children to be cared for in what they believed (often rightly) to be inadequate medical facilities in backwater towns like Chicoutimi.[58]

Was it better to be in a hospital or at home? That would depend. Some Montreal hospitals were relatively good. And many polio patients might have benefited from early hospital care. In Dore Schary's play *Sunrise at Campobello*, Eleanor Roosevelt speaks thus about her recently paralyzed husband Franklin Delano Roosevelt: "He should be in a hospital, getting the best care, the most modern treatment."[59] Franklin had had particularly bad doctors caring for him at Campobello. Nevertheless, judging from what we know now about the various treatments for polio at the time, it would seem that FDR might have had as good a chance out of the hospital as in.

In any case, for good or ill, I myself did not have the usual experience of the polio ward—with all its separation anxiety, opportunity for new friendships, and subsequent separation from a "hospital-school family." For other polios, such experiences were as life-shaping as trench warfare for the World War I generation, say, or college for privileged Baby Boomers of the 1960s. The polio wards of the 1950s have been much criticized—sometimes for having been run like military barracks and often for having treated young children brutally; they have also been much praised—as is the case with Warm Springs in Georgia, which usually took on patients older than I was. In either case, the polio wards usually provided inmates with tentative answers to such questions as "What is wrong with me?" and "What will become of me?" They also provided someone to listen to the young patient in a spirit of camaraderie (like a fellow patient in the polio ward, blowing straws) and someone to answer elementary questions in an empathetic (even believable) way. The celebrated Australian artist John

Perceval sympathetically sketches his own polio ward at Stonnington in 1938.[60]

I had no one with whom to speak about such matters. Turnley Walker begins his book about having had polio, *Rise Up and Walk,* with a chapter titled "Polio Is a Lonely Place."[61] One encounters something like the same sort of isolation in Jean-Jacques Rousseau's *Confessions* (1782–1789) and Edward Said's *Out of Place.*[62]

What's Wrong with Me?

Oh don't ask why
No don't ask why

—"Alabama Song," in Bertolt Brecht and Kurt Weill, *Rise and Fall of the City of Mahagonny*

While paralyzed, I asked my parents, "What is wrong with me? With my leg?" My parents told me, "You have a cold in your leg." I know now that this fib was not then an unusual parental tactic. Many child polios tell the same story. Geoff Lucas in Tasmania, for example, was put off, after asking the same question, with "nods, mumblings, and doctor stuff." The children of doctors who specialized in polio were fibbed to in much the same way, as in the case of Sheila Williamson, likewise from Tasmania.[63] (Such stories seem mostly to concern some such "far-out" places as Tasmania, the site of the world's all-time worst polio epidemic in 1937–38.)[64] Tenley Albright's surgeon father kept the fact of her polio secret from her when she contracted the disease in 1946 at the age of eleven in Newton, Massachusetts.[65] Most of these stories close with the parents telling the "truth" to their child after the polio attack is over. But in many cases the secret is kept for years. Mary Morgart, who got polio in 1916 and was twice orphaned because of her disabilities, tells in her *Abandoned Child* about asking one of her adoptive mothers, "Mama, why does my food all go down into one leg and leave the other one so thin?"[66] All Morgart got was no answer or else denial of the fact that her leg was thin.

Sometimes familial denial goes so far as to constitute blindness: no one in the family even knows that anything is wrong when a child is limping.

Many other Quebecers too were paralyzed by polio without anyone's ever noticing that they were paralyzed. One example from Montreal is Suzanne Martel.[67] That their disease was neither detected nor diagnosed one might attribute to the failure of individual doctors or the medical system of the time—or, in a few cases, to the carelessness, terror, or the sociopathology of guardians. A telling literary example is Theresa Dunn, the schoolteacher hero in Judith Rossner's novel *Looking for Mr. Goodbar*. (Theresa Dunn is the Diane Keaton character in the 1977 movie *Looking for Mr. Goodbar*.) Theresa's serious scoliosis is the result of a bout with polio never followed up with diagnosis or treatment. Theresa's mother and father "didn't look at her for almost two years and then it was too late. Besides, once they understood what had happened, there was nothing but guilt in their eyes so that when she saw them look at her she had to turn away in shame and confusion. If it hadn't been for her brother's death they might have realized sooner that she needed help." As Rossner makes clear, "Nobody noticed what was happening."[68] Like Morgart when she asked about the difference in size between her two legs, Theresa Dunn never got a real answer to her question about what was wrong with her.[69]

What made my parents think to tell me I had a cold in my leg? I had collapsed on the sidewalk outside our home. Unable to "arise and walk" without help, I told my parents about the incident. They said I'd soon get over it. This parental reaction to such fearsome symptoms was not extraordinary. Fred Davis, in his study of polio families carried out between 1953 and 1957, claims that half the polio families he studied did not "wholly admit that the child was ill." In some families, indeed, "parents questioned the legitimacy of the child's complaints; they believed he might be feigning or faking illness so as to win attention and indulgence."[70] (Michelangelo Antonioni's movie *Il deserto rosso* turns on a son's feigning polio.[71] Compare the "fake paralysis" in the 2000 movie *Where the Money Is*.) My own parents waited a long time to call the doctor, as did many other parents.[72] I exerted myself mightily for the next couple of days in the effort to walk to and from school. Another Canadian, Garth Drabinsky, who likewise contracted polio in 1953, has a similar memory. In his book *Closer to the Sun*, Drabinsky thinks back on how he might *not* have been quite so paralyzed from his bout with polio. He was told that his mother called the doctor right away but the doctor did not come soon enough.

Our doctor finally came on the fourth day, and only after my mother called him and said, "You've got to come now because Garth fell over while he was walking." Whenever I think of this now, anger floods my mind. Maybe, even if the doctor had come promptly, it would have made no difference. But maybe it would have made all the difference in the world. Maybe I would still have been able to run.

Everything would have been different.[73]

Many parents, when their first guess or hope about what was wrong—a cold—turned out to be wrong, nevertheless stuck to their mistaken initial diagnosis instead of accepting the illness. In *Passage through Crisis*, Davis writes of such families:

Some parents attempted somehow to assimilate the warning cue to the commonsensical diagnosis of the child's illness that they had held from the first. Thus, when they first became aware of muscular weakness or rigidity in some part of the child's body, they assumed that the cold had "settled" in the legs, abdomen, or feet, as the case might be. Their "migratory theory of pathology"—whereby an illness moves through the body and settles somewhere—had both a *denial* and a *rationalization* component.

According to Davis, college-educated couples acted much more swiftly than other parents—and probably also more wisely.[74]

Whence came my question? "What is wrong with me?" I know that it was not—it was not *only*—for such a word as *poliomyelitis* that I was asking.

I was *not* then asking for a mere name—although the "comparatist's dozen" in the list speaks to what I have now become. I was asking instead for "the ring of truth." What bothered me most in those terrible days was that I was being lied to. Like so many other young polios, I lost my trust in my parents. Not only was I now a ward prisoner in my body. I was also a prisoner in my "home."

Should I now, looking back on those days, dispense such advice to present-day parents with disabled children as "Don't lie to sick kids—especially since you can't get away with it"? Some polio writers like the

One Dozen Names for Polio

1. *Teething sickness*—what the disease was called when the novelist Walter Scott had polio. Throughout the nineteenth century, *teething fever* remained a commonplace English term for infantile disease involving paralysis.

2. *Debility of the lower extremities*—when Underwood wrote in 1789.

3. *Lähmungszustände der unteren Extremitäten*—Heine's term in 1840.

4. *Morning paralysis*—West's principal description in 1843.

5. *Paralysie essentielle chez les enfants*—the influential term used by Rilliet in 1851.

6. *Paralysie atrophique graisseuse de l'enfance*—which Duchenne de Boulogne called the syndrome in 1855.

7. *Spinale Kinderlähmung*—another term from Heine, in 1869.

8. *Tephromyelitis anterior acuta parenchymatose*—the unusual usage from Charcot, in 1872.

9. *Heine-Medin disease*—the name Wickman insisted, in 1907, that we give polio.

10. *Infantile paralysis.*

11. *Poliomyelitis.*

12. *Polio.*

Sources: 1. William Francis Collier, *A History of English Literature in a Series of Biographical Sketches* (London, 1861), 400: "A severe teething fever deprived him of the use of his right leg." 2. M. Underwood, *A Treatise on the Diseases of Children with General Directions for the Management of Infants from the Birth,* new ed. (London: Mathews, 1789). 3. J. Heine, *Beobachtungen über Lähmungszustände der unteren Extremitäten und deren Behandlung* (Stuttgart: Kohler, 1840). 4. C. West, "On Some Forms of Paralysis Incidental to Infancy and Childhood," *Medical Gazette* (London) 32 (1843): 829. 5. F. Rilliet, "De la paralysie essentielle chez les enfants," *Gazette médicale* (Paris), 3rd series (1851): 681, 704. 6. Duchenne de Boulogne, *De l'électrisation localisée et de son application à la physiologie, à la pathologie et à la thérapeutique* (Paris: Baillière, 1855). 7. J. von Heine, *Spinale Kinderlähmung* (Stuttgart: Cotta, 1860). 8. J.-M. Charcot, "Groupe des myopathies de cause spinale: Paralysie infantile," *Revue photographique des hôpitaux de Paris* 4 (1872): 1. 9. I. Wickman, *Beiträge sur Kenntnis des Heine-Medinschen Krankheit* (Berlin, 1907). 10. For fuller references, see Paul, *History of Poliomyelitis,* 5.

"psychologist" Garrett Oppenheim in his *Golden Handicap* sprinkle their accounts of having had polio with such bits of advice.[75] I cannot.

What If

> Flee for your life; do not look back.
>
> —Genesis 19:17

God's advice to Lot was "Do not look back." For looking back, Lot's wife was petrified into a column of salt. She was paralyzed. Jesus is onto something when, in a memorably short verse in the Gospel According to Saint Luke, he gives one of his very few outright commands: "Remember Lot's wife."[76] Can one remember without looking back?

Many polios look back on the moment they were petrified by polio and wonder, "Why me?" Many post-polios are swept back, over and over again, to the same question: "Why *me?*"[77] This is not only a religious problem in the tradition of theodicy. Oftentimes the issue involves matters of etiology and diagnosis. Thus, as we saw, Drabinsky wonders in his book *Closer to the Sun* whether a more attentive doctor, back in 1953, would have made a difference. "Maybe, even if the doctor had come promptly, it would have made no difference. But maybe it would have made all the difference in the world." And sometimes the ceaselessly tormenting and purgatorially mordant and remordant question revolves around what-if matters of long-past rules of prevention.

Among these rules were "Stay out of 'polio water'" and "Do not have a 'needless' tonsillectomy."

Many polios tell how they went swimming in the days before contracting the disease. I went swimming at the pool of the neighborhood Young Men's Hebrew Association (YMHA) in Snowden. In retrospect, it is easy enough to say that we shouldn't have. As we read in Devoto's novel *Last Days*, "These summers are so hard on us all. Hard because we don't know what's right or wrong. Shall we let our children drink the water, play in the pool, associate with someone who has had or might have polio? . . . The problem is, we can't let the fear end up being worse than the polio."[78]

Many polios also tell how they had tonsillectomies in days before contracting polio. Tonsillectomies were sometimes done in the belief that they would stop such illnesses as quinsy, rheumatic fever, and even polio. A few medical articles written around the time of the New York polio epidemic of 1916 had suggested that children who had had their tonsils removed did not get polio and that often children who had gotten polio had inflamed tonsils at the same time.[79] Miner and Kimball's memoir *Camilla* concerns a family in which the parents believed that removing the tonsils would help stave off polio.[80] And yet there was no really reliable evidence in the 1950s showing that tonsillectomy did that.[81] In fact, in 1915 Dr. M. Talmey showed definitively that recent tonsillectomy increased the likelihood that a child would contract polio—and that if the child did contract polio at such a time, it would more likely be the more serious, bulbar kind.[82] Dr. W. L. Aycock of Harvard endorsed this position in 1929. Soon thereafter the Talmey-Aycock thesis was proven correct both epidemiologically, by Drs. Thomas Francis and Gaylord Anderson, and experimentally, by Dr. Albert Sabin, in 1938.[83] *Polio and Its Problems,* by Dr. Roland H. Berg, sold widely after it was published in 1948. Claiming to report to the public "the sum of our knowledge" about polio, it told the story of the "Tragedy at Akron," about the K family in Ohio, which suffered mightily on account of a tonsillectomy. Tonsillectomy, concluded Berg, definitely increases both the frequency and the severity of the long-term paralytic effects of polio-myelitis.[84] Penicillin was able to ward off the very infections that had jus-tified widespread use of tonsillectomy in the first place. (All this says nothing about the "psychological" problems sometimes associated with tonsillectomy.)[85]

One might ask, therefore, why doctors and parents continued to favor tonsillectomies, even during the 1950s. They should have known that doing so would precipitate even more polio and more serious kinds of polio. The question Why seems now to be part of a *ghostly* legal brief masquerading as history of medicine. And the predictable responses to the question are desperation (especially on the part of parents), greed (especially on the part of doctors), and ignorance.

Desperation was dangerous. Polio doctors' desire for the "best" treat-ment for their patients often drove out their ability to do what was good for those patients. In 1953, the polio Edmund Sass was given injections of "the best curare" in order to reduce muscle spasms and allow for stretch-ing.[86] My Harvard colleague Diana Barrett was injected with cod liver oil in Mexico. Enid Foster was given massive injections of vitamin B.[87] William

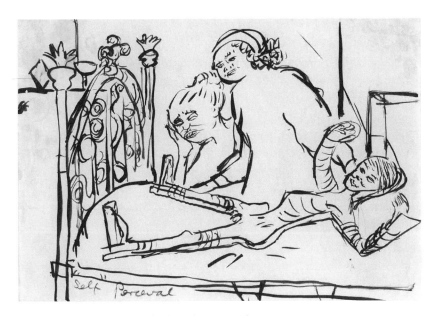

Self-Portrait in Bed with Polio, by John Perceval.

Haast, a poison researcher, provided polios with injections of cobra venom in Florida. Lorenzo Wilson Milam was given electric shock treatment, as he reports in his account.[88] Other patients, usually children, suffered the application of hot irons and firebrands.[89] Tens of thousands of other children went through numerous surgeries, many experimental or unnecessary.[90] At one time, many polios were put into nearly head-to-toe body casts. In Quebec, this practice was not unusual in the 1950s; and in Tasmania it was commonplace.[91] The artist John Perceval, himself a polio, records the usual casting process in a reed drawing, *Self* (1943), in the collection of the Australian National Gallery.

Thanks partly to the work of Sister Kenny—known as "the woman who challenged the doctors"[92]—some orthopedists eventually gave up such casts and came to believe that, after a period of total rest, the polio should have various sorts of hot packs applied. This method, with its notorious skin burns, was the "Sister Kenny method." Sister Elizabeth Kenny was the Australian author of *The Treatment of Infantile Paralysis in the Acute Stage* and, with Martha Otenso, of the nearly autohagiographical *And They Shall Walk: The Life Story of Sister Elizabeth Kenny.*[93] The National Foundation for Infantile Paralysis adopted Kenny's ideas in 1943, as discussed in Dr.

Pohl's *Kenny Concept of Infantile Paralysis and Its Treatment,* and the foundation's guidelines for both nurses and parents thereafter promulgated her methods.[94] In 1952, when Kenny died, she was the most admired woman in America—easily winning out over Eleanor Roosevelt.[95] That popularity was due partly to Rosalind Russell's portrayal of Kenny in the movie *Sister Kenny* (1946).

Some narratives written by polios compare the harmful treatment they believe they received in one place with the good treatment they believe they had elsewhere. Consider, for example, this passage from Lorenzo Wilson Milam's *Cripple Liberation Front Marching Band Blues* about his stay at Hope Haven, a polio recuperation clinic in Jacksonville, Florida:

> Permanent harm? Did I suffer any permanent harm from Hope Haven? Sure: I have a souvenir of Hope Haven that twinges me to this very day. Medical care—sensible, up-to-the-latest-technology medical care, available to those who could look for it in 1952—dictated total bed-rest for the post-polio for at least three months. And then—a gradual, gradual, gradual reeducation of the muscles.[96]

Milam blames the cupidity and stupidity of Hope Haven for his being more crippled than he had to be. Not until Milam got to Warm Springs, Georgia—he says—was he treated in a way that he believes was properly beneficial. Around that time, Eleanor Roosevelt herself was writing celebratory pieces about Warm Springs, such as her foreword to Turnley Walker's book *Roosevelt and the Warm Springs Story.*[97]

Rushing to declare a polio cured (whether as a result of "wise therapy" or "spontaneous recovery") often did great harm. Most properly educated doctors were in agreement already in 1949 that "the poliomyelitis child in the late stage needs to be seen twice yearly until full growth has been attained" and that, as Dr. Joseph Barr wrote from Harvard, exercise needed to be curtailed.[98] (Researchers—for example, Dr. R. W. Lovett's team at Harvard—had gotten the same results much earlier in the century, in 1908, 1915, and 1917.)[99] I was not seen at all.

A summary of informed belief about the need to be seen by medical experts is here produced from an article by Dr. W. J. W. Sharrard, which was published in 1955, less than two years after my bout with polio.[100]

Similar advice can be gleaned from most other experienced medical

Extract from Sharrard, "The Distribution of the Permanent Paralysis in the Lower Limb in Poliomyelitis" (1955)

The quantitative relationship between the loss of motor nerve cells and the residual power in muscles is particularly important in cases [purportedly like mine] regarded as a-paralytic in the acute stage of poliomyelitis. Although there may never have been any clinical paralysis, a considerable proportion of motor cells may have been damaged or destroyed. The nerve supply to some muscles, especially those supplied by short cell columns, may have been diminished by up to 60 per cent. Patients without paralysis are frequently allowed to walk within two or three weeks of the onset of the major illness [as in my case]. It is known that overstretching or over-fatigue can occur in muscles such as the hip abductors or *tibialis* anterior and may result in deterioration in power. Paresis, previously undetectable, may be revealed later by the development of a limp or a *valgus* foot. It is probably wise, therefore, not to allow the resumption of full activity in an a-paralytic case at too early a date, and to continue to look for evidence of paresis over a period of not less than six months.

In the management of the later stages—that is, after the first six weeks—the importance of accurate muscle testing has been stressed by Seddon and has been found to be of value in the prognosis of recovery in paretic muscles. If the results of muscle testing are also used to reconstruct the probable site of major cell destruction in the spinal cord, the clinician will have a much clearer idea of what he is trying to treat, and what the chances are of recovery in paralyzed muscles. The presence of associated paralyses . . . may also help to define the prognosis for recovery of a paralyzed muscle. Recovery can be expected in some muscles but the prolonged and uneconomic treatment of those that are beyond all hope can be avoided.

Source: W. J. W. Sharrard, "The Distribution of the Permanent Paralysis in the Lower Limb in Poliomyelitis: A Clinical and Pathological Study," *Journal of Bone and Joint Surgery* 37, no. B.4 (November 1955), 37. Reproduced with permission and copyright © of the British editorial Society of Bone and Joint Surgery.

consultants of the period. In 1954, Dr. William P. Frank advised that, in cases of nonparalytic polio, "patients should have an extended period of rest after deferescence [sic] and also subsequent examinations for signs of delayed muscle involvement," and he recommends the use of hot packs.[101] In the same year, 1954, Dr. Charles L. Lowman put forward the idea that

> About 75 per cent of all people have some postural fault. Hence, the large group of non-paralytic and mild paralytic cases which may have very slight degrees of muscular imbalance superimposed on pre-poliomyelitic postural deviations will have greater potential for later deformity than would otherwise exist. . . . The need for regular check-ups at 3-month intervals the first year, 6-month intervals the second year, and then once a year until full growth is obtained should be explained to the parents of young children. Advice about strenuous activities such as gymnastics, athletics, and summer camping is the responsibility of the physician who shares with the parents, supervision of the child's growth and development.[102]

Many child polios who are now in middle age can say truthfully that had they had proper testing of their muscles in the years following their polio—and, concomitantly, had they thereby gleaned more knowledge about their physical condition and received appropriate training in how to deal with their bodies—much of their present loss of strength and function might have been avoided.

So in many cases parents of polio children were right to keep their children out of the hands of medical professionals. Our doctors knew little, and they were psychologically unprepared to do what was good, partly because they fantasized about what was best. Writes Rudyard Kipling (1865–1936) in his pleasantly forgiving poem "Our Fathers of Old":

> Wonderful little, when all is said,
> Wonderful little our fathers knew,
> Half their remedies cured you dead—
> Most of their teaching was quite untrue—[103]

What if I had seen good doctors? "The *what-if* game, a futile exercise in hindsight," an Australian writer reminds us, "poses such unanswerable questions as *what if* Romulus and Remus had fallen foul of a hostile . . . wolf?"[104] What if young Susan McPherson had not had a tonsillectomy? What if FDR had not gone swimming at Campobello Island? What if FDR had seen a proper doctor earlier in the acute stage of polio? It is all but impossible to know whether Roosevelt, had he become ill with polio near a good hospital instead of on Campobello Island, would have been less crippled than he was—though that is one implication of Schary's play *Sunrise at Campobello*.[105] Likewise, one can hardly know whether, if he had not been so severely crippled by polio, Roosevelt would have become so great a president. What good does it do to wonder whether one would have been better off had Roosevelt been seen at Warm Springs like Milam? It's best to not look back.

At the same time, laying out how things might have happened otherwise often serves at least to map the ways taken—and the ways not taken—in a historical context. Laying out alternatives, one product of the comparative method, provides a cultural record of the past of some people (hindsight), while at the same time establishing guideposts for the future (foresight) of others.

Vaccination Day

Polio Vaccination Day in the 1950s was an emotionally complex time for young polios—and a favorite topic for photographers of the period (see the photograph on p. 127). One vexing problem is Why wasn't the vaccine there when I really needed it? It was especially acute for polios who were struggling to live in iron lungs or those like Eddie Bollenbach who were given a placebo instead of the vaccine itself.[106]

Another issue was Should I have the vaccine or not? This question greatly troubled Edward Le Comte in *Long Road Back*, Wilfrid Sheed in *Memory of a Recovery*, and Susan Terris in *Wings and Roots*.[107]

I was stumped in much the same way. I was a child, so I knew less than did Le Comte, Sheed, and Terris. And the various decisions could not be mine to make. In 1955, I was not given the Salk vaccine because, as my caretakers said, "You don't need it." I was too terrified to ask, "Don't I?" At the time, no one had even told me that I had had polio.

The question "Should I have the vaccine or not?" raised anxiety-producing thoughts for me again in 1960. At that time, the so-called killed Sabin vaccine was being distributed at Algonquin Elementary School in the Town of Mount Royal (TMR). First, I tried to determine whether or not my "cold in the leg" had been polio. Then I tried to determine (on my own) what would be the right thing to do if I *had* had polio—and if I had not had polio. What would happen if I had had polio and now received the vaccine? Could you get polio more than once? Would the vaccine trigger a return of polio? Might you get polio from the vaccine itself? Would I be one of these unlucky persons?[108] (Such "freakish" cases of polio play a key role in several children's books of both the fictional and the nonfictional sort. In Jerome Brooks's *Big Dipper Marathon,* the guilt-ridden parents, who had had their son vaccinated, try to keep secret from him the official fact that his "particular case of poliomyelitis need not have occurred.")[109] I also had to respond to one classmate whose parents thought that the polio vaccine was a bad idea for everyone, whether they had had polio or not. (Such booklets as Eleanor McBean's *The Poisoned Needle* and Mira Louise's *Protection from Polio and Animal Research* [1956] passed about the school-yard from time to time.)[110] Even so, I wondered what would happen if I had not had polio and did not now have the vaccine. Did having polio give you immunity only to the one kind of polio you had had? Having had polio once, could you get it again? In her *Polio Tragedy of 1941,* Virginia Acosta writes of calling up her polio doctor and getting the school nurse fired for telling Acosta that, since she couldn't get polio twice, she didn't need the vaccine![111]

Who Are You?

Five years after my bout with polio, I got up the nerve to ask my parents again whether I had actually had polio. At the time, my paternal grand-mother, Bubbie Rose (Selechonek) and one of my maternal uncles, Bennie (Cytrynbaum), had both told me that I had had polio. The oral (Sabin) polio vaccine was being distributed at school, so the issue was again a pressing one for me.[112] I wanted confirmation or denial from my parents of my having had polio. My parents admitted—"Yes—but a tiny case that left no blemish. You were not even paralyzed." I was admonished not to speak about the matter. *Why* not speak about the matter? Was having been paralyzed (as I still remembered that I had been) something to be ashamed of?

To have a child with polio was shameful in many ways. According to the sociologist David Riesman, it was actually even "un-American."[113] A child polio was the cause of family shame. But as it seemed to me, or as I hoped, my parents were not so much ashamed of me as lovingly worried about me.

The instruction to be silent about polio looms large in memoirs and much fiction about polio. Thus, we learn in Betty Cavanna's *Joyride* that the heroine "never spoke of her disability, even to her mother."[114] Thanks to just such early admonition, many polios were afraid to talk about their experience of polio and disability. Thus Roxane Frigon—who had polio in Abitibi, Quebec, at the age of three—reports that her interview in 1998 with Pierrette Caron and Gilles Fournier was the first time she had ever spoken of her disability. "This interview allows me for the first time in my life to really talk about my handicap."[115]

As for me, I usually followed the parental rule not to mention my polio. I also often wondered what the punishment was for being deformed by polio. I had read in Hillyer's *A Child's Geography of the World* (1929) about how Maria Eleonora tried to kill her infant daughter Christina Wazu because Christina had been born with a caul over her pelvis. Christina eventually became the great queen of Sweden. (*Caul*, referring to the membrane surrounding a baby before it is born, which may not rupture at birth, was a word I did not understand until, many years later, I saw the polio Francis Ford Coppola's *The Conversation* [1974]. This movie is a gloss on Alfred Hitchcock's *Rear Window* [1954]; the main character is the private eye Harry Caul, a polio survivor.)

"You were not even paralyzed." The effect of telling me that I had *not* been paralyzed affected my understanding of the special power of words and also of the limitations of their magic. Like many young polios, I felt a little like Alice disengaged from her body. Having changed her size, Alice says, "I'm not myself." Already she has been fed such questions as the utterly terrifying "Who are *you?*"[116] This exchange is from *Alice's Adventures in Wonderland*, by Lewis Carroll, who was a stutterer. The questioner is the Caterpillar, an animal that is a butterfly-to-be and therefore, at any given moment, is both itself and not itself. My parents' message seemed to be this: I was neither what I had been (paralyzed) nor what I was (weak). My

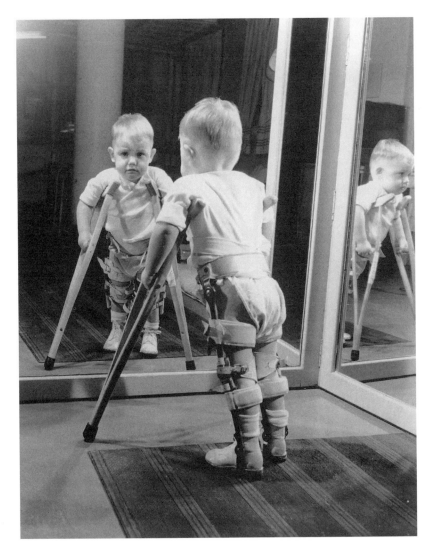

Polio at the mirrors.

condition was somehow merely *nominal*. Therefore a name change—like the transformation from Charles Lutwidge Dodgson to Lewis Carroll—could cure me. Alternatively, my problem was voluntary (instead of nominal). If so, then a change of will could cure me. These intellectual messages became fused in my mind with the name changes that actually marked my growing up as much as did bodily metamorphoses.

I had thought I was the lame little boy named Maier Selechonek. That is what my Hebrew-language Jewish birth certificate said my name was. But to me, my parents seemed to be saying, "Become now the whole-bodied young man called Marc Shell!" By 1961, when I graduated from Hebrew School, Marc Shell was already my de facto name—as on the certificate of graduation. I become de jure Mark Shell in 1967 by means of an official Order of Council. (Such name changes were not untypical among assimilating Eastern Europeans in Canada.) So it is that I have a multilingual set of first names: Hebrew Maier, French Marc, English Mark. Likewise, I have a set of equally malleable family names: the Hebrew ben Chaiim, the Yiddish/Czech Selechonek, the English-sounding Shell. I still don't know whether Marc was chosen to be my nominal "password" because it was Christian-sounding (as in "Saint Mark") or because it was Polish (Marek)—or both.

Would a nominal change (from Maier to Marc) work to change me bodily from what I was? The question recalls Shakespeare's *Romeo and Juliet*. Here a desperate Juliet wants Romeo to "be some other name!" She hopes that a name change (from Montague) might (also) change kinship, or blood-familial condition. That is to say, she considers that kinship, ordinarily understood as a matter of immutable biology ("in the blood"), is merely a matter of naming. Juliet even compares gaining or losing a name with gaining or losing a limb:

> What's Montague? it is nor hand, nor foot,
> Nor arm, nor face, nor any other part
> Belonging to a man.[117]

But, as I knew when I first read this great play, polio—of "any . . . part / Belonging to a man" is finally less mutable than kinship. It is only in cartoons and comic strips that a polio like me could become a superman by virtue of a name change—as does, for example, the superhero Captain America, born Steve Rogers (a polio), in the well-known comic book series *Captain America* (1941–1954).[118]

Why can't *I* fly like Captain America? This question is something like Dorothy Gale's question in *The Wizard of Oz*: "Birds fly over the rainbow, / Why then, oh why can't I?"[119] When I first saw *The Wizard of Oz*, in 1957, I noticed its matter-of-fact attempts to overcome paralysis. Oh sure, there

was the *superficial* appearance that *The Wizard of Oz* is merely about curing the "arthritis" of old Hickory. Hickory tells us that he is so *plagued* that
his joints feel rusted.[120] Hickory is finally cured, if at all, only in his fantastic persona as the Tin Man in Oz. And the paralytic condition from which
the Tin Man suffers is less like arthritis than like polio—a disease just getting its start as an American epidemic around the time that Frank Baum
was writing "The Rescue of the Tin Man."[121] Baum himself had seen the
rise of polio epidemics in New York State (where he was born), Chicago
(where he wrote *The Wizard of Oz*), and Kansas (where Dorothy lives).

The Tin Man, while just minding his own business, was, like me in October 1953, paralyzed (frozen by rust) one day.[122] It happened to him suddenly—as it does to a polio! Trapped in his metal body, the Tin Man has
become no muscle and all prosthesis. He is like a completely paralyzed human being imprisoned in the iron lung that keeps him alive. What is more,
the Tin Man can move so little that he can barely talk. He is like a stutterer—blocked. Yet the Tin Man manages to come out with the memorably ambiguous words *oil can.*

"Oil Can" was my first polio poem. The Scarecrow, one of Dorothy's
variously disabled friends, interprets the Tin Man's "oil can" to mean "oil is
able." And Scarecrow figures that Tin Man is stuck in midsentence, like a
stutterer blocking. The Scarecrow wants the Tin Man to complete his sentence and asks, "Oil can what?" The jest resides in the pun: *can* means not
only "is able" (the verb) but also "container made of tin" (the noun). So
now we can interpret *oil can* as meaning, among other things, "Oil can
cure my paralysis." So says the Tin Man, or the Man in the Tin Can. What
kind of oil can cure polio? Some doctors in the 1950s said it was cod liver
oil, taken by injection. But Baum's near contemporary George Washington
Carver (1864–1943) claimed that massage with peanut oil cured polio.[123] In
The Wizard of Oz, in fact, oil turns the Tin Man from a dumb person (stutterer) into a fluent speaker and—when taken in combination with physiotherapeutic manipulations by Dorothy and the Scarecrow—from a paralytic (stumbler) into a mover. Now at last, thanks to oiling, the Tin Man
can cancan.

When, after the great polio epidemic of 1916, Baum's *The Tin Woodman
of Oz* was published—with its tales of leg amputation and restoration, and
of voice reparation by means of oiling—it was an instant success.[124]

In the Family

Of all diseases, poliomyelitis is the one most dreaded by families.

—Elizabeth Rice, speaking at the First International Poliomyelitis Conference (1949)

Polios of almost all generations know Dinah Maria Craik's Victorian novella *The Little Lame Prince*. In this work, his family keeps the lame Prince Dolor secreted away in a prison tower. Such secretive family behavior typified the culture of denial and paralysis in the mid-twentieth century as that culture reveals itself in myriad historical, autobiographical, and aesthetic artifacts.

Bondage and Bandage

In regard to this widespread secrecy about disability and how it played out in the case of polios, I recall how two "invisibly" disabled members of our family were treated. Their treatment reveals something about the treatment of the disabled in the post-Holocaust, ambiguously Jewish culture in which I grew up, and I think it suggests how profoundly an experience like polio can affect a young child's thinking.

The first of these disabled family members was Usher Meller, a paternal cousin. Cousin Usher Meller had been "in Europe" during World War II. That war, like my illness, was something we were not supposed to discuss. In the beginning, when I first met Usher, I used to ask my parents why he walked as I had walked in the period after I had had polio. I was "shushed." To this day, I do not know for sure whether the etiology of Cousin Usher's symptoms involved torture in some horrible experiment by Dr. Josef Mengele or resulted from multiple sclerosis. No matter, both possibilities were apparently equally shameful—not to be s-s-s-spoken of. (I had by then developed the stutter I still have.) Whereas most everyone in our extended family treated me either as if I were "fully normal" or as if I were an ill-tempered hypochondriac, Usher was one of the few people who treated me as I was. People in my family were afraid of Usher and kept him as far away from us as possible. My brother Brian told me recently that he had recollections of being afraid of Usher. I was not afraid of Usher because I was a little like him. Had people not blinded themselves, or been blinded, to *my* disabilities—muscular atrophy, a short leg, and stuttering—would they not have been afraid of me too?

I hesitate now to draw any analogies between such traumas as those I experienced as a young polio and those Usher may have experienced as a Holocaust survivor, but at the time I was just a boy, and I had already been "prepped" culturally to make the conflation between the Holocaust and polio experiences. Certain cultural circumstances encouraged this conflation. To begin with, there were the visual comparisons. Alfred Eisenstadt's *Life* magazine photographs of polio wards, for example, famous at the time, made the wards *look* like concentration camps.[1] Hitler sent institutionalized polios to the gas chambers.[2] When I saw my very first full-length commercial movie, *Lili*, in 1953, at the neighborhood YMHA, I conflated the situation of the post-Holocaust orphan (played by Leslie Caron), whose only friend is a puppet operated by a cripple, with the situation of the crippled puppeteer (Mel Ferrer).[3] In addition, *Lili's* theme song—"A song of love is a song of woe / Don't ask me how I know"—reminded me of my own lonely situation.[4] In fact, the period of the 1950s was replete with stories of orphanhood, polio, death camps, and puppeteering (as in Tony Kemeny's *A Puppet No More*).[5] The polio Susan Hyun Sook Beidel, born in China of Korean parents, was also abandoned, in 1950, during the Korean War, and she tells the tale in her self-published autobiography *The Story of Susie Lee*.[6] A variant on the theme of polio survivor as Holocaust victim informs *Stephania,* by Ilona Karmel.[7] Karmel, who had been hospitalized in Sweden at the end of World War II for injuries received in a Nazi concentration camp, provides an account of a year in the lives of three patients in the same hospital room. One patient is a Polish refugee (modeled on Karmel herself) determined to have a normal body after the disfigurement of the ghetto and concentration camp. The second is a sixteen-year-old whose supposedly passive acceptance of infantile paralysis keeps her immobile.[8] The third is a provincial unmarried woman whose broken leg cannot bear the overweight of her secret feeding. From the Holocaust survivor's standpoint, Karmel's account points to some similarity between the Holocaust and the polio experience.

After all, I am not surprised that many other Jewish polios were tormented by the similarities between the nightmare of polio and that of the Holocaust. First-person Jewish polio narratives, like Elaine Strauss's *In My Heart I'm Still Dancing*, often mention that in the grip of polio's initial onslaught, the narrator imagined being in the power of the Nazis.[9] (The superman Captain America—once known merely as the weakling Steve Rogers—was cured of his polio by a scientist who had escaped from the Nazis.)[10]

The main similarity between polio and the Holocaust as framed in the sociopathology of the 1950s lay in the "silent treatment" and tough love accorded to polios and Holocaust survivors alike. (In his stage play *The Normal Heart,* Larry Kramer compares the silence about AIDS in the 1980s with the failure to remember the reality of polio and the facts of the Holocaust.) Polio survival was, in this respect, as taboo as Holocaust survival. From 1945 to 1960, for example, the Holocaust received short shrift in the Jewish-Canadian community: we Jewish children knew that *something* had happened "over there," but the adults purposely neglected it in conversation and in the Jewish press. Likewise, Jewish schools overlooked the Holocaust in Jewish history classes, claiming that the subject would traumatize the students. As Franklin Bialystok writes in *Delayed Impact,* "most Canadian Jews did not want to know what happened, and few survivors had the courage to tell them." "The Holocaust," says Cyril Levitt, a Jew whose ancestors had come over to Canada in the nineteenth century, was " 'a *disease* that one didn't talk about.' "[11] That was the world for the survivor Cousin Usher.

The other disabled person in my family was my maternal grandfather, Zeyde Joseph Cytrynbaum. Zeyde Joe had emigrated from Poland to Canada just after World War I. Zeyde had a paralyzed, twisted finger. For the most part, he kept it secret, or at least didn't make an issue of it. However, the story of Zeyde's life terrified me: his family abandoned him, and he mutilated his own digit. The story was that on the day of his bar mitzvah, Zeyde Joe had been ordered by his father Solomon Cytrynbaum to leave the house in Poland because the boy's stepmother no longer wanted him around the house. I wondered whether Zeyde had been ejected from the family because of his disability, much as the lame Greek God Hephaestus was by his mother, Hera. I was told several different stories explaining Zeyde's permanently twisted "trigger finger." My mother told me that Zeyde, when he was a young boy about my age, had accidentally injured himself—a little like the Tin Woodman—while chopping wood.[12] When I was eleven years old, though, Zeyde himself told a different story to a small group of us. My grandfather had been drafted to serve in the Russian army, but he did not want to fight, so he purposely cut the tendon in his trigger finger, in order to make the finger curl, so that he would be unable to fire a gun.

There was a good deal of laughter in the room when the story ended. The grown-ups probably knew that such automutilation was not an uncommon practice among Jews and others in the Hapsburg Empire. As for me, I remember wondering whether the adults enjoyed the thought of Zeyde's outwitting the Poles. Were *they* not bothered by Zeyde's voluntary self-mutilation and lifelong disability?

In much of the Jewish tradition, automutilation is as taboo as being uncircumcised.[13] Even normally disabled people are sometimes barred from being part of the minyan. That Saul commits suicide "lest these uncircumcised come and make sport of me," as the book of Samuel has it, is puzzling—especially when one considers his suicide in the context of the physical disability of his lame grandson Mephibosheth.[14] In any case, I did not ask anyone in the family how Zeyde's actions squared with Jewish law. Instead, I screwed up enough courage only to ask Zeyde about the pain: "Does it still hurt?" My mother told me, "Shaaa!" (Be quiet!).[15]

The stories about Zeyde's cutting his own finger remind me (now) of two events. I loved vacationing at my maternal grandparents' blue and white summer cottage in Val David: I especially enjoyed sliding down the rapids in the North River and spent hours exploring the woods there, with my mother, who often took with her a copy of *Exploring Nature with Your Child*.[16] These were the happiest hours of my childhood. One day, when I was eight years old, however, I cut my hand badly; we went to the local hospital, where it was properly bandaged. When I was bar-mitzvahed at thirteen, my memories of that bandaging came back to haunt me. That is the age at which, as a Jewish adult, I had to learn to put on tefillin every day. Now, the English phrase *leather bandages* was my peer group's slang term for these tefillin or phylacteries. These religious items themselves had for us an almost fetishistic quality—not surprisingly so, since the word *phylacteries* actually means something like "magical amulet." (The Greek *phylacteries* derives from a distinctly anti-Semitic usage in the New Testament.)[17]

The rule for wearing tefillin is that you are supposed to bind, or bandage, your hand *(yadcha)*.[18] Which hand? Scholars and rabbis often interpreted *yadcha* as meaning "the weak hand" *(yad kay-ah)*. That would mean that a right-handed person (like me) should put tefillin on his left hand, and vice versa; however, what if the person in question was ambidextrous, as my father was? More to the point: What if the person learning to put on tefillin, although right-handed (in the sense of writing naturally with his right hand), was actually much stronger on his left side—because, say, he had had polio on the right side? The point is What if the person was weaker on the right side, but everyone, including himself, all but denied the fact? Cantor Muhlstock, who taught me to put on tefillin, avoided the issue. He asked me, with his thick Yiddish accent, an intentionally rhetorical question, "You're right-handed, right?" I said, in Sephardic-accented Hebrew, "Kane" (Yes). I put tefillin on my left arm, although my right arm was the weaker.

One can make a paralyzed finger move by binding it to a nonparalyzed adjacent finger. So Zeyde taught me early about prosthetics and compensation.

Which Leg Was It?

Early on in the polio experience, I had asked my parents, "What's wrong with me?" They told me, "Forget it." I was a dutiful son. Pretty soon I had "forgotten" which leg had been paralyzed. But try as I might, I could not forget that one of my legs had been paralyzed. So one day I asked, "*Which* of my legs 'had a cold'?" They never answered. I do not know whether my parents forgot which leg had had the "cold." But if they had, this forgetting or denial would be much like the parental strategies I have encountered in the literature and historical polio narratives. In Jerome Brooks's *Big Dipper Marathon*, the parents hide polio-related mail from their crippled son, "mainstream" him in school, and deny that he is any different from anyone else—even though, in his case, he must use wheelchair and crutches. According to the plot, or argument, of this book, "they're locking *him* up in a vacuum so that *they* won't feel the pain. In a vacuum nobody hears screams." The boy, who narrates the book, writes, "Pater and Mater, who are really good at creating vacuums, they'll take care of the little things, like seeing to it that he goes to the dances." Throughout his youth, says this boy, he has dealt with "the Big Lie, . . . the vacuum some people try to keep their kids in."[19]

Did parents actually decide—make a compact—not to speak to their polio children about the paralysis because they did not want their children to favor "that" side? Or were they perhaps hoping to discourage the children from becoming attention-seeking hypochondriacs or manipulative malingerers?

I have heard of some families' never once discussing a *parent's* paralysis, as in the case of the family of Danièle LeBlanc. "We never spoke of polio in the family, certainly not! I tried to speak of it with my father during his last years, but it was a delicate subject, almost taboo."[20] (I do not, however, know of a single nonliterary case of a *child's* paralysis where paralysis could not be mentioned—except for my own case.)

Parents often fail to ask about, and sometimes they ignore or deny outright, their children's experiences. Consider the experience of the young girl, Beth, who had polio in the Australian Carol Mara's novel *Iron Cradles*—probably named with some such medical book as A. Barnett's *Iron Cradle* in mind.[21] Beth returns from a lengthy stay in the hospital; the mother did not ask her about her experience there. This experience included wetting herself and being punished for it. The mother "felt the urge to ask Beth what they had done if she wet her pants, but decided that she did not want the knowledge that might break her heart." The mother's desire to keep her own heart "whole" had the effect of fragmenting her bond with her child.[22]

Miracles

In the 1950s, people were fond of two notions, of dubious but not entirely doubtful medical standing, that tended to distinguish between "serious polio" (which was to be feared) and "not-so-serious polio" (which was to be hoped-for, once a diagnosis of polio had been made and accepted). First the view was that there was a paralytic kind of polio and a nonparalytic kind. This division of polio into two sorts is problematic from the scientific point of view, especially given the confusion between polio and polio-like diseases (for example, Wallgren's disease).[23]

The second view was that polio could be of the permanent kind or of the temporary kind.[24] This belief tended to ignore that all forms of polio damaged neurons, permanently. The damage was not reliably testable in living patients, even by means of electromyelograms (EMGs) or muscle biopsies. Nevertheless, beginning at least as far back as 1942, "autopsies on people who had non-paralytic polio, but who died from other causes, show nerve damage and some degree of neuronal death consistent with paralytic polio."[25] Such findings as these were being confirmed in the 1950s.[26] Nonparalytic polio was not different from paralytic polio in terms of the type of neuronal damage.[27]

Many parents professed belief in spontaneous recovery from polio. In so doing, they often mistook their own hopefulness that their children would recover—"a positive attitude"—for kindness to their children, who probably would not recover. In any case, just such recovery is described and prescribed in religious, or pseudoreligious, American books like Edward Doherty's *Saint of Paralytics*.[28]

Miracles were also still big business in Quebec. A few miles beyond Île d'Orléans, in Sainte-Anne-de-Beaupré, the Basilica of Sainte-Anne is a pilgrimage site, piled with crutches left after miracle cures; historians have it that the chapel, which houses the finger- and wrist-bones of Saint Anne, was already a site for healing paralytics when Marie de l'Incarnation visited in 1665! ("There is a church dedicated to Saint Anne in which our Lord performs great wonders through the intercession of this saint, mother of the Virgin Mary. We can see the paralytic walk," wrote Marie in letters of that year.)[29] I grew up in Montreal, very near just such a site of pilgrimage: Saint Joseph's Oratory. Here, the Crutches Room evidenced miraculous recoveries from polio—in the tradition of the various paralysis miracles overseen by Jesus and Saint Peter. (The latter's miracle is the subject of the polio Brother John Sellars's blues spiritual "He Came All the Way Down."[30] At the time, I knew of the seventeenth-century saint Margaret Mary Alacoque, the patron saint of paralytics, to whom James Joyce refers in his story "Eveline" in *Dubliners*. "Eveline" concerns what Joyce, referring to his experience of Irish culture, calls "the centre of paralysis" that is

Dublin.[31] But I read it as Montreal.) This room in the Oratory of Montreal was full of thousands of crutches labeled with the names of the paralytics who no longer needed them; the crutches demonstrated the miraculous powers of Father André at Saint Joseph's Oratory.[32] On the one hand, the doctors in 1953 were giving us crutches—as in Esther Bubley's brilliant but patronizing prizewinning photograph of 1953, later made into a National Foundation poster. On the other hand, the local priests were stockpiling the same prostheses for their Crutches Room.

The Catholic Church itself—if not Father André—was interested not so much in curing the body as in saving the soul. Pope Pius XII, in his French-language *Address to the Third International Poliomyelitis Congress* held in Rome in 1955, reminds his audience, "It would be an error to believe that moral and psychological balance can be restored more easily than muscular strength."[33] Would that Pius's audience had really understood—and acted upon—these words! As I later learned, even anglophone, non-Catholic Christian polios visited Saint Joseph's Oratory with an expectation of *physical* cure. One of these was the upper-class eight-year-old Mary Grimley Mason. Mason, who was eventually to study English literature at Harvard, writes in her *Life Prints: Memoir of Healing and Discovery* that God's failure to follow through on the deal she proposed to him at Saint Joseph's Oratory was the turning point in her life. "Let Nana live," she told God, "and forget about my ever being cured and able to walk."[34] God's "failure" to save Nana led to Mason's finally giving up on her father's unrealistic hope that his daughter would be cured of polio, hence also to her coming to terms with being crippled and getting on with her life.

In the United States, many Protestant polio cripples were encouraged to believe that they would reap a heavenly reward for enduring polio on earth: God would "make up for" the polio by giving them a mansion in a special "heaven for polios who die"—as Virginia Acosta puts it in *Polio Tragedy of 1941.*[35] Record albums of the period, with such names as *Cripples Reward* (Buddy Robertson's in the mid-1950s), put forward the proposition that, to polios, God would one day provide a "mansion in the sky."[36] Most remarkably, Warm Springs, Georgia, was a *Decameron*-like Mecca on earth for realistic East-coast polios—as Plagemann calls it in *My Place to Stand.*[37] There the patients themselves—who required realistic assessment of where they stood more than did the people who pitied or ignored their travails—often got together to dispel the idea of miracle cure. Plagemann

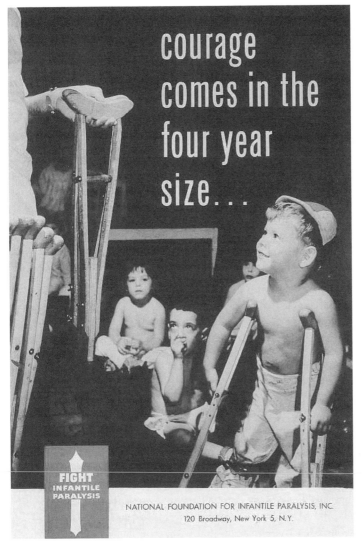

Courage comes in all sizes: crutches being handed out to children.

reports what I call the Drama of the False Polio Miracle, which was performed to trick visitors.

One of the healthy push boys [the men who helped the polios get
about] allowed himself to be put in a chair, wearing borrowed braces,

with a lapboard to support his arms across the arms of the chair, and crutches hung on the back. Then, when the visitors had arrived, standing, as was their custom, in silent awe, some distance removed, another push boy went reverently to the fountain, dipped a paper cup of water from it, and carried it to the pseudo-patient. After drinking greedily, the cup held for him, he began to shake, jerk, jump; a glad smile broke on his face, and with a shout of delight he leaped from the chair, shedding braces, and danced about the pool, crying, "I'm cured! I'm cured!", while the real patients sat all about him, helpless and weak with laughter.[38]

Parents' and well-wishers' belief in a spontaneous recovery often required, for its sustenance, that the child not see a polio specialist after that recovery. Certainly I did not see a specialist after the initial two weeks of polio. The specialist I did see was Alton Goldbloom, often photographed with Sister Kenny; he had written in his book, *The Care of the Child*, that no one really ever "fully recovers" from polio.[39] My mother and father, who were relatively well educated, might have been expected to peruse Goldbloom's book.[40] I rather suspect, therefore, that what kept them from asking Dr. Goldbloom to examine me later on was fear of being told that I had not had a full "spontaneous recovery"—or they might have felt the need to exhibit toughness in the name of love.

Tough Love

> [Poliomyelitis] leaves many scars on those who were affected besides the obvious physical handicaps. If this fact is recognized and the children and parents are given assistance at the time of the acute illness and during the convalescent period, the future of these children may be less impaired.
>
> —F. S. Copellman, "Follow-Up of One Hundred Children with Poliomyelitis"

Polio children experience a radical scission of mind from body, a harrowing separation from family and friends, and painful exclusion as handicapped persons. Institutions everywhere were compounding the trauma by ignoring and even denying the children's experience. Dr. D. B. Kidd, in her chapter on patient psychology in *The Physical Treatment of Anterior Polio-*

myelitis (1943), grandly announced her favorite rule: "No crippled individual must be left to indulge in his own thoughts."[41]

Doctors had at their disposal many ways to guard against such indulgence. One was to pay attention only to adult polios. For example, Dr. Visotsky and colleagues ask, in *Archives of General Psychiatry*, "How is it possible to cope with such powerful, pervasive and enduring stresses as those involved in severe poliomyelitis?"[42] But though the coauthors profess a professional interest in such subjects "as social services for children," they do not even once consider children.[43] Likewise, writers in the *Journal of Mental and Nervous Diseases, Psychosomatic Medicine*, and the *American Journal of Orthopsychiatry* were studying the traumatic psychological aspects of being in an iron lung, yet they paid no heed to children.[44]

D. B. Kidd's rule and others like it were part of a powerful ideology of the time: adult caretakers were not to think much about the child polio as a person in his own right. Most all the "scientific" literature concerned with the psychology of polio, while it pays lip service to the child's psychology, immediately shifts attention to the psychologically damaging effects of the child's polio on his or her adult caretakers. It is as if the tragedy of infantile paralysis were only that of the parents and not that of the child with polio. There are only a few exceptions to this ideology—Newell's study in the *American Journal of Orthopsychiatry*, for example, and a few articles in the scholarly journals of the time. The more influential writers followed the same general pattern.[45] Here is how Roland Berg, in a book sponsored by the National Foundation for Infantile Paralysis, typically deflects attention from the child patient toward the parents: "Physically the patient may make a fine recovery, but psychologically he may still be seriously ill. Polio may have a profound psychological effect not only on the patient but on his family as well. Frequently parents blame themselves for their child's illness. They feel . . ." The rest of the paragraph concerns only parents. It closes with an unreferenced statement that parents generally need far more psychological treatment than patients. "One doctor, well versed in the treatment of polio, once remarked that he found parents of polio patients in greater need of psychological adjustments than the patients themselves."[46] In this same vein, Elizabeth Rice, speaking at the First International Polio Conference (1949), is concerned basically with how "parents become upset if they see the child is not happy."

None of this is to minimize how a child's polio might affect the parents in various ways or how proper psychological help for the parents would have also helped their polio children. In fact, the problems faced by polio parents were extreme. Many polio narratives written from the viewpoint of parents of polios start off with some such words as these from Quebecer Paul Decoste: "We had dreamed of handsome and strong boys." Decoste goes on to ask this question: "How to describe to what extent this test was able to murder our hearts of young married persons?"[47] The family of Garrett Oppenheim falls apart after his polio. Garrett's first-person narrative, *The Golden Handicap,* quotes his father (James Oppenheim), as writing, in *Mystic Warrior,* that Garrett's crippling was "the symbol" of all James's familial failures.[48] Concerning such parental feelings of disappointment, the king in Craik's *Little Lame Prince* is "crushed" when Prince Dolor becomes a cripple.[49] Many a magazine included articles about how *financially* crippling a polio could be to his family; thus the *Financial Post,* popular in Canada, featured the article "Polio and Your Pocket Book: In the Rare Case, It Can Be a Financial Crippler."[50]

The greatest part of the literature that professes overt concern with the psychology of young polios focuses, however incongruously, on how and why to keep children and their medical guardians apart from their parents. Dr. Richard Young, in an influential article in *Mental Hygiene* (1940), argues against any visits, claiming that "the almost ritualized visits between parents and patients at the polio wards" (as Robert Hall phrases it) was more harmful than useful. (In his polio memoir *Through the Storm* Hall suggests a similar tension between parent and child patient.)[51] Sometimes "tough love" toward polios was directly encouraged, as a guiding institutional policy. There are three moments in the breakdown of the efficacy of such warnings against "coddling":

In 1938, J. D. M. Griffin and colleagues published "Mental Hygiene in an Orthopaedic Hospital" in the *Journal of Pediatrics.* They describe the various steps taken to help children cope psychologically while in a Canadian polio-convalescent hospital.[52] Nurses there were given a lecture, which emphasized having an "objective" attitude and warned that the "danger lay in allowing one's natural sympathies to get out of hand." During the first month of preliminary hospitalization, the rule was simple and strict: No Visiting. All children over four years of age were seen by the psychiatrist or social worker soon after admission for "a five or ten minute chat . . . to make the child feel that someone in the hospital was taking a special interest in him." Younger children were not seen at all. Parents were brought in for a training session before their child's discharge, during which the dangers of spoiling the child in their upcoming after-discharge existence were stressed. Griffin and colleagues noted that there were severe cases of homesickness at the hospital and attributed these either to the child's "abnormal" attachment to its mother or to the child's being unstable.[53]

In 1948, The First International Poliomyelitis Conference reported, "The psychiatry of polio is the least well understood segment of the problem."[54] In the same year, M. Seidenfeld published a relevant article in the first issue of *Nervous Child* about the psychological aftereffects of polio in children.[55]

In 1952, the *American Journal of Physical Medicine* (1952) warned nursing staff and other caretakers that the traditional management philosophy—not "spoiling" polio children—in reality increased the children's anxiety, dependency, and hostility. The *Journal* further counseled that newly admitted patients should *not* be left alone in isolation wards (as they had been ever since 1916) and that they should be given a nightlight. Nurses were advised to make rounds frequently and not to remove patients' call bells. In fact, the author said, once patients established that staff could be trusted to respond to their needs, they would reduce their demands markedly. Most important, nurses were encouraged to allow patients to voice their fears and to answer their questions.[56]

An amusing anecdote in a family where polio had struck may serve to convey the toughness and tenderness at work here. It concerns the first encounter, in 1950, between Basil O'Connor (chairman of the National Foundation for Infantile Paralysis and FDR's law partner) and Betty Culver, his daughter (the mother of five children), who had just contracted polio in 1949. When father visited daughter in the polio section of the hospital, reports Victor Cohn in *Four Billion Dimes*, the first words spoken were "You'd better pull yourself together."[57] Yet, these were not a parent's tough words to a six-year-old child recently stricken and paralyzed; they were the words of a thirty-year-old daughter to a too-pitying parent.

Some parents' tough reaction to their polio children's physical predicament arose from those parents' psychological limitations. (In the case of my parents, for example, both were still recovering from the deaths ten years earlier of their parents. My mother's mother, Lieba Cytrynbaum, née Goldfinger, had died of cancer and my father's father, Max Selechonek, of a strokelike incident. Each of my parents was twelve years old at the time of the parent's death.) In such situations, tough love followed from parents' attending more to their own desires—say, for the disease and the attendant problems simply to go away—than to their polio-children's need to deal with things as they were. Sometimes too the parents were merely exercising the doctrine of tough love (though they wouldn't have called it that).[58]

We know a good deal now about the psychopathologies of parents who have disabled children (or fear to have them) and about how their feelings themselves disable the parent-child bond.[59] In the 1950s, however, the main predisposition was to have parents and guardians do everything they could to guard against the supposedly natural tendency of polios to use their disability as a defense mechanism. This mechanism, said the Freudian analysts, would come to explain most failures in their lives and hence encourage the children to persevere in a life of disability even when they were actually able-bodied.[60] The same sort of theorizing led psychiatrists in the school of Alfred Adler to regard stuttering as "a devious means of preserving in fantasy inflated longings for prestige against wounding encounters with reality, in the sense of what they might have become, if they had not stuttered."[61]

Now, one can recognize, on the one hand, the great danger in pitying disabled children. Relevant here would be Charles H. Andrews's book *No Time for Tears* (1951), described on the dust jacket as "the story of a ten-year-old boy's desperate but successful battle to survive polio, and his family's role in guiding him back to a normal life."

But the rule "Do not pity" is hardly sufficient. Considered from this perspective, my experience during the extended period of polio convalescence was sometimes tough. One event I recall has many parallels in the first-person narratives I have read, in which difficult situations typically exacerbate a polio-child's sense of loss of bodily control. In order to get to the bathroom, I sometimes had to drag myself out of my bed and onto the floor, then elbow my way across that floor to the door, then reach up to turn the doorknob with my left hand, and finally drag myself over the threshold and across the hall. I must have "sidled" along toward the bathroom in the way I imagine that the polio Christina Olson seems to sidle along in Andrew Wyeth's well-known painting *Christina's World* (1948).[62] (Andrew Wyeth's sister Henriette was a polio.) Young polios, like Elizabeth du Preez (who died in 1953), seem to move in much the same way—as suggested by the photographs in her book (1957). In any case, oftentimes I did not make it on time all the way to the toilet—a common story in the polio narratives. At such times, I think, I might have benefited from a session with the unusually insightful and empathetic psychoanalyst Dr. Jacob E. Finesinger, who was soon to write "A Depression in a Six-Year-Old Boy with Acute Poliomyelitis."[63] J. G. Farrell is doubtless correct when he writes in his major polio novel *The Lung,* "People who have polio almost always go through a period of depression."[64] The problem was especially difficult when one was told, in the tradition of tough love, that one could do things that one actually couldn't do—or shouldn't. Parents' treatment of polio children as if they were able-bodied often made the strain of having been crippled by polio all the more difficult. *If* there was nothing physically wrong with a child to explain the trouble with his body, then what would explain the problem? Many a child felt that there *must* be something morally wrong with him. Because one had had the *pest,* had one now become *pestilent*—that is to say, "morally baneful or pernicious"?[65]

Sometimes parents went overboard on tough love because they believed that *not* to deny that their child was a polio would be the death of him or her. This attitude toward disability was typical of that self-protecting insensitivity bordering on the callous which one often encounters in the culture of the period. Being crippled by polio was "a grim terror more menacing, more sinister, than death itself": that was an accepted theme among physicians and the popular press in early twentieth-century Canada.[66] My mother was a sad victim of this propaganda. She used to tell me that she would kill herself if she ever got arthritis so badly that she was unable to walk nine holes of golf; in the early 1960s, she began collecting books from the euthanasia-promoting Hemlock Society and its instructions for "choosing a hastened death." She did not understand consciously how she might be arguing for the death of me. The adult polio Jane Boyle Needham tells, in her polio narrative *Looking Up,* how she overheard the doctor tell her husband, "It would be a blessing for her, for all who loved her, if she would die tonight."[67]

Many polio children who had partially recovered and could pass as non-polios were sent to summer camp. There were warnings, as in Dr. Charles Lowman's writings, *against* sending polio children to regular summer

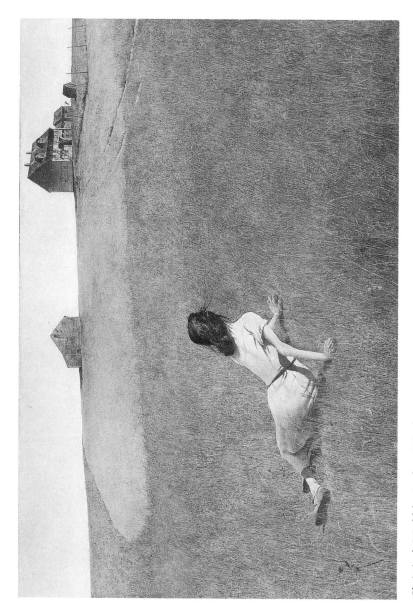

Christina's World, by Andrew Wyeth.

camp. Yet some parents desperately needed a vacation from their children—especially those who were sickly. (Jerry Bledsoe's *The Angel Doll*, set in the 1950s, describes a makeshift summer camp *especially* for polios.)[68] A few parents probably believed the camp brokers who told parents to send their young children away for the summer in order to get them out of the city during the polio season so that they would not get polio.[69]

When I went to summer camp in 1955, my parents told no one at the camp that I had recently had polio.[70] During that first summer at Camp Leawood, I wet my bed most nights for the first two weeks out of eight. (In the Australian novel *Iron Cradles*, the three-year-old polio Beth is punished for bedwetting during her hospitalization.) On camp visiting day, I did try to tell my parents that at least one thing was not fine. I said, I had been "seeing through" solid objects—or seeing double. My parent's responses were the usual ones: "There's nothing wrong," and "You are completely one hundred percent perfect." By contradicting my experience of my symptoms, they rendered further communication difficult. (I just came to believe that seeing double was normal and overcompensated for it, with often strange results.) I have long since learned that "double vision" was not unusual in polios. Enid Foster, for example, discusses it in her Rhodesian polio memoir. The Quebecer Suzanne Martel mentioned it, too, in an interview.[71] Ocular paralysis had been reported already by one of the great polio researchers, the Swedish doctor Ivar Wickman, and it appears prominently in the polio literature.[72] Sometimes the *superior obliquus* is paralyzed and the results are *diplopia* (the patient looks downwards and outward).[73] That was the case with me.[74]

I recall here that sometimes "trauma" is the result of lies or other dishonesties surrounding an incident—paralysis, say, or a sexual encounter. By way of an extreme example, consider Maya Angelou's *I Know Why the Caged Bird Sings*, which involves the rape of an eight-year-old girl. It is not only the physically violent sexual act, however egregious and damaging, that is traumatic and "ends childhood"; it is also the narratological structure imposed and the lies or denial surrounding it. Mary Vermillion thus remarks of Angelou's *Caged Bird* that the rapist, "after ejaculating on a mattress, tells her that she has wet the bed, and with this lie, he denies her knowledge about her own body and confounds her ability to make a coherent story out of his actions."[75] No wonder Mara Alper called her movie about sexual abuse *Stories No One Wants to Hear*.[76]

Many people, in what we sometimes call projection, blame the sick person for his illness; similarly, parents who fear that they did not properly care for a chronically ill child when she was little, sometimes claim, when she is older, that she does not care for others. Traumatized persons do *seem* sometimes to be emotionally uncaring or neutral, especially toward those who have traumatized them, as in the case of the post-polio hero in Judith Rossner's novel *Looking for Mr. Goodbar.*[77]

Sings the Tin Man: "If I Only Had a Heart."

Dependency and Isolation

These fragments I have shored against my ruins.

—T. S. Eliot, *The Waste Land*

"There's nothing and no one you can depend on, finally, but family." That's one of the rules my siblings and I were taught at home. The sentiment seems reassuring, a sort of declaration of love. But the axiom has its negative aspects. If there's no one you can count on but family, then what happens when you can't count on family? Then there is nothing and no one else. I could not depend on a family where denial, fear, and untruth had driven out trust; so the lesson meant now there would be nothing and no one. Were even self-reliance and independence out of the question? One way to encourage a child to love his parents, exclusively, is to remove everything and everyone else from him. In my case, just such removal exacerbated my already uncomfortable status as a physically dependent child polio who could not depend physically, psychologically, or intellectually on his parents. Most readers are able to recall well enough their own childhood attachments to one or another transitional object or beloved person, so I am bold enough to ask the reader's forbearance as I attempt to describe such removals in the case of a physically dependent polio seeking to determine what is wrong with him.

When I was home with polio, my first grade teacher Miss Bolotin was the only visitor I had from outside the family. During one visit, she brought me a school text, *Good Times with Our Friends*—one of the Dick and Jane readers in the "Health and Personal Development Series."[78] I was deeply distressed when, at age nine, I came home one day to discover that this book had disappeared. Such tales are usual in the polio narratives. Owen Dixson, in his first-person polio narrative *My Way with Polio,* tells of having various items taken from away from him because they would presumably remind him of the period when he had polio. Writes Dixson: "At any rate, when I later returned home from my new boarding school and asked for my photography they told me it had been broken and thrown away. It took me a long time to forgive my family for this."[79] Many polio narratives tell likewise of the disappearance of stuffed animals. Sometimes these transitional objects are destroyed to rid the home of germs, as in Margery Williams's *Velveteen Rabbit, or How Toys Become Real:* "'That?' said the doctor. 'Why, it's a mass of scarlet fever germs!—Burn it at once. What? Nonsense! Get him a new one. He mustn't have that any more!'"[80] Sometimes, though, polios' beloved teddy bears were discarded simply because they were manufactured by the very popular Steiff Company. Margarete Steiff, who had founded this company many decades earlier, was a wheelchair-bound polio—a fact much discussed in the magazines during the 1950s—and many caretakers believed that Steiff teddies would too morbidly remind polios of their difficult situations. So I lost my teddy bear, Mr. Doogie.

Many polios had their pets removed in much the same manner as their stuffed animals had been—presumably in order to help keep their environments free of dirt. Yet pets could be most important to polio patients. The dog named Mr. McPherson plays a key role in Ruth Sawyer's polio novella *Old Con and Patrick.*[81] The Scotch terrier named Fala was greatly beloved by Franklin Delano Roosevelt.[82] So did I love my springer spaniel, Buster. And as we shall consider, various relationships with animals, including outright identification with them, were often very helpful to polio patients.

I recall losing family members in a similar way. My maternal grandmother Bubbie Rose knew which of my legs was weaker and treated me kindly as a convalescent polio. Bubbie Rose used to carry me about on her shoulders; she was my "best vehicle"—even as Bob Cratchit was the "blood-horse" for his crippled son Tim in Dickens's *A Christmas Carol.*[83] Bubbie also pushed me on the kiddies' safety-swings and supported me on the children's seesaws in the public park. I loved the controlled feeling of *independent* weightlessness on the downswing when Bubbie Rose let go the opposite end of the seesaw's balanced plank. (At that point I had seen pictures of those seesawing rocking beds built to help bulbar polios breathe better. Louis and Dorothy Sternburg's *View from the Seesaw* discusses the rocking beds from the viewpoint of Louis, who got polio in 1955.)[84] There are many books about grandparents who help their polio grandchildren; one favorite was Ruth Sawyer's *Old Con and Patrick*.[85] But none could ever capture how crucial Bubbie's loving care was to me.

Soon after my polio convalescence, my parents forbade Bubbie Rose to visit with us at our home. This injunction had nothing to do with me, as far as I remember, but my mother did not get along with Rose. In any case, I saw Bubbie Rose far less frequently after we moved to our new house in the Town of Mount Royal in 1956–57. I regret that when Bubbie had her lower right leg amputated and was largely abandoned by family and friends at the Maimonides Hospital and Home for the Aged, I was already a student in California. During one visit to Maimonides, when my then relatively new wife, Susan, was visiting Rose with me, Rose pulled out the stump of her amputated right leg from under the covers and said to us, "Look what they did to me." I wish I understood then what I do now.

That we moved to the clean suburban Town of Mount Royal soon after my getting polio is not without its irony. It had long been supposed that diseases and viruses pitched their tents in the city environment.[86] And now politicians and real estate tycoons throughout North America exploited the fear of polio to sell people on clean suburban living.[87] In the nineteenth and twentieth centuries, such "urban blights" as typhus, cholera, tuberculosis, smallpox, and polio were frequently blamed on living in close proximity with the "filthy urban poor." Ebenezer Howard, for example, based his influential Garden City plans on a physician's design for a healthy city called Hygeia. Le Corbusier's designs for cities showed a similar obsession with knocking down "historic and tubercular" Paris.[88] Montreal itself had had a disastrous history of smallpox epidemics: the smallpox of 1885 killed 3,000 people out of a total city population of 150,000, and the reaction to it marked the beginnings of urban renewal and suburbanization in Quebec.[89] The irony here, though, is that that polio was a disease of essentially clean and middle-class environments—*more* suburban, in fact, than urban.

For me, moving to the suburbs was disappointing not only because Bubbie Rose was now barred from visiting us but also because I suddenly had difficulty sleeping and studying. Our new home had only one room for Brian and me, and we had to share the same double desk. I was usually unable to do my homework after Brian, my junior by four years, went to bed, and, like most recent polios, I was very sensitive to noise and needed more quiet than my rambunctious younger brother.

In fact, most polios have a need for relative peace and quiet in the five or six years following the initial attack. This is documented in the medical and first-person narrative literature, such as the account by Millie Teders, who got polio in 1942. Teders writes that after returning home from the hospital, she "started developing nervous mannerisms and twitching of the muscles" (subsequently said to be St. Vitus' Dance, or chorea, but actually another polio symptom). Teders remarks: "I couldn't live at home during this time, because I had five brothers and sisters, and I was supposed to have things very quiet. And aunt and uncle took me in to live with them for five months."[90]

After we moved to the Town of Mount Royal, I found a quiet place only in the winter months, when my parents graciously allowed me to spend time in the cavelike igloo I built in the backyard. This was a room of my own—candle, cot, and all—and I loved it.

I tried to run away from home the year after I had polio. Limping, I got only as far as the corner firehouse. At age seventeen I managed to "get out of that place" when I rented an apartment on Durocher Avenue near McGill University in downtown Montreal. I missed my sister Lieba. ("There's so many times I've let you down," sang Peter, Paul, and Mary in the song "I'm Leaving on a Jet Plane" by John Denver.) And I missed my brother Brian. But I just *had* to leave. The next year I left for California, where I had won a scholarship to study at Stanford University. ("I must take a trip to California" were words I recalled from "How Much Is That Doggie in the Window?"). I said my good-byes to my family and hugged my siblings. My passage to California was the sort of deliverance that American colleges often promise their students. I recall the first two pop songs I heard in California. One I heard at the first large rock-and-roll concert I attended—at the Cow Palace in San Francisco. This was the Animals (and Eric Burdon) singing, "We gotta get out of this place if it's the last thing we ever do."[91]

Getting out of Montreal was, for me, a delivery like Moses' exit from Egypt. I stopped stuttering so much. I studied comparative literature in

Stanford's Department of English as well as social thought in its Department of Political Science. Since the time I left Montreal in 1965, some twelve years after my polio, I have not been back there for more than a week or so at a time. Except for a summer (1969) spent trying to recover from an automobile accident and a few periods when my wife Susan was teaching at Concordia University (then Sir George Williams University) in Montreal, I have not looked back—until now.[92]

The Handicapped Family

Polio affected the family and its institutions in many ways—sometimes almost to the point where the contagion of kinship (if the spread of family membership is understood as a sort of epidemic disease)[93] and the contagion of kin (whereby family members sicken and die) become almost one and the same thing. "In the background of every individual handicapped child," writes Mary Sheridan in *The Handicapped Child, and His Home,* "there is always a handicapped family."[94]

Polio narratives often include discussion of the effects of polio when it strikes after marital engagement and before marriage or during marriage (when the strain on one or another spouse leads to a breakup.) The narratives also frequently include discussion of polio when the breakup of a relationship with a mistress is involved—a favorite theme in French polio memoirs, such as Heny Dory's *Sans Regret et sans honte* (1950s).[95]

Women polios are often so pleased to learn that they can have children, and their relatives so surprised to learn that they can, that their mutual happiness constitutes an important element in several accounts of parents and children and in polio narratives in general. An example would be the Australian Vivienne Overheu's *It Helps to Be Stubborn.*[96] Several other polio narratives, including the Canadian Viola Pahl's *Through the Iron Lung* and the American Anne Finger's *Past Due: A Story of Disability, Pregnancy, and Birth,* deal with women who contract polio while they are pregnant and the various difficulties, physical and psychological, that they face.[97] (Viola Pahl was in her seventh month of pregnancy when, in 1948, she contracted polio and was put into an iron lung.) Men have comparable fears related to having children; for example, I feared that I would be unable to hold my children and rock them in my arms or be a fully active parent. I wanted to

mother my children—become, as the Bible says of Moses, a "nursing father."[98] But I was afraid that I would be physically unable to do that.

Fear of contagion and contagion itself changed forever familial relations
both intergenerational and intragenerational. Because of widespread mis-
information about the disease, for example, many pregnant polios had
abortions, out of fear of "intrauterine polio." Moreover, in 1953, the *Ottawa
Journal* was headlining "[Scientists] Find Polio Virus in Unborn Child";[99]
and many publications were encouraging women—especially those in
whose homes a case of polio had been suspected—to have abortions.

Many nonpolio parents of polio children feared not only for children in
the womb but also for their still healthy children outside it, especially for
those close in age to the polio. In fact, examples of several persons in the
same family getting polio, and books with a focus on the subject, abound.
Take the story of the Tepley family, about siblings in 1952, for example,
and the circumstances surrounding Robinson's *We Made Peace with Polio*,
about siblings in 1953.[100] The studies "A Twin-Family Study of Susceptibility to Poliomyelitis," about acute polio infection in twins, and "Post-Polio
Syndrome in Twins and Their Siblings," a follow-up essay by other authors,
showed that contagion was common.[101] That is because 71 percent of twins
diagnosed with paralytic polio had developed PPS symptoms approximately thirty-eight years after infection and that 42 percent of twins *not*
diagnosed with polio had developed PPS-like symptoms approximately
thirty-eight years after their obviously affected twin was diagnosed with
polio. The 1951 study indicated that most of the "unaffected" twins actually
had subclinical or nonparalytic polio. Now two conclusions seem likely.
The first is that some siblings of polios, though never diagnosed with polio, have developed post-polio syndrome.[102] The second is that the likelihood of an apparently healthy child actually catching polio from a polio
sibling—fear of which affected family dynamics for years after "paralytic
polio" had made its first appearance in their midst—was not much greater
than the likelihood that the polio sibling had caught the disease from a sibling who had come down with a "mild flu" or "summer grippe" some
weeks earlier.[103]

Many adult polios have been afraid to have children because they are
afraid that certain aspects of their disease will be passed on genetically
from generation to generation. This apprehension could be especially
troubling for pregnant polios, who were often given incorrect information

by doctors. Similarly, children of people who have had polio still sometimes fear that they have inherited some aspect of polio;[104] and certain evidence points (incorrectly, as we now know) to schizophrenia as a side-effect of polio.[105]

Polio drastically changes relationships among the siblings in a family. It is not surprising that so far as siblings' relationships with polios go, some siblings are very supportive, and others are not. Consider, as examples of the first group in the polio literature, the cases of Diane Zemke Hawksford, who writes about her brother Ron Zemke in her self-published *Polio: A Special Ride,* and of Julie Johnston, whose *Hero of Lesser Causes* revolves about a twelve-year-old girl who wants to give her polio brother the will to fight for his life.[106] Not that all siblings were supportive. Many polios report, quite convincingly and believably, that their siblings were jealous or envious of them because of the apparent parental attention—even the material gifts—that the polios received; and siblings themselves report the same feeling.[107] In the Australian novel *Iron Cradles,* the young polio's brother is much bothered by the fact that his sibling has had polio. "I don't want to be in a crippled family. The kids at school tease me." He complains that his polio sibling receives a special bicycle (actually prescribed by the local doctor as a means to increase leg strength) from his parents before he does.[108]

Chimps with polio behave in much the same way as do humans. In *My Thirty Years with the Chimpanzees of Gombe,* Jane Goodall describes a conflict between two young chimpanzees at Gombe in Africa during a polio epidemic. One chimp, Figan, senses a new weakness in his older brother, Faben, after that older brother suffers an attack of polio in 1966. "When Faben was stricken by polio and lost the use of one arm," writes Goodall, "Figan managed to dominate his older brother. For the next three years, the two young males interacted very little. Indeed, had they not been equally drawn to spend time with their mother, Flo, they would probably have drifted apart."[109] Other chimpanzees died during the same polio epidemic.

Sometimes, in my family, sibling rivalry was intense. I felt I was a sort of Esau. In the Bible, Jacob comes out of Rebecca's womb "grabbing the heel" of Esau. Jacob *(ya-akov)* means "heel grabber," or "one who trips up," and in a typical biblical rhetorical reversal whereby the tripper becomes the tripped-up, Jacob was tagged as the lame one. This happens when Jacob later sustains an injury while wrestling with an unknown "creature."[110] The

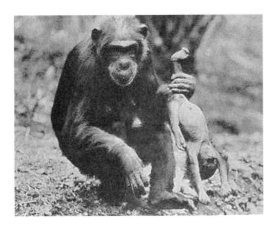

Olly's infant.

interpreters' identifications of that creature vary: Is it Esau? Is it an angel? Is it God? Previous and subsequent events in Genesis suggest that the creature is Esau. In any case, it was thanks to his wrestling match with "the man" that Jacob's name was changed to *yisrael* ("he who wrestles" [with God]). Jews, genealogically defined as *b'nai yisrael* (the children of Israel), memorialize Jacob's walking disability in the Jewish dietary rule that requires removal of the sciatic nerve from land animals before they are consumed.[111]

Mother Rebecca had a real preference for her younger son, Jacob—or an extraordinary hostility toward her firstborn, Esau. What bothered me, a firstborn son, was the apparent meaning of Rebecca's role in giving the "birthright" to Jacob. Reformation Protestants even believed that Rebecca so much favored Jacob that she actually encouraged Jacob to kill his older brother. (This is the gist of *The History of Jacob and Esau,* written in the sixteenth century.)[112] The boys' grandmother Sarah had similarly required that Ishmael—Isaac's older half-brother by the "concubine" Hagar—be abandoned to die in the desert.[113] Surely, relations between Brian and me did not have to end like that—I hoped!

In Mannon's mystery novel *Here Lies the Blood,* there are two brothers, one crippled from childhood by polio and the other able-bodied. One murders the other.[114] In reading such works, it was difficult for many polios, myself among them, not to fear for future relations with siblings. After all, on the day in Exodus when Aaron and Hur prop up Moses' weak arm in battle, God foretells to Moses that the descendants of Jacob (Israelites) will wipe out all the descendants of Esau (Amalekites).[115] Eventually, Samuel and his soldiers commit genocide on *all* descendant of Esau.[116] So much for Cain and Abel.

The disabled Franklin Delano Roosevelt, who could not walk without canes, makes a clever allusion to such intense sibling problems in this legendary response that he wrote out to a New York manufacturer of arches:

> *Question:* Can you walk without a cain *[sic]* or some assistants *[sic]*?
>
> *FDR response:* I cannot walk without a CAIN because I am not ABEL.

Roosevelt, ever polite, did not mail out this response to the arch manufacturer.

Brothers do often take advantage of each other's weakness. When it comes to polio, the sociopathology of relationships between human brothers, which often includes teasing and physical abuse with the aim of attaining a more dominant position in the family, is frequently no different from that of chimpanzees. All such behavior recalls, for me, Jane Goodall's description of the chimpanzee Figan, who practiced taking advantage of fraternal weaknesses and perfected his "charging behavior" just at the time that his older brother Faben became paralyzed during a polio epidemic.

> Even as an adolescent Figan was quick to notice and try to take advantage of any sign of weakness (such as sickness or injury) in one of the adult males. Then, while the higher-ranked individual was at a disadvantage, Figan hurled his challenge—his impressive charging display—again and again. Often he was ignored, even threatened. But sometimes his audacity paid off and the older male, at least until he had recovered, would hasten out of his way. Even a temporary victory of this sort served to increase Figan's self-confidence.[117]

If men are not much different from germs, as Mark Twain writes, then neither are men much different from chimpanzees.

The strain that polio put on a family was intense and hence resulted in long-term family scission. In many families, the children of women polios were put into orphanages or homes, as Needham tells in her *Looking Up,* because no one was at home to care for them.[118] The British movie *Long Day Tomorrow* has as its protagonist an athlete who is felled by polio.[119] When he comes home from the polio ward, he finds it psychologically impossible to stay, because his family pities him and otherwise fails to understand his new situation. He leaves his "family home" for a "home for the disabled" (a new family). There he falls in love with another disabled polio. (The movie, which stars Malcolm Macdowell in a role that seems to prepare him for the one he plays in Stanley Kubrick's 1971 movie *A Clockwork Orange,* is based on the remarkable 1964 book *The Raging Moon* by the polio author Peter Marshall.)[120] In *My Soul More Bent,* Allen Lee tells an anecdote that illustrates succinctly why a son, having contracted polio, might decide never to return home:

> I thought of Tom, who through war lost an arm, and bravely keeping it a secret from his mother in order to spare her pain for a while at least, he telephoned her when he docked in New York to say he would be home for Christmas.
>
> "But could I bring a friend of mine with me?" he added. "He's crippled, Mother. He lost an arm."
>
> Without a moment's hesitation her voice came back across the wires, cutting deep into Tom's heart, "Oh, no, Tom. Not at Christmas. It would spoil the happy plans I have made for us."[121]

Allen Lee never tells what happened to the relationship between his mother and himself. Where polio was all but unacknowledged, as in my own case, a straining of kinship is inevitable.

A great many polio narratives contain a chapter with some such title as "Other Members of the Family." Some have a section where each member of the family has his or her own say. Documentary films about polio, like *A Fight to the Finish,* are often arranged along similar lines.[122] Suppose, for example, that a parent has gone through "that land between life and death," as Elaine Strauss calls polio and recovery from it in her *In My Heart I'm Still Dancing.*[123] Then each surviving relative would write about the consequent change in the quality of the kinship relationship with the now crippled person. Various members of the same family write about what it meant that the woman of the family got polio. A son writes about how difficult it was when his mother returned from the hospital. A husband and father discusses the same issues from his spousal perspective. A daughter regrets that she can't remember anything before her mother had polio. And the daughter-in-law, who came into the family decades after the initial bout with polio, admires Elaine for her bravery.[124] Such works are quite different from Kathryn Black's narrative *In the Shadow of Polio*, which involves the effect of her mother's polio on the entire family,[125] but for all their difficulties, these purportedly multi-viewpoint polio narratives serve as fine memorials for the handicapped families that both produced and published them.

A Ghost of Him

> Oh give it Motion—deck it sweet
> With artery and Vein—
> Upon its fastened Lips lay words—
> Affiance it again
> To that Pink stranger we call Dust—
> Acquainted more with that
> Than with this horizontal one
> That will not lift its Hat—
>
> —Emily Dickinson, "Oh give it Motion"

A few fathers of polios write proudly about their sons having "conquered" polio, in the same manner as Scott Young in the chapter "Polio was a Killer" in *Neil and Me* about his son the Canadian singer Neil Young. A few fathers speak with their children about their polio: Pat Zahler thus says about her 1951 bout with polio that her father "was determined that there was not going to be anything I couldn't do . . . In fact, he said I'd probably do it better!"[126] But most fathers, and mothers, were silent.

In the book *Big Dipper Marathon*, the young polio believes that things might never clear with his parents: they have lied so long to themselves and to him about his condition and the fact that he is different that there is no longer any exit from the falsehood. "We've been lying to ourselves for so long, it's hard to get it out."[127] It was like that for me.

My own father did not once speak with me directly about my having had polio. It is terrible for me to recall that my father Chaiim added, to the not untypical pattern of intrafamilial denial and lies that I have tried to trace out, an element of physical violence. On a couple of occasions my father beat me with a leather strap on parts of my body that had been paralyzed and were still weak. Like many young polios, I was told to forget these beatings, and since I tried to be a dutiful son—one who obeyed the fifth commandment—I might well have done so.[128] But in order to know myself, I was all but compelled bodily to "pay attention to what they tell you to forget"—as Muriel Rukeyser puts it in her *Double Ode*.[129] There was something there that I did not want to forget. "Je me souviens" (I remember) is the motto of Quebec. Anyhow, I could not forget. The child that I was then counted on becoming this adult that I am now, who would try to write that child's polio memoir.

The accounting helps explain the oscillation in *Polio and Its Aftermath* between the viewpoint of the young boy with polio in the mid-1950s, as remembered by his grown-up self, and the middle-aged man with post-polio in the late 1990s who, forty years after the first onset, began to write the still ongoing, common story.

Fathers did sometimes strike out at their polio sons. Charles Ward's unpublished autobiography, "Crippled Thunder"—the most bitter of the first-person accounts that I know—thus begins with a description of his being beaten by his stepfather: "I only remember my stepfather hitting me once. Real hard. Right square on my rear end. The blow was hard enough to make me become airborne for just an instant. I flew, possibly, two feet before landing on my stomach. I remember I ended up with a mouth full of dirt. This momentary flight seemed like a mile."[130] Ward's "Crippled Thunder" includes several descriptions of his "saintly mother's" intervention with his violent stepfather.[131] Yet mothers too would sometimes hit polios: in some polio narratives, mothers claim they need to spank polio children who have been "spoiled" by hospital ward nurses and now need "tough love." (This is a major theme in Amy Gardner's book *Glynda's Bout with Polio as a Child*.[132] Another case in point is the polio Theresa in *Looking for Mr. Goodbar*, who suffers from scoliosis, and her relationship with her mother.)

What disturbs me now about my father's violence against me is my knowledge that, for all the love he bore me, Chaiim wanted to whip the demon out of me. What bothers me about my mother's role is that, far from intervening in the way Mrs. Ward did, my mother actually put my father up to it.

The Incorporeal Air: Dialogue

> Alas, how is't with you,
> That you do bend your eye on vacancy
> And with the incorporeal air do hold discourse?
>
> —William Shakespeare, *Hamlet*

Moi: I will make a ghost of him that lets me.

Be thou a spirit of health. Dad!
A question?

Ghost: Okay.

Moi: Well, it has to do with your whipping my legs when I was eight years old. I've tried to understand. I've read reports by psychiatrists who studied polio families between 1953 and 1957. I hoped to find a description of something like our family.

Anyhow, the research doctors reported that there were several ways North American fathers in the 1950s dealt with squabbles between a polio and his family members.

Some fathers had a sort of unwritten rule: when a controversy led to physical altercation between a polio and a nonpolio family member, the nonpolio might strike the polio, but never on the affected part of the body. (I know that from, um, Davis.) The rule had the beneficial result of protecting the recent polio from long-term physical harm to muscles and maybe even neurons. Sometimes, though, the rule gave rise to the unhappy situation in which a father might actually need to punish the nonpolio sibling—corporeally. Thankfully, this did not happen in our family. But if it had, I imagine that the non-polio-child might have felt that he had been treated unjustly. It wasn't his fault, was it, that his sibling got polio?

As it turns out, it was not so frequently the siblings as the fathers who hit crippled children—and at a far greater rate than they hit able-bodied children. (I know that from, um, Bruno.) How come?

Ghost: I'll be damned if *I* know, and damned if . . .

Moi: One theory was that fathers hit their polio-children out of frustration that their own dreams of having a healthy son had been shattered (owing to the ill health of those sons).

A second theory was that fathers were hoping to exorcise the illness from their sons by beating it out of them.

A third theory effectively combines the other two. It says that fathers were denying that there was anything wrong with their sons and, in order to show they were right, beat them.

In any case, here's my question: Why did you . . . choose . . . my *legs* to whip that day? This is the very coinage of your brain.

Ghost: Are you asking only to supplement your knowledge of fathers in the 1950s?

Moi: Yeah, sure.

Ghost: Sure, you are. I guess I believed that there was nothing wrong with your legs, Marc. There was no reason *not* to hit you in the legs. I didn't think about it beyond that . . . after that.

Moi: I'd have thought that you knew from your medical studies—from those books in the house written by Dr. Alton Goldbloom—that a polio's legs were weakened, sensitive, and prone to damage.

Ghost: Right. Well, let's say that *I* had a certain residual fear of the paralysis from which *you* were suffering. You alluded to that fear when you used the word "frustration." Let's say too I had an irrational hope that, by beating you on the legs, I might beat the polio out of you. I wanted to cure your body by means of corporeal punishment. I felt terrible about my inability to help you.

O, Marc! If only I'd been able to continue with my medical studies . . .

Moi: Greater men and women have tried and failed to cure polio. They still do. I am so sorry, Dad, that you were unable to accept me as I was. Please now help me understand better the tenor of those times.

Ghost: OK. I wasn't alone in my inability to accept a polio-child. The very first study of the psychosocial effects of having had polio showed that parents of rivalrous twins, one of whom had contracted polio, often became angry with their disabled child. (This was, er, Newell's gist in the *American Journal of Orthopsychiatry* in 1930.)

(continued)

A 1996 follow-up study—you see I follow these things—suggests that many polios in Australia suffered terrible rejection, especially from their fathers. Those fathers "were not able to accept a 'crippled' child." Moreover, 44 percent "of respondents described being cruelly rejected by their parents, particularly their fathers, who were not able to accept a 'crippled' child." (I know these things from Westbrook and, er, McIlwain.)

Many fathers could not even accept that the polio twin's poorer performance at school could be attributed to social factors, say, or to the fact that the polio had had to learn to write with his left hand owing to paralysis of his preferred right hand. So such a father concluded that the virus must have damaged his child's brainish apprehension.

When you were in your elementary grades, Marc, I was afraid of that. I was terrified that your brain had been affected. (Phillips warns about that.) That's why we brought you to the Gesell Institute at Yale University. You had a series of IQ tests there. Mom and I were there, "seeing unseen," as your Polonius has it. She and I observed you through a one-way rear window playing with puppets.

You knew we were there all along, didn't you?

Moi: Kinda.

By the way, why didn't *Mom* just slap me that day? She was angry at me for intervening in a violent squabble between Brian and Lieba, sure, but why did she ask *you* to hit me?

Ghost: Leave her to heaven.

Moi: O, answer me!

Ghost: Tradition. When Jewish men from the poverty-stricken Eastern European class—the group from which *my* parents had come . . . from which, Marc, you too came . . . when we arrived home from a hard day's work, we were expected to fulfill the day's threats to our children made by our wives. "Wait till your father gets home!" Tradition.

Moi: Yes. I remember. In Al Jolson's movie *The Jazz Singer,* Cantor Rabinowitz uses his leather strap to whip his thirteen-year-old son Jakie.

Jakie wanted to sing jazz instead of Kol Nidre. The cantor whipped his son on the Day of Atonement. The father drove the son to run away from home. I was too young, too weak, to run . . .

Ghost: I am so very sorry, Marc. They say that Eddie Cantor made up the phrase "March of Dimes" . . .

Let's move on. How is't with you? . . . I mean in your legs.

Moi: Okay, I guess . . . but it's not only my legs anymore. Did your father Maier ever beat you?

Ghost: Maier, my son! I am wary "to speak ill of the dead or to cast up their demerits." So should you be. *I* am compelled to keep the secrets of *my* prison-house. Do thou likewise.

I must go now. Adieu. Adieu. Remember me.

Moi: Chaiim! Did you want to beat Maier because you felt that he abandoned you when he died? You were only twelve years old . . .

Ghost: My hour is almost come. I must go now. Taint not your mind against your mother.

Let me too go. Goodbye.

I rise up, now. *Amen.*

Moi: And you, my father, there on the sad height,
    Curse, bless, me now with your fierce tears, I pray.

Sources: Shakespeare, *Hamlet*, 3.4, 1.4; Fred Davis, *Passage through Crisis: Polio Victims and Their Families* (New Brunswick, N.J.: Transaction, 1963), 130. See also Richard Louis Bruno, "Post-Polio Research: The State of the Art," in *Triumph: A Publication of the Greater Boston Post-Polio Association* (GBPPA) (Fall 2001): 4. H. W. Newell, *American Journal of Orthopsychiatry* 1 (1930): 61–80; Westbrook, "Early Memories": "Newell described a set of triplets consisting of identical twin girls and a boy (24). When they were two years old, one girl and the boy contracted polio and the latter died. The father blamed the girl for infecting his favorite child and her mother said that she 'forgot' to visit her while

(continued)

she was in hospital. Both parents favored the able-bodied twin. When studied at 14 years of age, the twin who had had polio was found to lack self-confidence, to feel inferior to, and jealous of, her sister and to be less cheerful and responsive toward other people than was her twin. Newell's reason for writing up the case was his amazement at the fact that twins, who were identical genetically, could differ in personality due to social factors (the parents' differential treatment of the twins)." Westbrook remarks also: "Nor did the writer speculate as to how other children growing up with a disability might be affected by their social environment." M. T. Westbrook and D. McIlwain, "Living with the Late Effects of Disability: A Five-Year Follow-up Survey of Coping among Post-Polio Survivors," *Australian Journal of Occupational Therapy* 43 (1966): 60–71: "Many survivors spoke warmly of their parents, e.g., 'I am now thankful my parents treated and accepted me, and polio, in such a positive way' but 44% of respondents described being cruelly rejected by their parents, particularly their fathers, who were not able to accept a 'crippled' child." E. L. Phillips, "Intelligence and Personality Factors Associated with Poliomyelitis among School Age Children" (Washington: Society for Research in Child Development, National Research Council, 1948); Shakespeare, *Hamlet,* 3.1; Glasgow Kirk Session Records (1604), in George MacGregor, *The History of Glasgow from the Earliest Period to the Present Time* (Glasgow: T. D. Morison, 1881 [1604]), 149. Compare Shakespeare, *Hamlet,* 1.5: "Taint not thy mind, nor let thy soul contrive / Against thy mother aught"; Dylan Thomas, "Do Not Go Gentle into That Good Night," in *The Collected Poems of Dylan Thomas* (New York: New Directions, 1957).

My father died of brain cancer on Saint Valentine's Day, 1977, at the age of fifty-three. Today, as I imagine the foregoing séance, I am fifty-three. The living one thus summons up the dead . . . within the book and volume of his brain.

In Hitchcock's *Psycho* (1960), Norman Bates speaks ventriloquially for his dead mother, whom he himself apparently killed and then preserved. His mother's ghostly spirit then paralyzes him as regards both speech and movement of his own. In the end, Norman's mummified mommy demands of Norman, "Put me down!" Norman cannot.

There are, of course, many fathers who grieve over a son's death from polio, as does the British composer Herbert Howells.[133] Howells's *Hymnus Paradisi,* composed in 1938, was not performed until 1950. I wept when, as a student in Cambridge in 1969, I heard parts of it performed at King's College Chapel. That was the same year I first heard Alban Berg's Violin

Concerto (1935), with its brilliant interpretation of Bach's chorale "Es ist genug" (It is enough). Berg's concerto, I knew, was inspired by the death of an eighteen-year-old polio—Manon Gropius, daughter of the architect Walter Gropius. Everyone in the chapel was entranced by Berg's sequence of three whole tones, or *tritonus*—the "Diabolus in music."[134]

Es ist genug.

3 A Polio School

A more frightful teacher than the plague, which swept over humanity with special fury in the middle of the fourteenth century, it is difficult to imagine.

—P. Dieppe, "Die Bedeutung des Mittelalters für den Fortschritt der Medizin" (1924)

During the summer of 1956, my parents were making plans to move to the suburbs. We were to move to the Town of Mount Royal (TMR) in January 1957. My parents decided that it would be best for me were I not to change elementary schools in the middle of the fourth grade, so I started off school that academic year (1956–57) at the Algonquin School in TMR instead of the Van Horne School in Snowdon.

Hippotherapy, or Trojan Horses

But come now, change thy theme, and sing of the building of the horse of wood, which Epeius made with Athena's help, the horse which once Odysseus led up into the citadel as a thing of guile.

—Homer, *Odyssey*

The decision to leave Snowdon meant that I had to commute during the first half of the school year—from September to January. There was no public autobus and neither of my parents was willing or able to drive me to TMR. My parents told me to use my bicycle—my friends used to call bicycles iron horses—in order to travel the eight miles each weekday from our home in Snowdon to the school in TMR and back. I had great physical difficulty making the trip. I could not pedal up the hill at the railroad underpass; I was often exhausted in school; and my right leg and hip often hurt. My bicycle felt like what French inventors had introduced in the 1790s as a "little wooden horse," with a fixed front wheel; the German baron Karl von Drais later improved upon that horse in 1817 when he added a "steerable" front wheel and called the contraption a dandy horse. In any case, my parents paid little heed to my condition and complaints about my "hobby horse." Mounting this iron horse without a horse-block—without what the polio-horseman Walter Scott in his novel *Waverly* called a "louping-on-stane"—eventually caused me serious harm. "For O, for O, the hobby-horse is forgot."[1]

Equally dangerous for me had been the roller skates that my parents had insisted I use after visiting the Gesell Institute. Why roller skates? On the one hand, Dr. A. Windorfer had suggested as early as 1941 that roller-skating was a good treatment for polio.[2] On the other hand, roller-skating was obviously difficult and hazardous for polios. Alberta Armer's novel *Screwball* depicts a polio's triumph in the use of a soapbox car. The Mickey Rooney movie *Fireball* (1950) features a champion roller-derby skater who gets polio; but improperly trained polios on wheels are a hazard to themselves and to others.[3]

At Algonquin School in TMR, I had other physical problems. Among these was stumbling in gym class: for example, I could neither run properly onto the springboard nor jump properly onto the wooden vaulting-block that my classmates called the pommel horse. That block became my Trojan horse—"a device . . . insinuated to bring about an enemy's downfall."[4] My inability to do the leap onto the pommel horse resulted in my receiving two failing grades in gym. One failing grade was for the physical subject itself (because I did not do the jump) and the other was for my psychological effort (because I had not tried hard enough).[5] I was ashamed of myself. Many polios have written about the humiliation that they felt when they tried unsuccessfully to do what their more able-bodied classmates were able to do or when they were asked, before an entire class of peers, to take gym classes separately from the "normal" children.[6] (Janet Lambert's *Introducing Parri* includes the story of a young man who, on account of having had polio in his childhood, has difficulty passing the physical examination at West Point Military Academy.) Most all of these polio authors had one psychological advantage over me: I did not really know what was "wrong" with me. Like the citizens of Troy presented with an equine statue, I lacked the knowledge of what it was—and hence how to deal with it. In the fall of 1956, I began to play hooky from school to avoid gym class.

The actual explanation for my failing gym was not polio. It was my lack of knowledge—quite typical for the young polio "passers" of that time. I did not know what had happened to me when I had had polio (the muscles of my inner thighs were affected), and so I did not know what I might do to make up for what had happened to me. Other polios compensated for their weak muscles in one area by purposely developing countervailing skills or muscle strengths. Often these polios had real success—on actual horses; for example, the polio Lis Hartel—the 1952 Olympics champion for performing on horses—knew exactly where polio had made her weak, and she managed her sport accordingly. Hartel used special devices, including a horse-block with two or three steps to mount the horse, which she could not do on her own.[7] Likewise, the young Walter Scott, whose parents encouraged him to ride a pony from an early age, became a tolerable equestrian. Sometimes he wrote on a desk strapped to his horse.[8] In this sense, at least, Scott was a polio-writer.

Like most young boys my age, I wanted to learn to ride well—like Gene Autry on his horse named Champion.[9] But I could not even stay on the horse—although I did spend a lot of time photographing them. Would horseback riding have made a difference to me? For those polios who had the knowledge to compensate for their loss of human leg power, horseback riding was like the power that Mephistopheles offers to Doctor Faust in the first part of Goethe's *Faust* (1808). Here are the famous lines about horse-power—I am tempted to call it hippotherapy:

> What, man! confound it, hands and feet
> And head and backside, all are yours!
> And what we take while life is sweet,
> Is that to be declared not ours?
> Six stallions, say, I can afford,
> Is not their strength my property?
> I tear along, a sporting lord,
> As if their legs belonged to me.[10]

Mephistopheles, ever the unwilling and unwitting servant of God, here promises Faust a perfect prosthesis in the form of superhuman horse-power. For many polios, the horse was as powerful as the prosthetic arms of Götz von Berlichingen—Goethe's dramatic version of whose story Walter Scott translated into English.

In some ways, the animation provided by animals is greater even than such "mechanical" devices as the iron leg prosthesis fitted on Queen Vishpla in the Indian *Rig-Veda* (ca. 3500 BC) in such a way that she returned to battle immediately after losing her own leg. So, the polio Franklin Delano Roosevelt loved to ride horseback; his methods of mounting are well documented. Moreover, Roosevelt in the 1920s had already outfitted his several multi-horsepowered automobiles with hand-controls.[11] Sometimes, if a wheelchair-bound polio could not settle in the saddle, the chair itself would become the saddle—as storied in Arthur Tarnowski's "realistic" polio-travel adventure book *The Unbeaten Track* (1971). William O. Douglas, of the United States Supreme Court, derived physical strength and exercise as well as spiritual replenishment from horseback riding in the aftermath of his life-shaping bout with polio, as described in the chapter "Infantile Paralysis" in his autobiographical *Of Men and Mountains*.[12] Edward Le Comte, who got polio in 1954, recalls in his memoir *Long Road Back* the joy of driving a car for the first time after having had polio.[13] Arthur Bartlett's early polio novel, *Game-Legs*, written for adolescent readers, tells how the hero's "handicap vanished when he was seated in a buggy behind a horse," as if that hero and his horse-driven buggy become one centaurlike automotive (self-moving) engine.[14]

An equestrian might think that he and his horse are one, in somewhat the same mysterious way that Saint Paul believes that man and woman become one flesh.[15] That is to say, the horse's legs *are* the equestrian's legs. Together, the horse and the human make up a single four-legged self-moving entity with more than either human or equine horsepower.

Horses are perhaps the most crucial animals for therapeutic kinesis. "Human therapy on horseback," say the hippotherapists, cures many ills—among them, the dysfunction in motor verbalization that is stuttering.[16] Small wonder that around the time of the polio epidemics, it was the Horsetrot that ruled the dance floors. It was also the movement of horses

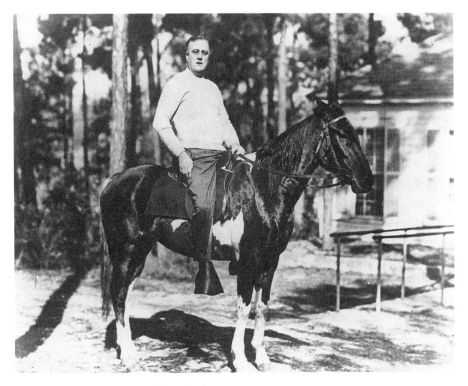

Franklin D. Roosevelt on horseback.

that became a central subject matter for still photographers who, like Eadweard Muybridge, used serial "stills" to understand movement and to make those stills seem to move cinematically.

Another factor that make horses helpful to disabled people also moves us beyond the notions of horsepower both for disabled people who want (that is, lack) legs of their own *and* for able-bodied people who want (that is, desire) the power of cars, bicycles, or roller skates. After all, human beings often perceive the tame horse as a cross between an inanimate object like a puppet or doll (for example, my stuffed dog Mr. Doogie) and an animate object like a human being or pet dog (for example, my springer spaniel Buster).[17] In the same way, the tame horse marks the boundary between humankind and non-human-kind and between familial and nonfamilial kin. The tame horse is perceived as a creature that loves without qualification and, more important, a creature that loves without pitying the loved one. (The "no pity" theme is an important one for polios and in the juvenile literature for them, as in Luis and Millar's *Wheels for Ginny's Chariot.*)[18] So human beings project onto horses their own fears and desires— thus representing, or projecting, those fears and desires outside themselves.

Projection of oneself onto such a social or domestic animal involves creatures other than horses, too. As far as cows go, consider the Disney movie *Tomboy and the Champ* (1961), which concerns an orphan polio's love for her steer on a Texas ranch.[19] Determined to prove her worth, the orphan (Tommie Jo) raises the angus Champ to compete in the U.S. champion fat-stock show; Champ returns the favor by helping Tommie Jo through polio and a climactic coma. A cow appears likewise in Acosta's first-person narrative *Tragedy of 1941*. In this work, the cow has the identical name that Acosta herself has. Another one of her pets, a dog, pulls her sled.[20] (My dog Buster used to pull my red wagon with me in it in just the same way.)

Yet horses helping polios is the common topos. Carolyn Baber's novella *Little Billy* tells about a polio training a mustang in the 1940s.[21] In Dorothy Lyons's *Dark Sunshine*, a buckskin mare helps a girl with polio overcome her illness.[22] Vian Smith's *Tall and Proud* concerns "a girl and her horse" and how together they "triumph over . . . pain." Lois Johnson's *God's Green Liniment* tells how the young daughter of a Swedish-American farm family recovers from polio, thanks to her parents' rubbing her with green horse liniment![23] In Hawksford's *Polio: A Special Ride* (1997), the sister of a polio-stricken boy takes him to ride on the carved wooden horses of a merry-go-round. After caring for her brother, this sister goes on to become a professional nurse specializing in rehabilitation. Another sister of a polio comes to her brother's rescue on horseback in Johnston's *The Hero of Lesser Causes*. That heroic sister says, "I was Keely the Connor charging forward on my silver stallion to save my brother from . . . what?" Emily Crofford's *Healing Warrior*, one of many children's books about the Australian Sister Kenny, shows on its front cover a representation of that nurse-heroine leading a horse toward the home of a polio-stricken patient.[24] (Kenny has been much represented in the polio literature ever since Rosalind Russell's portrayal of Kenny in the award-winning 1946 movie *Sister Kenny*.) The movie *Interrupted Melody* (1955) was based on the book of the same title (1949), written by the Australian opera singer Marjorie Lawrence after she got polio in 1941. Lawrence explains how she carried out Richard Wagner's specific stage directions when, in 1936, she portrayed Brunnhilde at the

Metropolitan Opera in New York in the immolation scene of *Götterdäm-merung*. She devotes the first chapter of her *Interrupted Melody* mostly to the incident where she rides on horseback into the flames. In fact, dozen of polio books featured photographs and pictures of similarly adaptive horses on their front covers and dust jackets, among them William O. Douglas, *Of Mice and Mountains* (1950), Dorothy Lyons, *Dark Sunshine* (1951), Vian Smith, *Tall and Proud* (1968), Diane Hawksford, *Polio: A Special Ride* (1997), Julie Johnston, *The Hero of Lesser Causes* (1992), Emily Crofford, *Healing Warrior: A Story about Sister Elizabeth Kenny*, Arthur Bartlett, *Game-Legs: The Biography of a Horse with a Heart*, and Arthur Tarnowski, *The Unbeaten Track* (1971), a polio travel-adventure book whose color jacket shows the author in a wheelchair—on horseback! Both polio books written by the Australian Alan Marshall are relevant here: the autobiographical *I Can Jump Puddles* (1955) (the posters for the 1981 movie based on the book shows a body with wooden horse), and the novel *Hammers over the Anvil* (1991), which was made into the movie of the same name, are horse-related.[25]

An early example of hippotherapy of the prosthetic type would be the above-mentioned polio novel by Arthur Bartlett, *Game-Legs: The Biography of a Horse with a Heart*. Here, the young hero, Jimmy, has lost the use of his legs: "An attack of infantile paralysis at an early age had left him paralyzed in both legs." Into his world is then born a lame filly that Jimmy calls his weak-kneed sister, with which the boy identifies to the point that he assures his parents that if they plan on killing the filly, then they may as well kill him too. In fact, his physician father has wanted the horse dead only so that his son would not be made unhappy by being reminded of the horse's "crippledom." So the boy adopts the filly; he calls it Sister and thinks of it as his kith or kin (*kind*, as in species). Eventually, the two creatures—Jimmy and Sister—become something like a centaur: "And now he had a horse whose life actually was blended with his own." The horse recovers from its lameness and wins races; after one of these, Jimmy throws away a crutch. Jimmy learns a good deal from the horse's treatment by the veterinarian: when the boy is taken to see the polio specialist in Boston, the treatment is a little like that which Jimmy himself administered to Sister: "'This is just what we did with Sister,' Jimmy grinned." In the end, Jimmy regains the use of his legs.[26]

Hydrotherapy; or, Fishmen

> The water put me where I am and the water has to bring me back.
>
> —Franklin Delano Roosevelt

It requires no expert balneologist, hydropathist, hydrotherapist, or philosopher of the bath to note that hydrotherapy works for many people with neuromuscular disorders—for example, when they "take the waters" at fancy European spas.[27] Using the buoyancy of water to relax, and its resistance to strengthen, muscles is what does the trick. John Summers, in his *Short Account of the Success of Warm Bathing in Paralytic Disorders* (1751), made the point long ago.[28] Water therapy takes advantage of water's unique properties to promote a course of physical exercise.[29] The reasons are simple enough: the body becomes lighter in water; also, water pressure helps stimulate various bodily processes, including blood circulation. And psychologically speaking, warm water is beneficial, for being in water enables the patient to do things that he or she cannot do otherwise.[30] You might not think there would be much disagreement about these things. But there has been—and still is.

Water therapy in the United States has a short history. It rises to prominence around the time of the polio epidemics; it declines with the advent of the polio vaccine. Only in 1911 did therapists and doctors first begin to use bathtubs in treating children with cerebral palsy. Soon thereafter, the need to treat war veterans helped bring hydrotherapy to the adult population as well. In 1924, the Spaulding School for Crippled Children in Chicago began to use Hubbard tanks as basins in which to exercise paralyzed polio patients, and Dr. Charles Lowman converted a lily pond in Los Angeles into a treatment pool for polio patients. Franklin Delano Roosevelt popularized pool exercises during his own convalescence, beginning with a 1922 swim at the home of Vincent Astor.[31] When Roosevelt's Georgia Warm Springs Foundation was established in 1927, Dr. MacAusland wrote, "The advantages of hydrotherapy in the treatment of poliomyelitis have been recognized only recently."[32] The Baruch Committee followed in the footsteps of Dr. Wilhelm Winternitz—a founder of early modern hydrotherapy—and finally endorsed hydrotherapy.[33] In 1953—the year of my encounter with polio—orthopedists generally came to agree that polio pa-

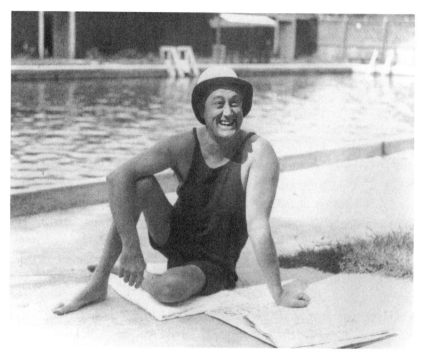

Franklin D. Roosevelt at the pool complex in Warm Springs, Georgia, on his first visit, in 1924.

tients should be given access to a warm pool from the very outset of their treatment.[34]

But once the polio vaccine was introduced in 1954, the water treatment became controversial—enough so, in fact, that research in hydrotherapy was soon all but shut down. Today, the dominant view of hydrotherapy in the United States—especially in the Northeast—is that in-pool aquatic therapy (AT) should be a desperate last resort, adopted only when land-based physical therapy (PT) has failed. Many major rehabilitation hospitals have not even one small pool.

What a change! At one time, New England could boast many hydro-therapeutic facilities. As early as the 1870s small-scale aquatherapy was common at treatment and research facilities in the Massachusetts towns of Florence (from 1856 on), Westboro (from 1845 on), and places in Vermont (from 1850 on).[35] Boston had its first aquatherapeutic facility by 1903.[36] Yet now New England—where much of the polio research had been done in universities like Harvard and Yale and where the study of polio once played an important role—has relatively few decent therapeutic pools.[37] How did this come about?

The introduction of the polio vaccine, together with concomitant factors encouraging denial or forgetfulness about the disease that we have already considered, is not the only explanation. Local reasons also exist for the relatively rapid demise of warm-water hydrotherapy in New England and elsewhere.

First, the local medical establishment could neither void nor avoid regional debates about the efficacy of dunking. In Boston, for example, a certain Puritanism vied with Methodist, Catholic, and Baptist views about the role of water in physical and spiritual life. Puritan doctrine argued against the use of warm water, which was believed to encourage lasciviousness, and instead endorsed cold-water bathing as good for both body and soul. To understand how the different religious groups can have arrived at such opposing viewpoints, we should observe that communal bathing has a psychoanthropological side and that for Christians hydrotherapy sometimes resembles, and is often compared or contrasted with, both Roman bathing ritual and Christian baptismal rites and practices.[38] Christians have both imitated and excoriated "pagan" bathing traditions, usually while claiming to transform them to heavenly ends, as in baptismal rituals.[39] The Boston Puritans thus often adopted an almost medieval-Christian condemnation of hot springs as a pagan *fons sanitatis*. They further opposed those Christian sects—Methodist, Baptist, and sometimes Catholic—that endorsed baptism by immersion (at the religious level) and tolerated public pools (at the secular level). The founder of Methodism, John Wesley, wrote a best-selling book endorsing hydrotherapy, and for many Catholic polio patients, the swimming pool pavilion at Warm Springs, Georgia, was like a cathedral.[40] Thus, Plagemann writes in his first-person memoir *My Place to Stand:* "My first impression of this closed pool was that it rather resembled a cathedral; further visits served to strengthen the feeling approaching religious awe which came over me when I first entered." Plagemann continues: "And for me, always, the pool was the temple where the spirit was, and Mrs. Schlosser [Plagemann's physiotherapist] her high priestess."[41] Warm Springs' famous hydrotherapy is probably not unrelated to its Baptist and Methodist environs in Georgia.

The Puritan prejudice against bathing was sometimes so intense that when polios tried to use the waters unencumbered by heavy clothing, they often met with aversion or were even arrested. Consider, for example, the well-known story about the "hydrotherapeutically restored" polio Annette Kellerman—whom a Harvard professor described as "the most beautifully formed woman of modern times" and whom Roosevelt, speaking extemporaneously at Warm Springs, claimed had "swum her way back to health."[42] When she appeared in 1907 in a one-piece bathing suit—scandalous at the time—on Revere Beach near Boston, she was arrested for indecent exposure.[43] Kellerman's arrest jump-started her silent-film career later documented in *Million Dollar Mermaid,* but it dampened enthusiasm for public hydrotherapeutic facilities in Boston from the beginning.

The second reason for the rapid demise of hydrotherapy in the New England area was its association with the treatment of mental disease.[44] Polios were often segregated as mentally deficient. (The so-called feeblemindedness and even insanity that accompany other forms of paresis had long been associated in the popular mind with poliomyelitic paralysis.) And polios were often housed in the same institutions as people with mental diseases. It is not surprising, therefore, that among the best pools for therapeutic purposes in New England is the one at Fernald State Hospital in Waltham, Massachusetts, which is thought of as an institution for the mentally retarded. (In the 1880s Fernald's official name was the Massachusetts School for the Feeble-Minded.) Dozens of unwanted, "orphaned" polios in Massachusetts ended up at Fernald, and also at Lakeville, in Rutland. Housing polios and the so-called psychopathetic together was not unusual even at major treatment centers like Rancho los Amigos in the Los Angeles–area Medical Center.[45] Only in 1957 did Rancho separate polios from mental patients.[46]

A third explanation for the demise of hydrotherapy involves one of the supposed causes of polio: dirty swimming-pool and sprinkler-truck water. Polluted waterways had been associated with contracting polio since well before 1915.[47] (Henrik Ibsen's Dr. Stockman in *Enemy of the People* [1882] seems to hint at the same issue.) New Englanders justified banning the baths by citing a deterioration in the hygiene situation and claiming that dirty swimming water spreads polio. (Americans often claimed too that bathhouses transmit sexual disease and encourage illicit sexual contact. They closed therapeutic bathhouses as if they were stews and bagnios.)

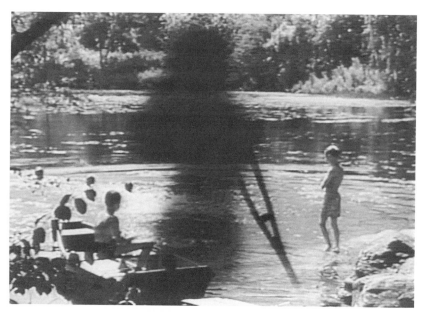

The shadow of polio in *The Crippler*.

Polio was allegorized in the popular press and cinema as the Crippler stalking children at the water's edge.

Many parents did not allow their children to go swimming.[48] Swimming was illegal during the polio season—a favorite theme of novels like Devoto's *My Last Days as Roy Rogers*.[49] Ponds and other bodies of standing water were called polio water.[50] (The usage still survives, as in Caroline Kava's short film *Polio Water*.) Though "cleanliness is indeed next to godliness," as John Wesley said, the Puritans claimed that the water in swimming holes was inherently dirty.[51]

Their claim contains a germ of truth. Water is not only a means to deal with the consequences of polio but often also the means by which the disease is transmitted in the first place. Many a polio memoir thus begins with a story about swimming in cold water. So begins the memoir of Ian Dury, who went on to write the song "Spasticus Autisticus" in 1981, to mark the Year of the Disabled.[52] Similarly, the Briton Dixson writes of falling into the princess of Wales' pond in Blackheath.[53]

And yet warm, clean water is also part of the remedy. Elaine Strauss says in her memoir *In My Heart I'm Still Dancing,* "Water is still the best therapy for any crippling disease."[54] In his novel *The Lung,* J. G. Farrell, who fell ill with polio after swimming, accurately describes what it feels like for a polio patient first entering the water: "An extraordinary feeling of euphoria stole over him at the sudden lightness of his limbs. The constant aching in his neck, back and shoulders disappeared magically. It was as if he had never been ill. This is ridiculous, he found himself thinking. What am I doing here? I'm perfectly all right."[55] In his drawing *Man on Crutches, Carlton* (1943), John Perceval displays the key tension between using crutches on land and using a ring lifebuoy in water.

As agent of therapy, water provides human beings with a modifiable whole-body prosthetic. It provides them, whether they are disabled or not, with an extension of the body. Some of us want to be winged bird-men (whether as Icarus or airplane pilot) and others imagine themselves as powerful horse-men (whether as Centaur or car driver). "At one time he wished for a horse," writes Goethe in *Wilhelm Meister's Apprenticeship,* "at another for wings."[56] Such polios as President Roosevelt and Supreme Court Justice William O. Douglas were horsemen. Others sought to become birdmen, since flying in the air appears as welcome a means to overcome gravity as swimming underwater. The polio Letty ponders the matter in Erick Berry's novel *Green Door to the Sea.*[57] The Stanford-educated psychiatrist Arnold Beisser poses the question in *Flying without Wings: Personal Reflections on Being Disabled.*[58] Stephen Meader's novel *Topsail Island Treasure* concerns a polio who is a bird-watcher.[59] The painter Frida Kahlo, who got polio at the age of six and eventually needed to have her lower leg amputated, asks in her diary, "Feet what do I need them for / If I have wings to fly [?]—1953." In Jerome Brooks's novel *Big Dipper Marathon,* the polio dreams of disconnection from gravity by means of trapeze artistry.[60] (When polios saw *Peter Pan* in the 1950s, they already knew how Peter Pan flies. No wonder the polio Ronny Yu of Hong Kong became an expert director in the tradition of invisible-rope leaping and dancing, as in his 1997 movie *Warrior of Virtue.*)[61]

For the polio in convalescence, the gravity-defying apparatus was not the swinging trapeze but elaborate physiotherapeutic paraphernalia. The "Guthrie Smith" came about as the result of the physiotherapist Guthrie

Smith's search for an adequate substitute for water in which to exercise paralyzed limbs. Enid Foster, in her polio narrative *It Can't Happen to Me*, describes the Guthrie Smith apparatus as a "queer array of ropes, pulleys, cleats, boards, springs, and slings that dangled above me, suspended from a metal frame."[62] All such contraptions aim at results more easily achieved by means of water.

Even as hippotherapy helped create a modern ideology of the centaur, so hydrotherapy created one of mermen and mermaids for polios who seem almost to accomplish an ichthyological merger with water. The transformation turns human beings who are more than normally disabled by gravity into powerful humanoid creatures who move through the water like birds through the air.

There are five types of fish-people. First are those "dolphinate" humans who show their "backs above / The element they [live] in" and swim their way back to health and toward celebrity.[63] These would include the merwomen-polios Barbara Hobelmann (who made All-American in 1951), Ethelda Bleibtrey, Nancy Merius, and Annette Kellerman.[64] The movie *The Million Dollar Mermaid* (1952), starring Esther Williams—who built a career making swimming movies—tells the story of how Kellerman survived childhood polio to become a world-renowned swimmer, water ballerina, and silent-film star as well as author and feminist.[65] Writes the clubfoot Lord Byron in his poem *The Island*, "Did they with ocean's hidden sovereigns dwell, / And sound with mermen the fantastic shell?"[66]

The second type of merpeople comprises the partly immersed, hippopotamuslike, bottom-bound walkers. In Berry's book *Green Door to the Sea*—one of a series of children's books about polios and water, a sixteen-year-old polio, Letty, is in Jamaica with her family, in order that she can get the benefits of both fresh- and saltwater therapies. (A more recent such story is Mary Towne's *Dive through the Wave*, 1994.)

Then, as she sank into the water, came that joyous feeling of having no weight; of being free, really free, *like a bird flying,* not like a human being crawling along the surface of the ground. She swam fifty stoke with her arms, letting her feet tiptoe *light as a ballet dancer's* along the bottom, across the shallow part of the pool and back again.[67]

In my secondhand copy of hydrotherapist Igor Burdenko's *Overcoming Paralysis: Into the Water and out of the Wheelchair,* the author has left a handwritten inscription. Burdenko writes: "To my dear friend Alison! May the wind always be in your sailing!"[68] The physiotherapeutic reverie involves transforming the patient from living in the air to living in the water.

The third kind of fish-man is the fully immersed bottom walker—like the Australian hand fish, which walks on leglike fins. Letty becomes such a one in *Green Door to the Sea.*[69] (The Fishwalk was a dance that became popular around the time of the first polio epidemics.) With a jury-rigged oil drum and breathing-hose, Letty walks along the sea bottom and does underwater painting:

> Oh, it was wonderful! Never had she walked like this before, not even before her illness. She took a little jump, floated upwards a yard, and drifted back again to the ocean floor as softly as a feather. Oh why hadn't she learned of this before! You were disembodied, you were a bird, a feather, a ghost without weight. It was heavenly. No wonder fish flitted about in the water with such skill and abandon. No wonder mermaids were romantic figures. She would prefer being a mermaid any day in the week to having to hobble along on dry land. Why, in fact, did that first fish ever choose to crawl out of the water onto the dry land?[70]

The fourth type of fish-man is the fully submarine creature who moves in water the way that birds move through the air. Human Aqua-Lungers of the 1950s likewise got along with their underwater breathing equipment, often depicted in popular magazines of the 1950s, along with iron lungs.[71] It is small wonder that polios seek out such an almost religious therapy as *Wassertanzen* (waterdance) and join such Aqua-Lung organizations as Moray Wheels.[72] By analogy, Waldo, crippled by myasthenia gravis in earliest childhood in Robert Heinlein's science fiction story *Waldo,* moves about freely in the weightlessness of space, where he invents remote-controlled hands and other prosthetic devices. Becoming Waldo is the dream of the post-polio sufferer Arthur C. Clarke. Clarke was writer for the movie *2001: A Space Odyssey.* That screenplay features a key paralytic moment, and Clarke himself, like all polios, loves "the delightful zero-gravity environments of the sea."[73]

A word is in order about how polios may feel the weight of air in much the same way that human beings in general sometimes feel water pressure. Thus, Jessica Yu's documentary movie *Breathing Lessons* begins with the sound of an iron lung breathing-machine.[74] Its resident, Mark O'Brien, then recites from his poem "Breathing" (1988):

> Grasping for straws is easier;
> You can see straws.
>
> "This most excellent canopy, the air, look you,"
> Presses down upon me
> At fifteen pounds per square inch,
> A dense, blue-glowing ocean,
> Supporting the weight of condors
> That swim its churning currents.
> All I get is a thin stream of it,
> A finger's width of rope that ties me to life
> As I labor like a stevedore to keep the connection.
>
> Water wouldn't be so circumspect;
> Water would crash in like a drunken sailor,
> But the air is prissy and genteel,
> Teasing me with its nearness and pervading immensity.
>
> The vast, circumambient atmosphere
> Allows me but ninety cubic centimeters
> Of its billions of gallons and miles of sky.
>
> I inhale it anyway,
> Knowing that it will hurt
> In the weary ends of my crumpled paper bag lungs.[75]

O'Brien in his breathing machine is borne down upon by air like a drowning man by water. On-screen we even see condors flying on the heavy blue air. O'Brien's breathing stops are audible—at once poetic and mechanical caesuras. We see and hear an air-pressure gauge like the one on Aqua-Lungs.

In the field of popular music, the rhythmic bellowslike sound of the lung is integrated into songs like Al Yankovic's "Mr. Frump in the Iron Lung" and Bush's "Insect Kin." The sound of the iron lung is also crucial to movies like *Star Wars,* in which the bellowslike breathing of Darth Vader (played by the stutterer James Earl Jones) matches Vader's cocoonlike mechanical support system.[76] In poetry, the lung is important in thousands of works—especially those which, like "Iron Lung" by the bulbar polio Omega Baker, employ the caesura, or breathing-stop.[77] In "The Man in the Iron Lung," Mark O'Brien thus alludes to the way in which any scream is "controlled" by the enforced caesuras, or breathing stops, mandated by his yellow iron lung:

> I scream
> The Body electric,
> This yellow, metal pulsing cylinder
> Whooshing all day, all night
> In its repetitive dumb mechanical rhythm.[78]

At the same time, O'Brien refers to that other paralyzed American poet, Walt Whitman, who wrote in 1888, "Of me myself—the jocund heart yet beating in my breast / The body wreck'd, old, poor and paralyzed."[79]

A fifth group of fish-men would actually change, chrysalislike, from fish to man. We sometimes say that ontogenetic "birth" is the individual mammal's progressive passage from the saline amniotic fluid to the air; in just the same way, we often claim that the phylogenetic passage of species-from water to air—as symbolized for us by the mudskipper or the climbing perch of Southeast Asia—is a triumphant moment in evolution. But when we call that crawl onto the mud evolution, do we not take the side of land-based PT against water-based AT?

Roosevelt said, "The water put me where I am and the water has to bring me back."[80] Roosevelt was probably right to think that the cold sea-water in which he had been swimming at Campobello Island in the Bay of Fundy had something to do with the severity of his paralysis. But he was probably wrong if he felt that the virus might have been transmitted in the sea water. When it came to water therapy, though, Roosevelt definitely knew his way around.

Dance Therapy; or, Paralyzed Dancers

> Nothing sadder than a washed-up dancer.
>
> —Ana Castillo, *Peel My Love Like an Onion* (1999)

The term *dance medicine* generally means "medicine to cure dancers' problems." These are "problems that afflict professional dancers more often or more acutely than other people." Dancers, of course, are often afraid of the time when they will no longer be able to perform "properly" that "rhythmical skipping and stepping, with regular turnings and movements of the limbs and body" which is dance. (That is how the editors of the *Oxford English Dictionary* define *dance*.)[81] My aunt Susan Lee's scholarly essay "Is It the Last Dance? Ballet Dancers at Age 30" considers the matter from the viewpoint of normal aging.[82] W. Schweisheimer in "Watch Out for Your Hand!" warned musical performers about potentially more serious and unpredictable conditions of "temporary paralysis"—stasis, as opposed to kinesis.[83] Dance medicine, which has a long history of its own, sees and treats the dancer as a type of athlete, and it treats general medical problems—like degenerative joint disease, scoliosis, various sorts of lower-back pain, upper-back and shoulder pain, and spondylosis—with special concern for the dancer.[84]

The term *dance therapy*, on the other hand, generally means "use of dance to cure many types of medical problems"—including, but not limited to, dancers' problems.

Here we need to move beyond the dictionary definitions of *dance*—and likewise of *dance medicine* and *dance therapy*—as movement per se and toward an understanding of dance in light of dialectical and nondialectical oppositions between stillness and movement—oppositions that better define a philosophical understanding of dance and better interpret those pathologies of movement with which dancers, both as medical patients and as therapists, are concerned.

The principal dialectic is that between stasis and kinesis. Paralysis—the end of polio—is the bodily stasis defining one pole of dance. Consider here the performers known as human statues, or living statues—whose work was popular in the 1990s as street performance.[85] "Living statue" performers pretend to be petrified as permanently as Lot's wife. Their art is, in some ways, an art of trompe l'oeil (fool the eye)—linked with *nature morte* (dead nature), or still life. The usually surrealist painter Frida Kahlo makes the relevant visual pun in her *"Naturaleza" bien muerta!* (A very still "still life"!), which is part of her *Diary*.[86] Her painterly *still*-life rendering of vegetation suggests the theme of death-in-life or life-in-death.

Seen from the viewpoint of a teleology at once biological and aesthetic, "living statue" performers are indistinguishable from stone statues (that represent actual human beings), from petrified human beings (like Midas' daughter turned to gold),[87] and from paralyzed living persons rendered altogether motionless.

Whether a person who cannot move can *still dance* is a problem approached by dance therapists like Brandfonbrener in his "Music of the Heart" and by such paralyzed polios as Elaine Strauss in her self-published memoir *In My Heart I'm Still Dancing*. (She dreams of dancing with Fred Astaire.)[88] In the polio survivors' support groups, the subject that tends invariably to make the most stoic of polios cry is . . . being unable to dance.

The advice to "face the music and dance" may seem helpful. (This is the refrain of Irving Berlin's song adapted to the dance routines of Fred Astaire and Ginger Rogers in the movie *Follow the Fleet*.) But what if one cannot dance? I recall here that, during my convalescence from polio, my parents removed my favorite gramophone recording from my room. This record featured Dinah Shore singing Berlin's "Dance to the Music of the Ocarina," a routine from *Call Me Madam*, a movie made in 1953. Was it because Dinah Shore was a polio and they didn't want me to identify with her? Or was it because the song's injunction to dance distressed them . . . because I had been stilled?[89]

The simple polar opposite of perfect stasis is perfect kinesis, often associated with the physician's *perpetuum mobile* or the musician's or dancer's sometimes choreic *moto perpetuo*.[90] For a few people, therefore, the cure is Saint Vitus' Dance. Richard Burton, in his *Anatomy of Melancholy* (1621), writes, "S. Vitus Dance . . . they that are taken with it can do nothing but dance until they be dead, or cured."[91] Many polios have therefore been interested in dance therapy. One such is Professor Carolyn Bereznak Kenny; another is FDR in Schary's play *Sunrise at Campobello,* especially when, grimly humorous, he does "the Roosevelt slide."[92]

> *FDR: (Sitting on his haunches and using his hands to move his body, he slides backward on the floor and towards the floor. As he does,* ELEA-NOR [ROOSEVELT] *and* [LOUIE] HOWE *stand frozen. FDR continues speaking)*
> This method of locomotion I shall call the Roosevelt slide: half waltz, half foxtrot. Easy on the feet, placing all the wear and tear on the derrière.[93]

Choreographers would argue that dance can cure stillness by means of motion. That is also the general idea behind the dance called the tarantella. It might cure the disease called tarentism by means of its six-eight time, great rapidity, and "perpetual motion." So propose composers like Daniel-François-Esprit Auber, in his opera *La Muette de Portici* [The Mute Girl from Portici (1828)], Carl Maria von Weber, Franz Liszt, Frédéric Chopin, Sigismond Thalberg, and César Antonovich Cui (in his Suite Concertante, op. 25). During my convalescence from polio, the radio often played the song "That's Amore" as interpreted by Dean Martin in the movie *The Caddy* (1953). Its dark reference to the diseaselike dance the tarantella explains the use of the song in Hitchcock's *Rear Window,* where a strangely amatory Jimmy Stewart, cast as the hero opposite Grace Kelly, suffers from partial lower-body stillness.

> Hearts will play tippy-tippy-tay, tippy-tippy-tay
> Like a gay *tarantella*

At the time, two great ballerinas of the twentieth century were struck down by polio: Tanaquil LeClercq and Elizabeth Twistington. Both published works touching on their polio ordeals and dance disorders.

Twistington's autobiography (1969) is aptly named *Still Life.* The title suggests both life without motion and a state that remains alive despite its stillness. Compare Strauss's title, *In My Heart I'm Still Dancing,* with Christopher Reeve's, *Still Me,* and with that of Frida Kahlo's drawing *"Natur-aleza" bien muerta!*[94]

Twistington's dancing ended abruptly when she got polio in 1953; the disease suddenly rendered her almost completely paralyzed.[95] Before polio (BP) artists had done sketches and paintings of her with such names as *Elizabeth in Action.* Now, Twistington spent her nights (and most days) in an iron lung. She went on to lead a remarkably active life. Besides her various travels and interviews, Twistington wrote books by means of arm rests, ropes resembling those used to manipulate marionettes, and an elec-tric keyboard; she also made mouth paintings and drawings—some of "still life" and some of action dancing.[96] (She was the United Kingdom's most active member of the Association of Mouth and Foot Painters.)[97] Twistington choreographed from a respirator and wheelchair, producing a tarantella for eight girls (1971), and she founded the Chelmsford Dancers.[98]

Twistington's other work involves the theme of "still versus moving pho-tography," including double exposure. At first most dance photographs were staged shots, or "still" portraits, but Merlyn Severn changed that with her "action photography," including the photos for *Still Life.* A movie about Twistington's life, *The Dance Goes On* (1980)—narrated by Rudolf Nureyev—depends for its effect on this tension between still and moving photography.

The second dancer to be stricken with polio is Tanaquil LeClercq. LeClercq had actually played a polio victim onstage in a brilliant produc-tion of *La Valse* (1951). The Specter of Polio had figured "allegorically" on the ballet stage several times before, but nowhere more brilliantly than as imagined by (her soon-to-be husband) George Balanchine in this brilliant, quasi-surrealistic production of Maurice Ravel's work. Ravel had written *La Valse* around the time of the first major French polio epidemics (1911, 1912, 1920).[99] And, in fact, this work concerns the fulfillment and destruc-tion of the waltz as dance form. (Ravel said that his piece was "a sort of apotheosis of the Viennese waltz . . . the mad whirl of some fantastic and fateful carousel.") Balanchine interpreted his *Valse* as the destruction of Dance itself (played by Tanaquil LeClercq) by Polio (danced by Balan-chine). In 1951 various early productions came to fruition at the New York City Ballet, and the work is available as a movie.[100]

Balanchine renders *La Valse* in the tradition of Edgar Alan Poe's tale *The Masque of the Red Death* (1842). In Poe's story, informed by legends about a

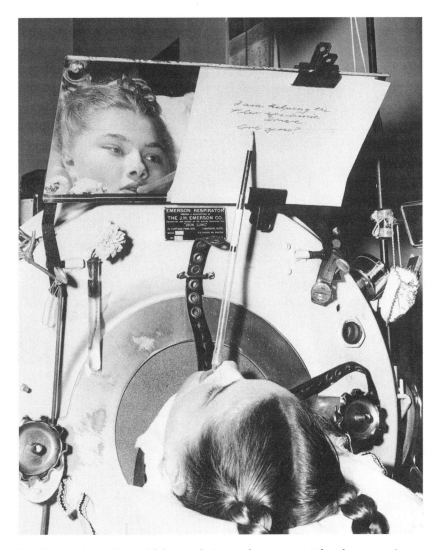

Paralysis victim writing with her teeth, September 12, 1949. After three years in a respirator, Carolyn Sandin, eighteen, of Arlington, Virginia, is shown in an iron lung at Children's Hospital School, Baltimore, writing: "I am helping the polio epidemic drive. Are you?"

ball held in Paris during a cholera epidemic in 1832, people retire to a castle to avoid the epidemic, much as they do in Boccaccio's *Decameron*. During a masquerade, masked ball, or "dumb show" with ballet dancers and mummers, an uninvited figure enters the castle hall. This "angel of death" takes the life of the lead woman.[101] Balanchine took it that Ravel's music conveys "some indefinable though unmistakable sense of a *danse macabre* or *Totentanz* . . . almost a frenetic energy about it which carries more than a hint of doom."[102]

Tanaquil LeClercq, who married Balanchine in 1952, got polio in 1956, at the age of twenty-seven, when she was at the height of her career and of her powers. From that moment until her death, LeClercq did not dance again.[103] Her "dancing spirit" comes through, however, in an unusual autobiographical book of photography for cat lovers that she wrote, *Mourka: The Autobiography of a Cat*. This book is ostensibly written by the couple's cat Mourka, but the photography makes it clear that Tanaquil LeClercq's authorial strategy involves her psychological projection into Mourka's body. For *Mourka*, in fact, Balanchine did the choreography.[104] LeClercq identifies with that cat in much the same way that child-polios identify with their horses and dogs. The photographer for *Mourka* was Martha Swope. Like Merlyn Severn, she specialized in stop-action still photographs. (Swope went on to collaborate on Kenneth Laws's *Physics and the Art of Dance: Understanding Movement*.)[105] In *Mourka,* the kinetic cat, which is always visible, and the static human, who is always invisible, do a pas de deux in which the two of them are one.

Most true-to-life books and movies about polio-dancers have unhappy endings. Consider G. W. Pabst's film *Rosen für Bettina* (1955–56)—a more extended treatment of the theme of polio than his earlier *Paracelsus* (1943)—in which a ballerina (Elizabeth Muller) succumbs to polio just as her career peaks. The climax of *Never Fear* has the heroine dancing to Ravel's *Bolero*. Consider too Joan Clarke's autobiography *All on One Good Dancing Leg*.[106] Nevertheless, there are a few happy stories, mostly fictional, in which professional dancers come back to "top" careers, after having been struck down by polio.

A currently popular example in the realm of literature would be Ana Castillo's *Peel My Love Like an Onion*, a realistic tale in which the main character, Carmen La Coja (literally, Carmen the Cripple), is a polio who finds strength in flamenco dancing and, in post-polio syndrome, finally

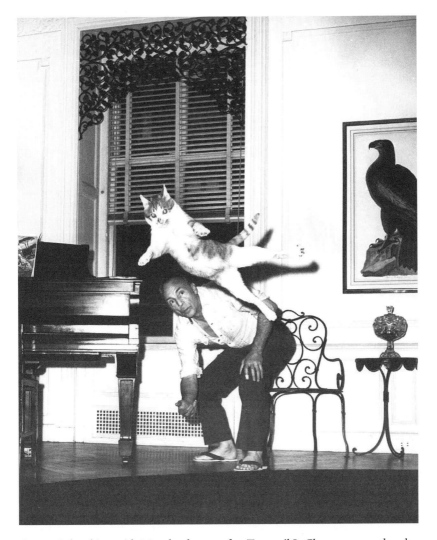

George Balanchine with Mourka the cat, after Tanaquil LeClercq was paralyzed.

discovers weakness. "No other skills but to dance as a gimp flamenco dancer."[107]

In Mary MacKey's best-selling novel *A Grand Passion* (1986), Tatiana Trey inherits her mother's talent and passion for dance. On leaving the New York City Ballet for Hollywood with her choreographer husband, Tatiana is struck down by polio. With courage, she fights her way back to her feet. Eventually she stars in movies during the heyday of such movie ballerinas as Moira Shearer, who played the suicidal ballerina in *The Red Shoes* (1948), and Cyd Charisse, who appeared with Gene Kelly in *Singin' in the Rain* (1952). In Liebe Wetzel's fantastic puppet show *Brace Yourself,* shadow-puppet choreography captures the relationship between dance and polio. Wetzel tells thus the story of her father's polio using a few pairs of shoes, some wheels, a purse, and a leg brace.[108]

Sometimes the polio-dancer's return to the top is due only to the public's wanting to see a disabled person "dance"—as in the documentary film *The Goddess Bunny* (1994), with its strange tap dance sequence. All such happy tales about polio-dancers are fictional—unless they involve such compensatory dance work as informs "Crutchmaster" Bill Shannon's "Art of Weightlessness."[109]

Many movies focus on polio's stilling the art of human movement that is dance. In the 1950s three standouts toed the boundaries of the genre: *Lili* (1953), *Never Fear* (1950; sometimes called *The Young Lovers*), and *The Five Pennies* (1959). All use cinema to explore the themes of human kinesis and stasis. During the 1950s I saw them all.

The closing sequences of *Lili*—the first feature-length commercial movie I ever saw—show the puppets, which Paul (Mel Ferrer) had "animated" and for which he had ventriloquized, come alive and *really* dance![110] Paul had been a onetime great dancer and choreographer who lost the use of his leg from an accident in the war. It seemed to me that Mel Ferrer played Paul as if Paul were a polio. Only in the 1960s did I learn that Mel Ferrer—who had been a Broadway-musical dancer in the 1930s—had had his own bout with polio before becoming an actor.

Ida Lupino, the onetime actress who directed *Never Fear,* wrote about her own bout with polio in *Photoplay.*[111] Her movies often include a polio. *Not Wanted* (1949), for example, features a lame hero who marries an unwed mother. (Lupino hired the polio John Franco to advise the scriptwriter about the matter.)[112] In *Never Fear,* a small masterpiece, a dancer gets polio. Her dance partner wants her to fight the disability, but she becomes bitter and reclusive. She spends time in a rehabilitation clinic. Much of this documentarylike movie was shot on location in a Santa Monica rehabilitation unit—a practice that the director Fred Zinnemann copied when he made *The Men* (1950), with Marlon Brando. Finally, Lupino's dancer breaks out of her depression and gets on with her life.[113]

The major scene in *Never Fear* shows wheelchair-bound patients staging a square dance that would appear to normalize the polio world. The Wheelchair Dance is, after all, a comment on the Paralysis Dance, the benefit for polios that the National Foundation for Infantile Paralysis hosted yearly. Not until Flanders and Swann would the wheelchair become again so important a dance prop onstage.

Paralysis Dance was the name given to FDR's annual birthday parties.[114] Dr. Paul De Kruif came up with its motto "Dance so that others may walk" when he was effectively the leader of the President's Birthday Ball Commission.[115] (Variants on the motto for the presidential balls included "So we may dance again." "Strong legs run so that weak legs can walk" was the Shriners' motto for their fund-raising all-star football games.)[116] The irony of the name was not lost on polios. After all, many movies from the early twentieth century had already made fun of (and profit from) disabled people trying to dance. Among these was *The Deaf-Mutes Ball* (1907).[117] Polios understood at once the political and financial rhythms of Glen Miller's musical piece "At the President's Birthday Ball."[118]

The third movie, *Five Pennies* (1959), concerns the relationship between polio and the "handi-capitalist" process of raising money. As such, *Five Pennies* follows in the footsteps of *The Leather Saint* (1956), in which a pugilist priest boxes in order to raise money to fight polio.[119] *Five Pennies* is based on the true story of the bandleader Red Nichols (Danny Kaye) who changed career directions and formed a band, the Five Pennies, after his daughter Dorothy came down with polio in 1942. The story was broadcast in 1956 in an episode of Ralph Edwards's television series *This Is Your Life*. (Elizabeth Twistington had appeared on another episode.)[120] *Five Pennies* includes scenes dealing with the stages in the life of Dorothy, who progresses from an iron lung at the age of six to foot-ankle orthosis; as a teen, Dorothy eventually goes to a single ankle-foot orthosis. At the end is a "triumphantly" touching scene where Dorothy *dances* with her father Red without any mechanical support. Danny Kaye, who plays Nichols, had been named the first traveling ambassador of UNICEF in 1954 and was already famous for raising money for polio-children.[121]

Another ambassador for polio and the dance was Grace Kelly, who in Alfred Hitchcock's *Rear Window* plays the woman who cares for the ambiguously disabled Jimmy Stewart.

Writing

> Had successful dedication of medical and educational buildings.
>
> —Franklin Delano Roosevelt, letter to Eleanor Roosevelt, December 4, 1938, written
> from Warm Springs

Depending on a polio victim's age, the initial severity of the illness, the longer-term consequences of that illness, and local medical and legal customs mandating particular treatments, the polio might be isolated from family, friends, and the community. After release from the hospital or rehabilitation institution, polios usually also isolated themselves from one another. They had internalized the doctrine that they should not "fraternize" with one another after discharge but instead should get on with normal lives.[122]

Most communal institutions for polios were partly rehabilitative and partly academic and social. They also included a brace shop, orthopedic surgery, and job training for the tens of thousands of usually young polios who resided in them, sometimes for years. These schools were "like a . . . family"—as Virginia Acosta describes her life at Warm Springs, Georgia, in *Polio Tragedy of 1941*.[123] They were also a college. Lorraine Beim's first-person narrative *Triumph Clear* thus opens with a letter of acceptance to Warms Springs—instead of one to Wheaton College, where Beim had planned to go "before polio" and where, eventually, she did go. "Warm Springs," writes Beim, "is in many ways like a college."[124] Allen Moore suggests much the same thing in his biographical *Growing Up with Barnardo's*, about Dr. Barnardo's School.[125]

Residential polio institutions have been largely excluded from the history of rehabilitation and from disability history.[126] Yet the polio wards were a key part of the hospital-school system in Progressive Era America. After all, the original development of the hospital schools during the years preceding the Great War was contemporaneous with the polio epidemics of the 1890s.[127] The American polio wards brought together polios from various economic classes. (The polio Arnulf Erich Stegmann suggests the counterpart opposite German experience regarding politics and class in his painting *Arm und Reich* [Poor and rich], the frontispiece to Part 3.) Friendships were formed in those communities, even in the huge iron-lung wards housing dozens of patients. Personal accounts bespeak a group spirit resembling that of wartime platoon narratives.

Historians of medicine have rarely made use of literature written in the polio wards. The amount of material is enormous, and much of it is still in archival format. Myriad newspapers were published in the hospital schools. (Sink's *The Grit Behind the Miracle* includes an illustration of one such newspaper.)[128] There were literary publications and scores for musicals, including reports on performances by the Poliopolitan Opera Company, and various scripts.[129] Among the scripts are skits written for the benefit of Franklin Delano Roosevelt at Warm Springs, as reported in Beim's *Triumph Clear*. One such play was *The Skeleton, the Fat Lady, and Franklin Roosevelt*. The president took notes during this skit, and his speech afterward—a presidential version of literary criticism—was a great hit among the inmates.[130] Another skit was *The Spirit of Warm Springs*, performed during Roosevelt's forty-first visit to Warm Springs (November 27 to December 17, 1944). Polios there were inspired by FDR and "understood" him—and "the pain in his voice."[131] Writes Acosta, who met Roosevelt at St. Luke's Hospital in Marquette, Michigan: "Only we could sense the endless tedium of his days, the being lifted in and out of chairs, of bed, bathtub, pool. And know that war and politics and the glory of his fame and career were outside of all this, strung like beads on the thread of the waiting days."[132] Another such "FDR play" (inspired and written by Beim—as she tells it in 1946) was *The Story of Warm Springs*, which, again, the president attended as a theatergoer.[133] Roosevelt visited such facilities around the country and apparently had much the same reception everywhere. Oftentimes the polios would do Shakespeare. (Compare Beim's description of her production.)[134]

A few digressive remarks on literature—letters, scrapbooks, various manuscripts, and above all, actual published books—written by polio-children are in order here. All such polio literature by children still awaits collection and archival records. Historians of medicine and students of literature have generally ignored this material, not only because they tend to ignore child-authors (a factor I discuss in *Elizabeth's Glass*, about the nine-year-old author Princess Elizabeth Tudor) but also because they are reluctant to read polio memoirs in particular.[135]

In fact, polio has almost never been seen from the child-patient's view-point as expressed in his or her own words. The historian Naomi Rogers, in *Dirt and Disease: Polio before FDR*, admits, "My study of polio and the public is not presented from the *patient*'s perspective," and she explains the total omission of the child-patient's perspective by reminding us, "Most polio patients before 1920 were not yet five years old." Rogers encourages "historians who study the health and illness of very young children . . . to fashion new ways to study relations between these important 'objects' and their healers." Some historians try to repair the situation by studying the letters sent by polio-parents to their children.[136] Very few, however (not even Rogers), look at the letters sent by children. Such letters are *not* inaccessible. Among them are the epistles sent by Emma Elizabeth Retan (born 1907) of Massachusetts to her friends and family, and the letters sent by Yvonne Greatwood Louise (1910–1997) of Buffalo, New York, together with her comments about the Reconstructive Home for Infantile Paralysis in Ithaca, New York, and her thoughts on being rejected for a teaching position.[137]

It is time that scholars looked into such writings by children and others. Sick and crippled children are hardly an unexpected minority, as they have been called by such scholars as Gliedman and Roth in *The Unexpected Minority: Handicapped Children in America*. Especially during the first half of the twentieth century, these children made huge efforts to make known their experiences.[138] (Myriad polios kept public "scrapbooks" and the like.) Considering the odds, what remains is remarkable. After all, many child-polios died soon after the onset of the disease, so they never had any chance whatever to write; of those who survived, only those possessed of literacy education, health, and leisure could write; of these relatively lucky ones, many did not want to revisit their pain but instead aimed only at getting on with their lives; of those who did write, only a few had their work preserved by way of publication or reliable conservation in a family or public collection; of work so conserved and accessible, very little has ever actually been seriously read.

One example of work conserved and published is the book by the polio Elizabeth du Preez, of Cape Town, South Africa. Du Preez died at the age of fourteen, in 1953. Her works were edited and published by her parents in the book *Elizabeth Sings*. Among her poems is "The Wonderful Healer"

(March 1953): "He healed / the sick and palsied; / He helped / the blind and the lame."[139]

The most politically prominent child-polio who wrote about his experience was the seven-year-old French *infante:* Louis-Auguste de Bourbon, duc de Maine (1670–1736).

Was it actually polio from which Louis-Auguste suffered? Medical historians are still undecided whether certain epidemics of the past were polio or not. The *baccach* (lameness) recorded for 708/709 CE in the Annals of Ulster: was it polio or not?[140] Likewise ambiguous is the condition from which suffered certain ancient Egyptians; Moses, a prince of Egypt, suffered from poliolike disabilities that affected both how he walked and how he talked.[141] Similarly, much controversy about polio surrounds the personages depicted in Masaccio's great painting *Saint Peter Healing the Cripple with His Shadow.*[142] Scholars also argue about the lameness from which the Roman emperor Claudius suffered: Robert Graves in his first-person, partly fictional narrative *I, Claudius* opted for the polio thesis.[143] Even the nature of Walter Scott's illness is uncertain. And yet when I first read about Louis-Auguste in Hillyer's *Child's History of the World,* I was sure little Louis had had polio. The second time I read about him, as an eight-year-old memorizing Jean de La Fontaine's poem devoted to the already eight-year-old Louis-Auguste, I was surer still.[144]

Louis-Auguste was one of the dozen or so legitimate and illegitimate children of the "Sun King" of France. (Many of the wise men in France hoped that he would become king, and still more later came to regret that he did not.) In any case, Louis-Auguste was also the "youngest author of France"—as he says in the book *Oeuvres diverses d'un auteur de sept ans* (Diverse works by a seven-year-old author, 1678), which was printed under the direction of his tutor, Le Ragois, who ran a sort of hospital school for the young cripple.

Most polio-writers got their start in writing or the performing arts in the polio hospitals. Among those who "graduated" from the hospital schools was Jim Marugg, a patient at Rancho los Amigos, who went on to a career in journalism; his *Beyond Endurance* is a first-person account of polio and hospital writing.[145]

For some polio patients, the act of writing was physically difficult. A few polios learned to write with their teeth (holding the pencil) in much the same way that Elizabeth Twistington learned to paint. Others used various machines. Ruth Ben'ari from Warm Springs wrote her novels, including *Prelude to Love,* as well as a best-selling typing manual (still in press) for all would-be touch typists.[146] Songwriters and singers from the polio schools include all three members of the reggae trio Israel Vibrations (patients at the Mona Rehabilitation Center), Ray Peterson (a patient who began his career by entertaining patients at Texas Warm Springs Foundation Hospital and wrote "Tell Laura I Love Her" in 1960), Brother John Sellars, and Joni Mitchell, who later worked with jazz pianist Charles Mingus when he had Lou Gehrig's disease (ALS).[147]

Some writers and performers from the polio colleges found transition to the outside world difficult owing to the prevailing conditions of isolation, denial, disorientation, and depression. It often happened that when the polio moved from the now familiar hospital environment to his consanguineous family, a certain shame or denial—a tension between the necessary dependence and the desire for independence—set in. As her daughter Kathryn Black reports in her *In the Shadow of Polio* (1996), the polio Virginia Black of Arizona, who had written a good deal for the *Vital Capacitor* at Seattle's Northwest Respirator Center, lost her will to live when she returned to her young children in Boulder.[148]

Do the residential polio institutions help explain the existence of a particular sort of writing following discharge from the residential institutions? A polio "school of literature"? Literate polio patients thought so. Thus, Bentz Plagemann in his memoir *My Place to Stand,* writes:

> As a younger man, reading Chatterton, Keats, D. H. Lawrence, Stevenson, my sympathy and admiration had gone out to the tubercular school of literature. I had not known of a polio school . . . , which was now suddenly invested with something of the same aura of uniqueness. And I have wondered since if a psychiatrist, for example, might approve of that identity with a special group [polios] which Miss Plaistridge was holding out to me.[149]

Alice Lou Plaistridge, the intelligent nurse and physiotherapist to whom Plagemann here refers, was director of physiotherapy at Warm Springs; she wrote articles for Warm Springs' *Polio Chronicle*.[150] (As Plagemann points out in his later memoir, *An American Past,* Plaistridge wrote the entry on poliomyelitis in the *Encyclopaedia Britannica*.)[151] We ought not immediately to reject the factual truth of her opinion about polios—or to discount the psychologically therapeutic effectiveness of her positive rhetoric for polios, many of whom went on to becomes writers, artists, and political leaders. Plaistridge's greatest admirer was Franklin Delano Roosevelt.[152]

In *Falling into Life* (1991), the polio Leonard Kriegel says, "As a writer, I am a creation of disease." He goes on to insist that "the writer who discovers his voice in disease or accident makes a corollary discovery; he finds that he has become a victim of the reality he assumes."[153]

Textbook Readers

The most widely read books about childhood-onset polio in the 1950s were the official school readers authorized for classroom use by local school boards and state offices. These readers included health class manuals and textbooks.[154] The readers usually featured a child who had had a disease that had left him crippled. The disease almost always went unnamed, but almost everyone knew that it was polio. One of these school texts is *Growing Pains,* in which Jack has had an unnamed disease and now limps, like Clara in *Heidi,* and wears a leg brace.[155]

Another such school text was *The Girl Next Door,* a standard fourth grade reader at my school. *The Girl Next Door* told the story of Susan, a new girl in the neighborhood, who had been paralyzed by an unnamed disease. (In the "health lesson" sections interspersed throughout *The Girl Next Door,* many diseases are named and discussed. The illustrations of quarantine signs include practically every disease of the time except polio.) Susan cannot attend school because she is in a wheelchair: no explanation is given for why being wheelchair-bound should preclude schooling. The children in *The Girl Next Door* take lessons in how to be polite to crippled people. Eventually, a doctor notices that there is something in which Susan can participate with the other kids: swimming! Thanks to hydrotherapy, Susan is able to gets out of her wheelchair and resume a "normal" life. All the textbooks have the same sort of happy ending.[156]

I identified with Susan. After all, I was the new boy in the neighborhood,

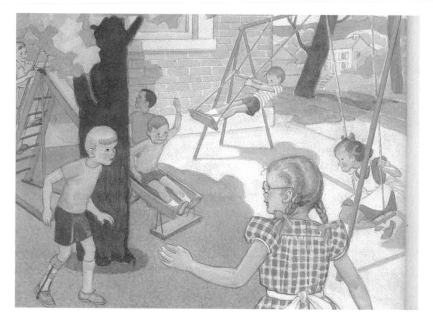

Growing pains: illustration from an official elementary school textbook used in much of anglophone North America.

I had been paralyzed by this disease whose name my parents feared to mention, and my "mainstream" public school did not admit students with braces or wheelchairs.

Caesura: Tales from inside the Iron Lung

> To be buried while alive is, beyond question, the most terrific of these extremes which has ever fallen to the lot of mere mortality.
>
> —Edgar Allan Poe, "The Premature Burial" (1844)

In famous studies of the mechanism of repression and its expression, Sigmund Freud discusses the feeling of the uncanny one has when confronting " 'doubts whether an apparently animate being is really alive; or, conversely, whether a lifeless object might not be in fact animate.'" Freud considers such "objects as dolls, doubles, statues, mechanistic automata, and, in extremis, phantasies of live burial." Later he builds on this idea: "To some people the idea of being buried alive by mistake is the most uncanny thing of all. And yet psycho-analysis has taught us that this terrifying phantasy is only a transformation of another phantasy which originally had nothing terrifying about it at all, but was qualified by a certain lasciviousness—the phantasy, I mean, of intra-uterine existence."[157]

In the 1950s in the United States, fear of live burial centered on the iron lung prescribed for victims of bulbar polio. The concomitant fear of and attraction to iron lungs tapped directly into the American gothic tradition. An exemplar of that tradition is Edgar Allan Poe, who was extremely popular among school-age children in the 1950s. Poe's general fascination with epidemics is evidenced in "The Masque of the Red Death" (1842), and with cripples in "Hop-Frog, or The Eight Chained Ourang-Outangs" (1850).[158] Poe's approach to paralysis is exemplified in "The Premature Burial." Here he provides an evidently nonfictional history of living inhumation, offers "a hundred well authenticated cases" of "living burial," "premature interments," "living inhumation," and "suspended animation"—all of which involve "temporary pauses in the incomprehensible mechanism" once "some unseen mysterious principle again sets in motion the magic pinions and the wizard wheels." Poe's "Premature Burial" brings into play vaguely "hysterical" conditions like lethargy, insensibility, stupor, apathy, numbness, syncopy, and swooning. It also presents the tale of the narrator's own trancelike catalepsy ("a tendency to trance"), together with a paralytic "binding of [his] jaws" that leaves him the mute witness to his own burial. During the burial, the narrator feels the pressure of the earth: "I endeavored to shriek—, and my lips and my parched tongue moved convulsively together in the attempt—but no voice issued from the cavernous lungs, which oppressed as if by the weight of some incumbent mountain, gasped and palpitated, with the heart, at every elaborate and struggling inspiration." The involuntary caesura, or breathing stop, informs much later poems in particular about the iron lung, but here, under the weight of earth instead of air, the stasis promises to cut off human life altogether. Those who witness these living-burial events are themselves always "paralyzed with awe."[159] In the popular literature of the mid-twentieth century the counterpart was contemplation of the "living" grave that is the iron lung.

Iron lungs played other roles in the political culture of the twentieth century; for example, iron lungs were important to defining technical aspects of public health care in relation to public funding and private medical philanthropy.[160] They played a significant role in histories of inventions, which now included Alexander Graham Bell, whose son died of respiratory problems; John Haven Emerson, who was the New York City health commissioner during the 1916 New York City quarantine; and Philip Drinker, who served at the Harvard School of Public Health.[161] Iron lungs are still used in medical wards today, in larger numbers than one might expect.[162]

In the literary sphere, there were dozens of first-person iron-lung autobiographies. Most were dictated from inside the lung. A few were written by polios who had "emerged" from the lung: the Kentuckian Regina Woods's *Tales from inside the Iron Lung and How I Got out of It,* Richard Chaput's *Not to Doubt,* Ann Armstrong's *Breath of Life,* Leonard Hawkins's *The Man in the Iron Lung,* Jane Boyle Needham's *Looking Up,* Phyll Western's *I Haven't Washed Up for Thirty-Five Years,* and Paul Bates's *Horizontal Man.*[163] The New Zealander June Opie wrote the iron-lung narrative *Over My Dead Body;* then, some four decades later, she published a post-polio sequel, *Over My Dead Body Forty Years On.*[164] Mark O'Brien, who spent some four decades in an iron lung after his 1953 bout with polio, wrote autobiographical poetry, including *Breathing, Love and Baseball, The Man in the Iron Lung,* and *Sonnets and Strikeouts.*[165] This last title recalls both Leonard Hawkins's first-person narrative about bulbar polio *Man in the Iron Lung* and the celebrated "man in the iron mask"—the hero of Alexander Dumas's novel—who historians believe was Louis-Auguste's rival for the French throne.

The topos of live inhumation pervades the work of polio-painters like Frida Kahlo, with her paralytic's "worm's eye view" of human interment. It also informs novels like Wallace Stegner's *Crossing to Safety* (1987).[166] Many people who have bulbar polio, focusing on the "claustrophobic intensity" of their lives, conceive of their iron lung as a grave or coffin, within which their once cinematic lives are now static deaths.[167]

Stasis and Kinesis

The kinema-drama raises some of the most fundamental problems of art.
—Alexander Bakshy, *The Path of the Modern Russian Stage, and Other Essays* (1916)

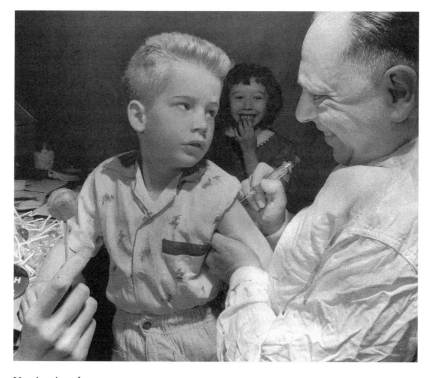

Vaccination day.

4 PARALYTIC POLIO AND MOVING PICTURES

I think [polio] was perhaps the most important thing that happened to me. [It] formed me, instructed me, helped me, and humiliated me. All those things at once. I've never gotten over it and I am aware of the force and power of it.

—Dorothea Lange, interview

During my convalescence from polio, Uncle Bennie gave me an American-made, battery-driven toy crane. This was the best gift ever. With its "joystick," operating a three-foot-long arm, I moved things around the room "prosthetically." A little later, Bennie gave me a green and red British-made Meccano set with an electric, clockworklike motor and instructions for making other toys. I designed automated trucks and drawbridges and tripods—and then assembled them. Other polios had such toys. In Great Britain, for example, sixteen-year-old Lord Snowdon (Tony Armstrong Jones) was hospitalized with polio in 1946; "his Uncle Oliver, who had been designing for Covent Garden and Glyndebourne, sent [Lord Snowdon] copious and detailed instructions for model-making, and Tony amused other patients by raising whole stage sets on his coverlet."[1]

Was model-building appropriate play activity for polio children in recovery? This was a serious question for therapists of the times. According to some thinkers at the time, No. In 1952 there was even a good deal of psychoanalysis-inspired writing about the proper play to prevent a child from even contracting the "partly psychosomatic" disease polio. Playing the game "This little pig went to market," for example, was supposed to keep polio "at bay." (So argues Francis J. Mott in *Play Therapy and Infantile*

Paralysis.)[2] Such thinking absurdly misses polio-children's simple need for access to prostheses and a chance to build something.

Unable to stand on my own two legs during my convalescence, I gradually came to understand Archimedes' dictum "Give me a place to stand, and I will move the earth."[3] I first read this dictum in V. M. Hillyer's *A Child's History of the World* and *A Child's Geography of the World*. Thanks to these two books, I reacted to my enforced time at home by reading about other times and places.[4] I daydreamed about traveling in time and space. On that account, I got in contact with consulates and government offices around the world and asked them to mail me maps and other topographical information about their countries. For me, Her Majesty's Postal Service became a sort of prosthesis. With my collection of maps and history books, I felt like the young boy with a spyglass whose picture adorns the frontispiece of Hillyer's *Child's Geography*. This child sits, Archimedes-like, on nothing; but he is able to see everything. The inscription on the frontispiece reads, "Just suppose you could go way, way off in the sky, sit on a corner of nothing at all, and look down at the World through a spyglass."

Delayed Shock and Double Exposure

When I had sufficiently recovered, Uncle Bennie helped me to deal with the paralysis. He began by teaching me about lenses and still photography. I understood photography as a prosthetic eye with a capacity for memorializing. (The polio-photographer Dorothea Lange wrote: "You put your camera around your neck along with putting on your shoes, and there it is, an appendage of the body that shares your life with you." Lange's follower Helen Nestor, also a polio, thinks much the same way.)[5] Many polios took up photography: angled or telephotographic lenses bring closer what a paralyzed person cannot reach. In this way it is now possible to shoot or capture those scenes and objects. Cornell Woolrich's short story "It Had to Be Murder"—the main literary source for Hitchcock's *Rear Window*—suggests that his largely immobile hero *depends* on his camera just as if it were a prosthetic part of his own body. As Woolrich makes clear, the paralyzed person "shutters" his own eye, as if he and his camera (lens) were one and the same.[6]

Lord Snowdon first took up photography while in the polio ward.[7] Other polios who did so include wheelchair-bound Bert Kopperl, as he describes in his wonderfully named book *With Two Wheels and a Camera*, and Dorothea Lange, one of whose many specialties was photographing lower legs and feet.[8]

Cripples, usually the victim of voyeurs and "rubberneckers," could turn the tables on the observers thanks to the camera. Allen Lee, an alumnus of Warm Springs, tells one relevant story about a photographer at Warm Springs in his book *My Soul More Bent*:

> There was Leroy who must spend the rest of his life flat on his back. Sometimes the curious ones would make so bold as to stand directly above him. Without a word, they would stand and stare.
>
> Photography has long been Leroy's hobby and he decided that a splendid opportunity has come to get unusual shots. Slightly concealed in his clothing so that no one would suspect, he planted his candid camera. Now let the curious ones come!
>
> Slowly, as before, they approached his cot. Now they stood beside him. Now they were bending over to *really* get a look. Eyes were opened wide. The jaw had dropped a bit. Then *click* went the camera. And bewildered, nonplussed onlookers fled speedily away.
>
> What a collection Leroy must have now![9]

Uncle Bennie inspired me to take up the camera and eventually to set up a darkroom in the "cold storage room" of our new home in TMR. From the ages of about eight to fourteen, I had a few photographic "specialties." One was photographing such clipped waterbirds as swans and such land birds as peacocks at Montreal's Lafontaine Park whose wings had been clipped.

I tried, in the tradition of Eadweard Muybridge, to make serial still photos of unclipped birds moving in flight; however, I lacked the proper photographic equipment to do it successfully. I did not have a still-picture camera with fast enough shutter speeds and large enough F stops; nor did I have a moving-picture camera. Using the British Meccano set that Uncle Bennie had given me, I tried to manufacture a sort of latter-day, Cirkut camera tripod that rotated, with the help of a clockworklike motor, in such a way as to allow me to take successively superimposed shots from slightly different angles.[10] In the end, though, I began to develop a more formal or ideal interest in cinema, in kinesis. Also, I began to make relatively simple double exposures instead of taking more complex panoramas.

The double exposure superimposes one image "onto" another sequentially on the same negative (using the camera to make two or more exposures on film) or on the same positive (using the enlarger to make two or more positives on paper). For me, such superimpositions, with their focus on time and movement, became photographic puns and visible stutters. My forays into this arena usually showed two images of the same subject side by side that at the same time suggested the subject's movement. "The good pun makes a double exposure on the mind."[11] Twistington's book *Still Life* includes a fine example: from static negatives, the ballerina Twistington, though struck down by polio, could produce, by means of superimposed multiple exposures, an aesthetic kinesis.

My more theoretical interest was cinema—moving pictures. The first movie I saw was the homemade travelogue that Uncle Bennie had made during his trip to Florida in 1952. Other young polios had access to actual moving-picture cameras; for example, when Francis Ford Coppola came down with polio at ten, he amused himself by creating puppet shows and making an eight-millimeter movie. That was, explains Coppola, when he first formed his long-standing interest in technology and "became obsessed with remote control."[12] I was fascinated by the puppet-controlling war cripple in the movie *Lili* (1953); I sensed intuitively that the actor Mel Ferrer, who played a bitter wounded soldier, was actually (in real life) a polio. The polio *qua* puppeteer is a subject of Tony Kemeny's *A Puppet No More* (1963).

My second specialty in photography was delayed action. *Delayed action* refers to "the operation of the shutter some time after the release is depressed, often due to the action of a built-in delayed action timer."[13] For years after the shock of polio, I would take photographs of myself or others swimming, weightless, in the water, like clipped waterbirds.

Delayed shock was a near synonym for trauma in the medical literature. It referred to "severe physical or mental disturbance, of which the symptoms occur a considerable time after the injury or mental impression is received."[14]

Delayed action and delayed shock, taken together, are the real keys to understanding such movies from the 1950s as Hitchcock's *Dial M for Mur-*

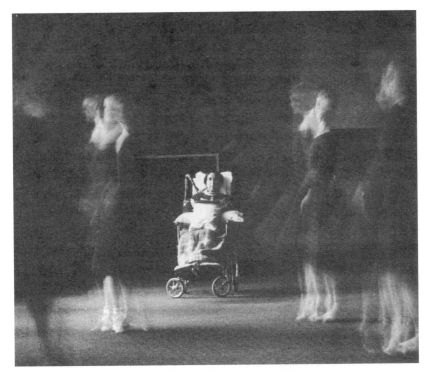

Double exposures showing the almost totally paralyzed dancer Elizabeth Twistington in a wheelchair.

der and *Rear Window.* In fact, Cornell Woolrich's story "Rear Window" takes up surveillance as a symptom or cause of paralytic disease and explores delayed action as a leading photographic trope.[15] Woolrich published his story, sometimes also called "It Had to Be Murder," in *Dime Detective*—that is, in the same magazine and during the same period (1939–1942) in which Bruno Fischer was publishing such stories about the polio-detective Ben Bryn as "Flesh for the Monsters."[16]

Polio and Cinema

Recent books about disability and the cinema suffer from a failure to consider the simultaneous advent of popular cinema (with its focus on kinesis) on the one hand and the epidemic of polio (with its enforced

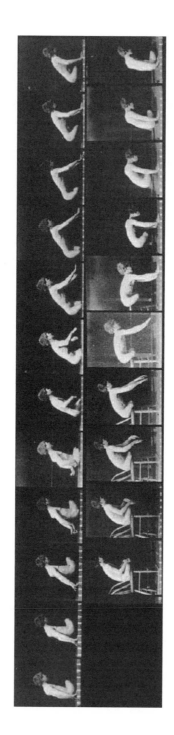

Serial photographs of crippled boy in motion, by Eadweard Muybridge.

stasis) on the other. Not only does poliomyelitis appear as an epidemic disease around the same time as the cinema; it also involves similar theoretical and technical issues of movement and prosthesis. Explaining (and eventually correcting) that omission from cinematographic historiography of this aspect of photographic history will adumbrate examples of the cultural "forgetfulness" about polio in twentieth-century culture.

The origins of cinema in the 1890s have to do partly with transforming still pictures into moving pictures or creating them from scratch; however, there are other ways to conceptualize this transformation. One might think of it . . .

1. As part of an intellectual revolution leading from anatomy, understood as the study of still life, or *nature morte* (dead nature), to physiology, understood as the study of life in motion, or

2. As an ideal (sometimes aesthetic) makeover of wholly paralyzed images of human beings to create moving images of them, or

3. As a "real" medical cure whereby paralyzed human beings become moving human beings—a cure documented by the ideal makeover aforementioned and sometimes even triggered by it

Relevant to understanding the cinema as this sort of motive spring or trigger (point 3) would be the precinematic photographic archives of nineteenth-century medical researchers like Jean Charcot. Also pertinent would be the serial photographic records of Eadweard Muybridge. He took photographs in quick succession, in order to study how animals move. Muybridge's freeze frame studies of movement are collected in such works as *Animal Locomotion* and *The Horse in Motion*. *The Human Figure in Motion* seems almost a study of how a polio might move.[17] Muybridge was interested not only in static images and how to animate them, but also in paralyzed beings—and how they might be made to move (again).

With the arrival of cinematography at the turn of the century, the link was clear between aesthetic re-creation through cinema and the medical restoration of kinesis. The first movie houses were "therapeutic" sites of *restauration* (recreation), and the early peep shows were properly called kinetoscope parlors. Many early movies were thematically and formally interested in the disabling and reenabling of motion in living creatures; for example, the first Western, *Cripple Creek Bar-Room* (1899), though only a minute long, has most of the Aristotelian elements of plot and complete action necessary to render clearly the topos of ability versus disability and health versus illness. A "likker'd up" man, disabled by too much "red eye," stumbles into the barroom. After having one more drink, he causes a ruckus. Other customers help remove him from the building. For thus restoring the community to its original health, these customers are rewarded with a drink on the house. This starts the pseudotragic cycle of crippling and reenabling all over again. The endless repetitiveness of the cycle is the reel and real creek—in the sense of "artificial contrivance"—of *Cripple Creek Bar-Room.*[18]

One widespread view nowadays about the origin of cinema is that early cinema involved an attempt to reproduce the effect of looking out the picture window of a moving railway car.[19] That is an attractive idea as far as it goes, but there are similar parallels one might draw. More important, it does not deal with the aesthetics and technique that originators of the cinematic medium themselves believed they were dealing with: the animation of the immobile.

Still photography itself, as these early technicians knew, demands a paralysislike stillness; moving photography cures that stillness. Early still photography as such involved photographic subjects' posing, or "sitting," without moving, sometimes for forty minutes or more. The relevant variables here are worth rehearsing.

Photography, "the production of pictures by means of the chemical action of light on a light-sensitive 'film,'" prefers a paralyzed subject.[20] Five technical variables explain why. These variables are the posing time, shutter speed, lens aperture, film speed (or sensitivity to light), and available light. The longer the posing time for which a subject remains still (seconds, minutes, hours, days, and so on, toward infinite stillness), the slower the shutter speed can be; and similarly, the smaller the lens aperture can be (F-3.5, F-5.6, and so on, toward infinitely small) and the slower the film speed can be (ASA-200, ASA-64, and so on, toward infinitely slow). The essential variable here is available light. On the one hand, the photographer (or "light writer") requires his subject "to freeze" really, in order to extend the posing time. On the other hand, the photographer "freezes" a moving subject ideally (or aesthetically) by restricting the shutter speed. All other things being equal, still photography becomes technically better and better, ad infinitum, according to the interactions of these five variables. A perfectly paralyzed thing or being is thus at once the best subject and the preferred purpose of still photography. The best living human subjects are therefore paralyzed ones.[21]

So much is suggested also by the cinematographic work of the polio Stephen Dwoskin. He specializes in making documentary-style moving pictures of paralyzed bodies.[22] Dwoksin, who had polio at age ten, has made the human body his special topic of study—bodies considered beautiful as well as those considered deformed. In moving-picture shots, often lasting for minutes, his camera investigates the details of a body and waits for the reactions in a face. The viewers become voyeurs even as the "actor" talks directly to them. Dwoskin's *Behindert* (1974), *Outside In* (1981–82), and *Pain Is . . .* (1997) all focus on Dwoskin's own polio.[23]

Moving-picture photography is dependent on the same general rules as still photography. Early movies thus made even "normal" people look odd when they walked—Charles Chaplin's quasi-stumbling gait is still celebrated. Thanks to the slow rate of shutter intervals in early movies, even nonparalyzed walkers seem to suffer from the same walking disorder that the French neurologist Jean Charcot had photographed and described in his paralyzed walkers. If still photography paralyzes moving people, moving pictures seem to free them from their partial paralysis. Cinematography cured the paralytic disease that still photography caused and from which it suffers.

This fact helps explain why so many early movies are concerned either with the comedic or the tragic curing of actual people or with the promise to do so. *The Automobile Accident* (1904) is an early French example. This trick-effect movie uses two look-alike actors, one an actual double amputee and the other a man with both his legs. After the protagonist's legs are cut off in the "accident," the victim picks up his dismembered limbs, sticks them back on, and simply walks off. The same amputee-actor played in *The Cripple's Marriage* (1909), a comedy about the nuptials of "a cripple minus his legs and a tall spinster," and starred in *The Legless Runner.*[24] In the "documentary" movie *Fighting Infantile Paralysis* (1917), produced with assistance from the Rockefeller Institute for Medical Research, the message involves not merely how to avoid paralysis but also how to overcome it.[25]

When I lay paralyzed in bed—a picture of motionlessness—dreaming about prosthetic mechanical devices to build with my Meccano set and planning various telephoto graphics, I came across a relevant cartoon in my copy of *A Child's Geography of the World*. It read, "Hollywood is the greatest moving-picture place in the wide World."[26]

HANDI-CAPITALISM AND CINEMA BUSINESS

5

> "Spirit," said Scrooge, with an interest he had never felt before, "tell me if Tiny Tim will live."
>
> —Charles Dickens, *A Christmas Carol* (1843)

Polio paralyzes its victims; but it then leaves most of them alive, in large numbers, as visible, feared, and pitied spectacles. Moving-picture artists and medical practitioners alike saw an opportunity to do well by doing good. Paralysis was the perfect aesthetic subject matter and object of medical treatment. It allowed the practitioner to weigh out fear and pity alternately in varying Aristotelian proportions, depending upon the genre. Charles Mee, who had polio my year (1953), writes in *A Nearly Normal Life:* "I think it is intact people who like to experience the feelings of sorrow and loss and bitterness over and over again—and who always ask injured people about these feelings, to conjure them up and experience them vicariously."[1] Polio wasn't the only cause of paralysis and deformity. Paralytic disability could also stem from other causes: injury and wars, for example.[2] Soldiers often got polio as well, as President Roosevelt discussed during a secret visit to Warm Springs on April 15, 1943.[3] It was often unclear to onlookers on the street just how a particular wheelchair-bound person had become crippled. The cause of the disability might be domestic or military, but the War against Polio knew no international borderlines. One illustration of the possible confusion can be found in the documentarylike movie about veterans *The Men* (1950; also called *Battle Stripe*), in which Marlon Brando plays a veteran-amputee struggling with the problems of his amputation. *The Men* harks back to *King's Row* (1942), in which Ronald Reagan plays an amputee, and to *The Best Years of Our Lives* (1946), which stars the actual amputee Harold Russell. In *The Men,* one of Brando's hospital ward mates dies of a suddenly contracted disease whose symptoms resemble those of polio. Moreover, the apparently true-to-life rehabilitation scenes are much like those in the rehabilitation movie *Never Fear* (1950; also called *The Young Lovers*), directed by the polio Ida Lupino, who set her work in actual hospital wards.

That's Entertainment

In such cases, the subject matter of rehabilitation cinema (which sets human stasis into motion) corresponds to the form of the medium of cinema (making still pictures move). Like the customers in the barroom at Cripple Creek, the early patrons of the movie houses gave their financial support to the new establishments. At the same time, under the aegis of Hollywood, donation of private funds toward the eradication of paralysis found encouragement. The orthopedic institutions, too, saw an opportunity, in the promise to make crooked children straight *(orthos)*.

Polio was a useful condition for raising money: it invoked the specter of sudden family catastrophe and usually left behind a permanent visible reminder of its crippling pediatric handiwork. That was one of polio's attractions as a subject for movie houses as well as cinematographers. Even if the movie houses lost money when they had to be closed down during polio season, polio as subject matter became the movies' most profitable drawing card during the rest of the moviegoing season.[4] At the same times as the movie houses collected ticket prices for their show of kinesis, they collected funds for the National Foundation for Infantile Paralysis (NFIP), in order that the foundation might cure people of their paralytic stasis.

In screening rooms, the public was often first shown a documentary movie (a "flyer") about polio. Then came a song or two. "Brother, Can You Spare a Dime?" (written for the Broadway musical *New Americana* of 1932) went to the top of the charts. In the 1950s, the song was still played in Zeyde Joe's cinema hall to encourage people to give to the war against polio.[5] Only after the hat was passed around did the feature movie start. Thus, Yip Harburg's song about unemployment came to assist the NFIP's

March of Dimes. Beginning in 1946, more than one third of all funds donated to the foundation came from monies collected in the theaters—much in the style of collections in American churches. Many novels of the period include descriptions of the foundation's various fund-raising rituals. We read in Devoto's later *Last Days:* "Now there appeared on the screen a man telling everyone that if they gave their money to the fundraisers who would pass among them, the money would help find a cure for polio." The next thing the movie shows is a man in an iron lung pleading for money as the hissing of his iron lung punctuates his sentences. The same movie included a version of the song "You'll Never Walk Alone" (1945).[6]

"You'll Never Walk Alone," from Rogers and Hammerstein's stage musical *Carousel* (1945), was used by many charitable polio organizations in order to publicize "walkathons."

> When you walk through a storm,
> Hold your head up high,
> And don't be afraid of the dark,
> At the end of the storm is a golden sky.
> And the sweet silver song of a lark.
> Walk on through the wind,
> Walk on through the rain,
> Though your dreams be tossed and blown,
> Walk on, walk on, with hope in your heart,
> And you'll never walk alone.
> You'll never walk alone.

To us polio-children, the words of this love song meant both that we would never be able to walk without braces and that we would always be dependent on someone to lean on. When young polios performed the song before audiences—as did Glynda at an early telethon hosted by the celebrity Lorne Green—the adults' tears would flow along with their money.[7]

Tens of stars from the big movie studios lent a hand in the movie theaters. They spoke after the showing of relevant flyers or trailers. Celebrity cult figures like Judy Garland, Mickey Rooney, Danny Kaye, Mary Pickford, Ida Lupino, Mel Ferrer, Marilyn Monroe, James Cagney, Jack Benny, Humphrey Bogart, Zsa-Zsa Gabor, Myrna Loy, Veronica Lake, Linda Darnell, and Alan Ladd came to the cinema houses. Liberace was a frequent visitor during the 1950s at Rancho los Amigos, where Ronald Reagan used to crown young polio victims with the title "Miss Breathless." Helen Hayes, likewise, was often photographed with iron-lung patients. The very name March of Dimes was supposedly invented by the popular performer Eddie Cantor, who always told people that sending a dime to President Roosevelt would cure polio.[8] Jimmy Stewart and Grace Kelly—the co-stars in Hitchcock's *Rear Window* (1954)—played unique roles in fund-raising.

The Miracle at Hickory (ca. 1944–1952), one of the flyers or trailers at the theaters, told the real-life story of a North Carolina town struck devastatingly by polio, which then miraculously recovered. (The story was also the subject of a book written by the NFIP.[9] In recent times, the polio narrative anthology *The Grit Behind the Miracle* came out of a patients' reunion at Hickory in 1990.)[10] Greer Garson, who narrated the movie for MGM, had starred in the movie *Madame Curie* in 1943; thanks to her celebrated role in *The Miracle at Hickory,* she went on to play Eleanor Roosevelt in Dory Schary's polio stage play and movie *Sunrise at Campobello.*[11]

Polio did not just make the news; it was the news: the March of Dimes displaced *The March of Time.* (The radio show *Hollywood March of Dimes,* which began in 1942, was a weekly staple, like many war broadcasts.) Among the most memorable television episodes of all times was Edward R. Murrow's live newscast on April 12, 1955, on which he provided in-depth coverage of "the end of polio." Using entertainment cult celebrities and private foundations proved both successful in its time and influential through the rest of the century.[12]

The NFIP, although a *private* foundation, assumed many of the financial and health functions that we associate nowadays with *public* health. The institution and progress of Roosevelt's once-tiny Warm Springs Foundation helped shape the functions of the private and public health sectors in America for the next half century. Sporadic private donations—rather than dependable public support—became a way of life. The NFIP itself, which had also been founded by Roosevelt, was "a new type of American institution, a supposedly permanent self-sustaining source of medical research funds, a voluntary health foundation based on small individual contributions, not the largesse of a handful of wealthy patrons."[13]

Where there was cooperation between the private and public sectors, of course, there was often also corruption, as the following example demon-

strates. Cinema joined hands with public medicine in the halls of government as soon World War II ended. On September 5, 1945—the first day
that Congress convened after the Japanese surrender—President Harry
Truman asked the House and Senate to take back $3.5 billion of the 1946
appropriations authorization for the war agencies. That same day, Truman
met with Nicholas M. Schenck (head of MGM) and Basil O'Connor (president of the NFIP).[14] The three men worked out a deal whereby MGM and
Loews would continue their work on behalf of the NFIP but only in return
for leniency with enforcement of the Sherman and Clayton antitrust regulations.

Fear and Pity

Although influenza killed tens of millions of people during the influenza
epidemic of 1917–18, it was quickly forgotten.[15] Tuberculosis too took myriad victims, but they were often kept in sanatoriums; and since "when a
man is out of sight, it is not too long before he is out of mind," they too
were quickly forgotten.[16] The effect of polio was different from that of influenza and tuberculosis: polio left tens of thousands of people as visible
objects of fear and pity. Not for nothing was polio called the Crippler. As
such, it was personified on screen as a gigantic shadow stalking the land,
seeking child-victims.[17] Polio *was* "the Shadow": T. S. Eliot, in his poem
"The Hollow Men," wrote about "paralyzed force, gesture without motion," when "between the motion / And the act / Falls the shadow."[18] Polio
was the sculptural artist that shaped and stilled moving human bodies in
the public sphere. Robert F. Hall begins his polio narrative *Through the
Storm* with these words: "Polio is spectacular, the way it strikes, the way it
kills, the way it leaves its trademark."[19]

   This oft-observed parallel between the artful sculptor and polio—that
both are "re-creators" of the human body—partly motivates the aesthetic
work of polio survivors like the painter Frida Kahlo. Kahlo, who got polio
at the age of six, as mentioned earlier, created such relevant works as *The
Broken Column*. (There are two series of works with this telling name: first,
variously painted orthopedic corsets and casts; second, paintings in which
Kahlo depicts herself as a spinal column and the nails in her body as stig-
mata.)[20]

The Aristotelian dialectic of fear and pity here works in concert with that of fear and hope. On the one hand, *hope* that an uncomfortable condition will be cured or go away—encouraged by the Christopher Reeve Paralysis Foundation, which promulgates belief that a solution to almost all paraplegia is just around the corner.[21] On the other hand is the *fear* that the condition will not go away—as acknowledged by the Hemlock Society, which backs suicide for the chronically ill.[22] In many cases, though, it seems not to matter to the viewing public whether we get our catharsis from the imitation of a crippling or from an actual crippling. After all, often the same people who go to see public spectacles like *Oedipus Blinded* and *Christ Crucified* on the stage or screen vote to keep both tuberculosis patients and crippled war veterans squirreled away in almost invisible institutions.

Seeing wounded soldiers rolling about in wheelchairs generally makes people feel bad, even when a wheelchair is skillfully integrated into a comic routine onstage, as in *Flanders and Swann.*[23] The confounding of aesthetic play stage with political or military "obscenity" is a disturbing commonplace of the public sphere.

In order for Aristotelian catharsis to work, the main event in tragic drama needs to be narratologically explicable or morally comprehensible. Of pity or fear, Aristotle says that "the effect is heightened when [events] . . . follow as cause and effect. The tragic wonder will then be greater than if they happened of themselves or by accident."[24] Things work out best when the tragic victim is somehow the author of his own downfall.[25] Consider here how polio as the victimizer was often regarded in Protestant America. If the patient in the polio ward "recovered" from polio, then it was thanks to God's grace—or, just as likely, it was owing to a donor's having graciously given money to the NFIP, or March of Dimes. Sometimes, it was also thanks to the polio's own hard work. If, on the other hand, the polio patient did not recover, it was because of God's damnation—or, just as likely, it was owing to someone's damnably not having given enough dimes. Sometimes it was thanks to the polio's not having worked hard enough. Chance, they usually said, had nothing to do with it.

Only the winners made it onto the March of Dimes' posters, which featured modern-day Tiny Tims. That is how the commonplace infantolatrous Americanism "Do it for the children!" became the hallmark of sentimentalized American politics—and remains so up to the present day.[26]

"Crippledom" was a good thing for the March of Dimes. It furthered money collection and a cure. It allowed telethon masters to use polios as distinctly dehumanized and deformed money collection props in the tradition parodied in Bertolt Brecht's *Threepenny Opera* (1928). Polios were likewise definitively *commodified;* thousands of children became naked patient demonstrators in surgical theaters and orthopedists' advertisements. This exploitative practice was the origin of Live Aid: the studios, and later the celebrity community, raising funds in the private sector, seemed to make the public sector both weak and unnecessary. Of the benefit concert, Paul McCartney said, "Often you find your musicians do more bloody good than your government does. Certainly on Live Aid they did."[27] McCartney merely mistook the effect for the cause.

Defective Detectives

Not all medical conditions are curable. Because a physician cannot heal himself does not mean that he is not a good physician. Who (but God) lives forever? Seen in this universalist light, Jesus Christ's taunt to the doctors "Physician, heal thyself!" seems inappropriate.[28] Even he can only do resurrection. Moreover, it is often when a physician knowingly suffers from a disease or disability which he knows he has that he has gained the insight to diagnose and to deal with that disease in others. Milton Erickson (1902–1980)—the subject of John C. Hughes's adulatory "The Wounded Healer" —suffered considerable physical disability as the result of polio, which he contracted in 1919, for example. Erickson's work on hypnosis and psychosomatic theory concerns the association or disassociation of mind and body and his refusal to mask that "alienation." Was it not that early experience of disassociation that helped make Erickson a healer—and indeed an interested diagnostician, or detective, of disease?[29]

Many crippled people try to act in public as if they are not disabled. Among actors themselves, Sarah Bernhardt is a famous example.[30] Yet some actors do the opposite. When Lionel Barrymore became crippled, he jumped at the chance to play a crippled physician in the *Dr. Kildare* movie series.[31] When Barrymore died in 1954, he was the best-known crippled Dr. Leonard Gillespie. Barrymore was known for doing movie publicity that benefited polio research. In the 1960s, though, television dropped the topos of the crippled doctor like a hot potato: the series *Dr. Kildare* and *Ben Casey*, which both ran from 1961 to 1966, made their doctors able-bodied. Not until the television series *ER* in the 1990s did a polio come to the small screen in a series—and even there, typically for polio, the disease is never named. (Laura Innes, the actress who plays Dr. Carrie Weaver in *ER,* is good at imitating the psychological and physical qualities associated with having had polio because, as she says, her sister is a polio.)[32]

What is true for lame physician-diagnosticians (Dr. Gillespie, Dr. Weaver in *ER*) is also true for "defective detectives."[33] The topos of the defective detective harks back to that original lame detective, Oedipus. Oedipus is able to rid Thebes of its plague because his disability, which requires him to use a staff when he stands or walks, gives him sufficient knowledge of human beings to detect one partial answer to the riddle of the Sphinx. (The answer is partial because, although he knows what a human being is, Oedipus does not know who he is. He can cure others but not himself.)[34] In American popular fiction during the polio epidemics, there were hundreds of defective detectives. One pulp writer in the genre was Bruno Fischer, whose stories feature the explicitly polio private eye Ben Bryn.[35] Crippled by childhood polio, Ben Bryn has developed a strong upper body and a strong mind. Fischer's "Pray for the Creeping Death" puts it like this:

> For twenty years of his life, those legs had been useless appendages as the result of infantile paralysis. His youth had consisted of pushing himself about on a wheeled platform and selling newspapers and shoelaces. That had placed strength in his shoulders and hands and iron in his soul; and when a series of exercises he had evolved had eventually developed his legs to normal, that strength and that iron had made him the most feared criminal investigator in the state.[36]

Ben Bryn was, in fact, a toned-down version of Calvin Kane. Kane was a private eye whose "severely deformed body made him look like a refugee from a side-show attraction."[37] With his withered right leg and twisted body, Kane had to crawl along the floor, using his extremely powerful arms. This earned him the nickname of "Crab Detective." *Crab-walk* became a common term used by doctors in the 1950s to describe the way that their polio patients moved. Enid Foster's *It Can't Happen to Me* (1959?) reminds us, in quoting Dr. James, the orthopedic surgeon in Rhodesia: " 'O Lord, another crab-walker!' he said, referring to my queer method of perambulation with the right leg always a good ways ahead of the left."[38]

Ben Bryn was the literary ancestor of Ironside, the police detective who, having been paralyzed from the waist down (supposedly as the result of a gunshot wound), becomes a private detective in a wheelchair. Ironside was usually played by Raymond Burr. (In Hitchcock's *Rear Window,* with its wheelchaired protagonist, Burr played the role of the invalid-murderer Thorwald.)

These days we keep our defective physicians and detectives in the closet. The sight of such persons would seem to make us uncomfortable, recalling all too vividly the physically threatening conditions that menace all human beings, and reminding us of the wish to keep such people out of mind once and for all.

Kill and Cure

> *King Claudius:* Do it, England;
> For like the hectic in my blood he rages,
> And thou must cure me.
>
> —William Shakespeare, *Hamlet,* 4.2

What should I do with an apparently disabled person who makes me uncomfortable? What can I do with myself so that a disabled person does not make me uncomfortable?

The answer to the first question seems obvious. I can cure the person of his disability (through therapy or medication, for example) or remove the disabled person from my presence (through distance, as was done, say, when lepers or the insane were isolated in colonies or madhouses).

The answer to the second question likewise seems evident: I can learn to tolerate comfortably another person's disability. Yet the very essence of toleration, "putting up with what we dislike," is a psychologically and intellectually painful process for most people. Might we then love the disabled person but not his disability? Toleration is difficult insofar as a person's disability may be an inextricable part of the person. (After all, Adam's descendants cannot simply extricate themselves from his "original" sin. Am I *able* to love the sinner but not his sin?)[39] If *a* polio (the person) is one who suffers from polio (the disease), then I cannot cure the disease without eradicating the person.

If toleration (which is good) is difficult, then universal love (which is best), may be impossible in the political arena. And insofar as the best is the enemy of the good, the injunction to love everyone the same may be more politically dangerous than even an injunction to cure or kill some people. If *all* people are my brothers, then it is all too easy to believe that *only* my brothers are human beings.

Can I cure one person by killing another? This option involves substitutive scapegoating as a means of rehabilitative therapy and lies at the bottom of both Greek tragedy and Christian doctrine. Whether you kill the person who has the disability or kill the disability that plagues the person, you accomplish the same thing: you rid the community of the intolerably disabled and hence discomforting persons.

Cinema, we have seen, prefers to cure bodily diseases *ideally*. That is true for more conditions than those involving paralysis and stasis. In early silent movies, blindness was the frequent subject of semi-miraculous cure. Many comedies and science fiction movies were organized around re-attaching limbs cut off or otherwise lost to use. Sometimes the cure comes about by means of divine miracle, as when Jesus cures the paralytic in such movies as *King of Kings* (1961) and *The Greatest Story Ever Told* (1965). Sometimes the cure is fraud, as with the Frog in *The Miracle Man* (1919), a movie made soon after the New York polio epidemic, in which a young woman rises out of a wheelchair.[40] (*Frog-boy* was a common slang term for a polio as late as the 1950s.)[41] Sometimes the cure is associated with raising money, as in *The Leather Saint* (1956), which features a priest who, in the tradition of the March of Dimes, raises money to help kids in braces and wheelchairs. Sometimes the cure is associated with family pets, as in *Lad: A Dog* (1962) and *The Littlest Hobo* (1958).[42]

An early influential movie involving a cure was *Polyanna* (1920), which seems a commentary on widespread effects of paralytic polio. In *Polyanna*, a young girl—played by Mary Pickford—has been paralyzed by an automobile accident.[43] As early as *Stella Maris* (1918), though, Pickford had been playing paralyzed girls like the ones crippled by the polio epidemic of 1916. In *Stella Maris*—a Pickford Film Corporation film based on the novel by William John Locke and written for the screen by Frances Marion—Pickford actually plays two interrelated roles.[44] First, she plays the heiress

Stella Maris—a beautiful, crippled, and bedridden girl. In the care of her guardian, Stella is kept unaware of all the unpleasant realities of life. Second, Pickford plays the orphan Unity Blake—an ugly servant who had been adopted and employed by Stella's guardian and has suffered from the harsh realities of life. (In the 1950s, Pickford came to play a prominent role in the March of Dimes, although she had already begun in the 1920s doing publicity for various foundations for infantile paralysis.)[45]

Mary Philbin's 1926 remake of the same story contains a good deal of innovative split-screen and double-exposure work. In the style of the double-exposure tradition described earlier, Philbin punningly links the two women: the one disabled, or static, and about to be cured, and the other able-bodied, or kinetic, and about to die.

The sacrificial victim in most such tales is as likely to be a god in human form (like Christ) or a humanoid animal (like an ape) as it is an ugly orphan servant. Beginning in the 1920s, apes were actually being experimented upon and dying by the tens of thousands, as part of human beings' search for a cure to polio. In the aesthetic realm, the "sacrifice" of the apes was often a theme for comedy. In Howard Hawks's *Monkey Business* (1952; also known as both *Be Your Age* and *Darling, I Am Growing Younger*), sacrifice helps human beings to cure age-old ailments. Sometimes, the quasi-simian sacrifice is genuinely grisly. *The Ape* is a Frankensteinian horror shocker with grave robbers. It concerns a doctor (Boris Karloff) who discovers a cure for polio that requires taking spinal fluid from human beings.[46] The doctor, dressed as a gorilla, kills and experiments on some human beings, in order to save the paralyzed legs of a wonderfully deserving girl.[47]

In the film *Rear Window*, to which we turn in the next chapter, the question "What am I supposed to do with a disabled person who makes me uncomfortable?" has two answers. On the one hand, "Murder the disabled person!" Murder his bedridden wife Anna (Irene Winston) is presumably what Lars Thorwald has done. The perhaps temporarily wheelchair-bound photographer L. B. "Jeff" Jeffries (Jimmy Stewart), who identifies with Anna, remarks that Thorwald might like to "run out on her," but then adds ominously, "Sometimes it's worse to stay than it is to run." On the other hand, "Cure the disabled person!" Cure Jeffries is what fashion model Lisa Carol Fremont (Grace Kelly) and insurance company nurse Stella (Thelma Ritter) are apparently trying to do.

6 THE CAST OF *REAR WINDOW*; OR, CINEMA AND AKINESIA

"What's the matter with me?"
The doctor's eyes left his own for moment, descending to the bed.
"A virus infection of some sort . . . polio perhaps."

—J. G. Farrell, *The Lung* (1965)

Soon after the Korean War ended, on December 1, 1953, John Michael Hayes submitted the "white script" for *Rear Window* to Paramount Pictures.[1] That day, I was lying at home paralyzed from polio, wondering what had happened to me. There was a wheelchair beside the bed.

What Happened to You?

"What happened to you?" This was usually the first question addressed to wheelchair occupants in the 1950s. The usual answer in the 1950s would have been "Polio." But there were always complications.

Polio Detection

How could one tell for sure what was the cause of a person's being in a wheelchair? As touched on earlier, not all cases of paralytic stillness result from polio, just as not all cases of polio lead to paralysis. Certainly you can't tell reliably that a person in a wheelchair is there as the result of a bout with polio. Captain Ahab (John Barrymore) in *The Sea Beast* (1926) has lost his lower leg, so we might figure that his situation is that of an amputee. But what if he is tricking us? Or what if amputation were a treatment for polio? How would we know for sure? In *West of Zanzibar* (1928), the legs of the magician Dead Legs (Lon Chaney) "become paralyzed from the waist down after his wife's lover . . . (Lionel Barrymore) pushes him off a balcony."[2] Is it the wife's fall from chastity that paralyzes the magician, by triggering a certain hysteria? Or is it rather his own fall from the balcony that actually paralyzes him? Or should we, like psychoanalysts, link Dead Legs' fear about his own loss of virility with his fall from the balcony? In the case of actual infantile paralysis contracted when an infant, the lame person may not know how he or she got that way. And in some artworks about paralysis, it doesn't even matter. In Alice Munro's story "Open Secrets" and Catharine Marchant's novel *House of Men*, the lameness of the polio survivors is merely the external sign of moral weakness.[3] Consider too Mickey Rooney's polio movie *Fireball* (1950).

What the occasional difficulty or irrelevance of a polio diagnosis means for us here, as we begin the study of Alfred Hitchcock's *Rear Window,* is that a movie or stage play that says it is about polio may not be essentially about polio. A case in point would be Kramer's *The Normal Heart* (1986). In this stage play, Dr. Emma Brookner is said to be a polio, and Kramer means her to be one, but Brookner's symptoms—especially her inability to have sexual relations—are not those of a real polio. They merely reflect playwrights' and theatergoers' usual sociopathology about disability and their ignorance of poliomyelitic paralysis. When it comes to polios, Kramer follows the usual pattern of assuming that polios do not have sexual desire or ability—and of course the plot's requirement for a celibate mother encourages him in that direction. That neither Kramer nor any one of his reviewers ever acknowledged the mistake says something about the pervasiveness of misunderstandings about polio.

In *The Normal Heart,* Kramer makes a sorrowful point about AIDS, but only at the expense of forgetting or denying the facts of polio.

Certain movies, like *King's Row* (1942), do not claim or seem to be about polio, but they are often better able to portray the polio experience than those which do make that claim. These are often postwar movies. *The Men* (1950) as well as *Coming Home* (1978) and *Born on the Fourth of July* (1989) are typical examples.[4] Dalton Trumbo's novel *Johnny Got His Gun* (1939) is an extreme version of the genre.[5] Largely suppressed from the time of its original publication until its republication in the late 1950s, this novel became a movie in 1979. Later on, it was brilliantly illustrated by the Spanish film director Luis Buñuel.[6] Concerning such movies and novels, where the position of war veteran and polio is easily confused, Bentz Plagemann tells in *My Place to Stand* (1949) how, when he returned from the war paralyzed by polio, he felt like an imposter because people took him for a veteran wounded in military action. "'What action were you in when they got you?' he asked me. 'My leg is paralyzed,' I said, 'I was not in any battle.'"[7] The Briton Paul Bates, author of the polio memoir *Horizontal Man*, contracted polio while on patrol in the Malayan jungle in 1954. Bates writes of his experience in an iron lung, beginning with his military time in Kinrara, much as Wendell Phillips, in his *Qataban and Sheba* (1955), writes of his polio experience while in the military in 1945.[8] The invalid wartime photojournalist L. B. "Jeff" Jeffries (Jimmy Stewart) in *Rear Window* seeks out the dangers of a similarly ambiguous war zone: "Didn't I tell you that'd be the next place to blow?"

We should not overlook so-called hysterical paralysis, as Freudians call it, and which the makers of *West of Zanzibar* imply. Polio often presents to the diagnostician as a disease that is "merely hysterical." Reluctance to acknowledge that certain symptoms arose from the polio virus meant overly quick diagnosis of the patient as hysterical. Doctors made this error from time to time—as did Freud in the case of cerebral palsy. Novelists and cinema directors were similarly reluctant to come right out and say that someone had polio. The case of the little lame prince in Craik's novella of 1874 is relevant here.[9] So too is the work of John Davys Beresford, in whose novel *The Early History of Jacob Stahl* (1911) the hero is lamed in childhood by an "accident"—like the little lame prince. (Ironically, Beresford himself was a polio: "'owing to the carelessness of a nurse' (said he), 'Beresford contracted infantile paralysis.'")[10] Confusion between hysterical and poliomyelitic paralysis is also at the crux of Arthur Miller's play *The Broken Glass*, set in the 1930s.

What is the specific character of the immobilizing injury that put L. B. "Jeff" Jeffries (and Jimmy Stewart) into *Rear Window*'s central cast? In answering this question, we recall what scriptwriter Hayes rightly calls the motivating leg art in *Rear Window*. "I hope I didn't take *all* leg art," says Jeff.[11]

By the term *leg art,* Jeff means in the first instance "girlie pictures" that show women's legs.[12] These are the sort of still photographs that the voyeuristic Jeff might have taken, along with detective Thomas J. ("Tom") Doyle (Wendell Cory), in some such helicopter reconnaissance and girl-spotting mission as that with which *Rear Window* begins. However, Jeff's reference to leg art also recalls the artfulness of Jeff's plaster cast and the writing on it: "Here lie the broken bones of L. B. Jeffries." It recalls as well the "theatrical casts" that Jeff observes in the rear windows, so similar to stage settings, of his neighborhood and the movie cast of *Rear Window* itself.

As we shall see, the leg art of *Rear Window* has to do with variously permanent, short-term, or delayed dissociations of body from mind. Just at the historical moment before the widespread introduction of the polio vaccine, the ambiguity surrounding Jeff's cast in *Rear Window* arises from —and casts light on—popular hopes and fears about invalidism and paralysis in the age of still and moving photography.

Immobilizing Casts and Moving Pictures

It is almost a general trope in the cinema that polios use plaster casts like Jeff's. It is important to distinguish here, however, between polios' putting on casts that they need for the care of bones, muscles, tendons, or nerves and their putting on casts that they do not need for those particular purposes. When polios put on casts that they require medically for the care of bones or muscles, they do so for at least three reasons. First, some polios need casts in order to avoid scoliosis and the like.[13] That is an important theme of *Looking for Mr. Goodbar,* in which the heroine's torso had been encased in a plaster cast for more than a year.[14] Second, polios break bones (many do, in fact) and require plaster casts. Let me make two important qualifications here.

First, as Dixson reminds us in his polio narrative, *My Way with Polio,* a polio, whose muscles do not work properly, can never be certain whether his bones will knit. "After a week at Charing Cross Hospital I was removed to Ashridge Hospital, Berkhamstead, where I was later examined by the visiting surgeon, Mr. Trevor. He was blunt and anything but optimistic: 'The broken bones of polio cases do not knit easily, if at all, and your age of forty-three is against you.' He thought it unlikely that I should ever walk again—we would have to wait to see."[15] If we assume that Jeff's walking dysfunction arises from a broken leg, then he (probably) will walk—maybe even in a week. However, if the "lie of the broken bones" betokens something other than broken bones—say, physical paralysis or hypochondriacal or hysterical paresis—then his medical prognosis, which is almost the same as *Rear Window*'s aesthetic end, would be different from that.

Second, permanently disabled polios with casts on can sometimes "pass" as only temporarily disabled people. Their casts can offer short-term liberation from society's general disapproval of permanently disabled persons—and hence, also, from the polios' disapproval of themselves. In *The Affair*, for example, Courtney (Natalie Wood) is a thirty-two-year-old polio-crippled songwriter who, because she feels unattractive, has her first love affair late in life. (In the same way, the polio Joan McDonnell in *A Spring in My Steps* feels attractive thanks to an epistolary love affair that keeps her otherwise obvious limp invisible to her correspondent.)[16] Many polios who have similarly felt unattractive come to feel appealing after putting on a plaster cast.

This last observation leads to a third reason that some polios put on casts: they hope thereby to come across as sexually more attractive. In Eduard Molinaro's movie *Just the Way You Are* (1984), the polio Susan Berlanger (Kristy McNichol) arranges to have a fake cast put on her paralyzed leg; then she goes to a French ski resort, where she has a love affair. Also, a polio with a real (needful) cast for a really broken leg may appear relatively normal or attractive. The main narratological device of Ben Lewin's movie *Lucky Break* (1994; also called *Paperback Romance*) involves a young woman, Sophie (Gia Carideas), crippled by polio. She writes erotic tales professionally,[17] but she herself has little active love life and refuses to go on dates. One day, while following a man with whom she has fallen in love at first sight, Sophie trips and breaks her paralyzed leg. That leg is put into a cast, and when the leg has healed, she hesitates to have the cast removed.[18] She then camouflages her permanently crippled polio self as an athletic woman recovering from the temporary effects of a ski accident. Everything goes well for Sophie—just so long as she can keep her lover from discovering the secret and keep her doctor from removing her cast. Once the cast is removed—a week later than the doctor had anticipated—Sophie has her regular polio brace put on again.[19]

Stasis and Kinesis

Akinesia is defined as the "loss of the power of voluntary movement; paralysis of the motor nerves."[20] *Rear Window* is an artwork about the ambiguities of stasis and kinesis in the realms of both image photography and bodily paralysis. The wheelchair-bound Jeff is a still (and static) photographer who uses his flash camera, or "flashgun," serially to try to freeze action. He has apparently attempted this on the racetrack, where he has failed to stop a race car. Jeff calls the resulting collision an accident. From the standpoint of the formal requirements of the plot in relation to cinematography and paralysis, however, the war photographer Jeff's supposed automobile accident (*accident* meaning literally how things "fall out") would seem to be anything but accidental. In the end, not only is Jeff unable to emerge from his cocoonlike case, but after being cast out his own rear window, his movement-inhibiting (plaster) cast is bigger than ever.

Jeff goes on to try to freeze action in his apartment, where he fails to stop a walking murderer (Thorwald) who appears as a photographic negative image. Jeff also uses his camera more or less inadvertently to do detective work, when he tracks the growth of flowering plants by means of sequenced diapositives. (He takes sequential photographic slides and compares them with each other. That allows him to guess that Thorwald is hiding something under the ground.) Detective Doyle is likewise interested in stillness and movement: he studies the painting in Jeff's apartment because its abstract subjects seem to move.[21]

When Detective Doyle (called Coyne in Hayes's script) asks Jeff, "By the way—what happened to your leg?" Jeff ambiguously answers, "Jay-walking."[22] His answer reminds me of a passage from Christine Brook-Rose's *Language of Love* (1957): "She jay-walked through the traffic-jam of St. Giles, vaguely hoping to be run over."[23] Jeff, who usually seeks what he himself calls the status quo (in his conversation with Lisa about their amatory relationship), was injured while he was "stand[ing] in the middle of that automobile race"—so he tells us.[24]

We are reminded of the freeze-frame technique of Jeff's profession throughout the movie. At the beginning of *Rear Window*, for example, the first artwork we see (according to the script) is a ten-by-fourteen photographic positive print showing the "split second" of the explosion of an artillery shell during the Korean War as it freezes men and equipment.[25] Near the end of the movie, too, Jeff uses his "flashgun" to shoot Thorwald (to render him static), but instead the sequences only make for animation (cinema). When Lisa—who is a model for still photographers at a fashion magazine—sees these elementary attempts at moving photography, even she is "frozen with panic."[26] So Jeff's immobility and disability are not so much the end of a careless accident as they are the aesthetic end of the photography that is Jeff's profession. (D. H. Lawrence referred to "a cinema-camera, taking its succession of instantaneous snaps" at around the same time he was writing partly about physical paralysis and emotional impotence in *Lady Chatterley's Lover*.)[27]

When we first meet Jeff, he is sitting in a director's chair that recalls the cinematic thesis of *Rear Window*. *Rear Window* alludes not only to the immobility of the spectator in the movie house, who ordinarily cannot join the action, but also to the immobility of the cinema director who ordinarily directs others to act for him.[28] (Sometimes, the director joins in that action—as in the case of Hitchcock, say, who shows up in *Rear Window*, or of Jeffries, when he takes his fall out *his* rear window.) Consider the case of the movie director Francis Ford Coppola, a polio himself, and of his character the voyeur Harry Caul, a polio turned private eye, in his movie *The Conversation* (1974). During his polio convalescence at age ten, as we have seen, Coppola created puppet shows and made an eight-millimeter movie. That was, explains Coppola, when he formed a long-standing interest in technology and "became obsessed with remote control." It was his polio too that attracted Coppola to making the movie *Jack* (1996).[29] The character of Harry Caul is based on Coppola himself. In a central dream sequence, Caul follows the wife of the "director" and tells her how he was struck down by polio and was paralyzed for six months. Caul has become, since his polio convalescence, a surveillance expert, in the tradition of *Rear Window*.

The Lie of the Broken Bones; or, L. B. Jeffries in a Cast

> Who said I was getting rid of it?
>
> —Jeff to Editor Gunnison, in Hitchcock's *Rear Window*

The celebrated long shot at the beginning of *Rear Window* all but ends with the grimly humorous epitaph of Jeff's medical case written on his plaster cast: "Here lie the broken bones of L. B. Jeffries."[30] To judge by the role of similar inscriptions in other Hitchcock films—among them the inscription engraved in the ring in *Shadow of a Doubt* (1943)—*Rear Window*'s opening graffiti should be scrutinized carefully. After all, *Rear Window* revolves about people laid up with broken bones (the invalids Mrs. Thorwald and L. B. Jeffries) and how to deal with them or to dispose of them while they are living and also once they are dead. To understand Jeff's case, we need to return to the question "What happened to you?" that Detective Doyle asks wheelchair-bound Jeff. Jeff says that he has a broken leg. Is he correct? Might he be "mistaken" about why the cast is there? After all, a cast is not only "a type of medical device," it is also "a type of aesthetic trick," a sort of spell.[31]

What would it mean if in the fiction that is *Rear Window* the real lie of the broken bones is that the bones are not really broken? What if they instead both hide and reveal another condition, uncannily present in the film—yet also submerged—a condition that might suggest another reason for Jeff's being in a cast and for his reluctance or inability to leave that cast?

Rear Window certainly seems to say that Jeff, *encased* in plaster, suffers from a temporarily broken left leg he suffered in an accident, or fall. Yet there is plenty of evidence that Jeff is also suffering from a bout of some form of transferred or hysterical paralysis,[32] even a sexual dysfunction recalling ostensible childish presexuality or adult impotence. The first words in the film suggest as much: the radio in the apartment of the composer-songwriter (Ross Bagdasarian) announces, "Men, are you over forty? When you wake up in the morning, do you feel tired and run down? Do you have that listless feeling?" Consider too Lisa's words to Jeff as he appears to awaken from a trancelike dream. "Is there anything else . . . ?"[33]

One might wonder then (I wondered when I saw this film in the 1950s) whether Jeff's more essential problem is not that his bones are broken, but rather that he suffers from one or another kind of failure of nerve. That "nerve disease," it would seem, involves anxiety about sexual impotence or marriage. His nervous condition might help explain why, like some hysterical paralytic, Jeff might want to remain in his plaster cast and so seem chaste. Jeff might well call his being less than accidentally cast from his rear window a "lucky break"—because, like a sibling-incest taboo, it keeps him from marrying the strangely sisterly Lisa. (John Lydgate played on *cast* and *chaste*: "To serue Diana that was the cast goddesse / That Venus had with them non intraunce.")[34]

Despite the circumstantial evidence regarding some connection be-

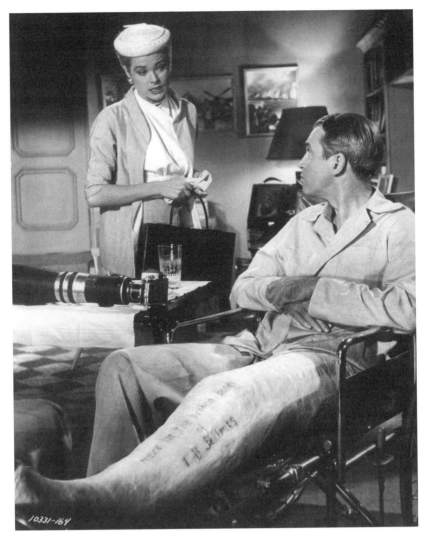

"Here lie the broken bones of L. B. Jeffries" (inscription on the plaster cast),
Rear Window.

tween broken bones and sexual dysfunction, might Jeff not (also) suffer
from a permanently paralyzed leg that he got from, say, paralytic polio? (So
I wondered in the 1950s.) After all, Grace Kelly (Lisa) was almost as well
known for her work with the Mothers March of Dimes as was Sister Kenny
for her work with polios. Kelly was also a favorite cover girl for magazines

such as those recorded in *Rear Window*'s opening shot: *Life* magazine for April 26, 1954, shows Kelly as its cover girl for an issue with stories about George Eastman's static photography and Hollywood cinematography.[35] The January 11, 1955, *Look* magazine likewise has Grace Kelly as its cover girl: right on the cover of America's foremost magazines, Kelly makes her prediction for the coming year—"Polio will be on the way out." (Kelly maintained her interest in polio long after 1956, when she married Prince Rainier of Monaco.)[36]

Rear Window works to suggest certain problems relating to polio and yet to hide them—to shutter the eyes to them. Consider again the famous opening shot of *Rear Window*—the one apparently from behind Jeff's rear window. The very first person in *Rear Window* is neither L. B. Jeffries nor any of the many foils (counterparts or analogies) whose stories we follow in their rear windows. The first person is a young child, apparently a girl, on a rear balcony. She is in a moving chair with her parental-seeming caretakers.[37] Is she sitting in a rocking chair, like Norman Bates's stilled mother in *Psycho*—she who plays the dummy to Norman's psychotic ventriloquism? Or is she in a fancy wheelchair, like the one usually prescribed in the 1950s for polios—the very kind in which, at the close of the same long shot, we soon see L. B. Jeffries almost as if he were a paralyzed film director in a moving seat?[38] Children and infants are an intermittent seen and heard presence in this film, but this child, who introduces *Rear Window,* seems preeminently a sign of the disease most prevalent among children: polio.[39]

"What happened to you?" Throughout the twentieth century, as we have seen, much about polio, or infantile paralysis, was ignored, denied, or unseen. No wonder, then, that viewers of *Rear Window* fail to remark *Rear Window*'s paralyzed infant, the static child, in the most famous long shot in this midcentury movie. No wonder too that Hitchcock, in the directorial "catbird seat," uses thus the ambiguity surrounding the cinematographic aspects of paralysis in the 1950s.

What might we learn about Jeff's condition from his medical staff and their attention to Jeff's body temperature? First, *Rear Window* rather unusually provides no doctor for its main invalid (Jeff) but only an insurance company nurse and a wooer. In the historical context, the doctor's absence suggests that the orthopedic medical profession, then largely male, has not

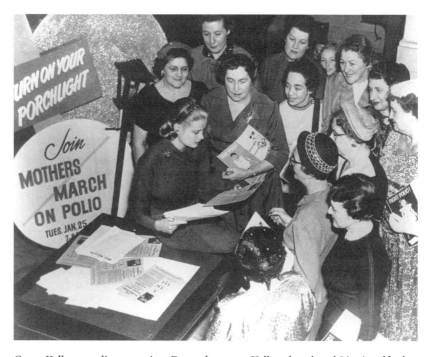

Grace Kelly on polio campaign, December 1954. Kelly, who played Lisa in Alfred
Hitchcock's *Rear Window* (1954), here contributes materials to leaders of the
Mothers March on Polio in Philadelphia.

quite ruled on his actual condition. In Woolrich's story "Rear Window," Dr.
Preston ministers to Jeff, but in Hitchcock's *Rear Window* Jeff himself
has to ask about the fate of Anna Thorwald: "Where's the doctor?" Hitchcock does not even provide us with a medical X-ray image of Jeff's bones.
This is especially odd: *Rear Window* includes many other kinds of photographs—the negative image of Lisa (which is as close to a cast as the art of
photography allows), her positive image on the cover of magazines, and
her first actual appearance as if out of a delirious dream.[40]

Second, Jeff has an unusual nurse. Jeff's counterpart in Cornell Woolrich's story has an official male attendant (Sam). However, Jeff in Hitchcock's *Rear Window* has a female nurse from the insurance company. Even
when Jeff falls from his rear window, Stella insists that she alone attend to
him: "Don't let anybody touch him. Get my medical bag upstairs."[41] Not
only does Stella consistently side with women (Grace Kelly) in the battle of
the sexes; she also stands in as a masseuse of the Sister Kenny sort. As ev-

eryone knew in the 1950s, Kenny had successfully taken on the male ortho-pedic establishment and transformed the treatment of polio by means of hot towels and massages. Kenny was, in fact, "the most popular woman in America" in 1952. And she was the heroine of Rosalind Russell's movie, *Sister Kenny* (1946).

Third, there is the issue of fever. Why does Nurse Stella always take Jeff's temperature so frequently? Why does Jeff perspire so much? It is not (only) an internal problem of sexual frigidity or impotency. Stella does joke, though, "You've got a hormone deficiency." Nor is it (only) the tempera-ture of the external air.[42] Yet cinemagoers in 1954 would recall how hot the previous summer had been, and likewise how that heat had been blamed for the polio epidemic at that time. Thus, Garth Drabinsky—author of a book on the business aspects of motion pictures—begins his autobiogra-phy by recalling the same hot summer of 1953: "I remember one day, in the torrid summer of 1953 when I was only three, running through the sprin-klers my father had set up on the lawn, joyous in the innocent way children are joyous, shrieking in childish glee, and then . . . sometime later, I re-member . . . falling down. *And waking into a nightmare.*"[43]

Whence else Jeff's fever? Broken bones—the usual diagnosis—rarely make for high fever of the sort Jeff suffers after his accident (or "falling out") on the racetrack. Polio does, of course. However, high fever in itself is not the only relevant symptom. Another is the tendency to lose track of time, as in a delirium.

Jeff says that he's been in his room for only six weeks. There is a differ-ence between the length of time that Jeff has been away from work (seven weeks)—which Gunnison would be likely to know—and the period dur-ing which Jeff has been in a cast (six weeks). On the one hand, Jeff has had no fever for a month. ("Those bathing beauties you've been watching haven't raised your temperature one degree in a month," says Stella.)[44] On the other hand, he had a high fever five or six weeks ago—of the very sort that polios usually had.

Timing is crucial in this detective film: the film's suspenseful plot is a clock being wound up tight—by Hitchcock, who makes his cameo appearance as a clock-winder—alarm clocks go off from time to time, Jeff watches his watch, and so forth. But the main temporal question is When, if at all, will Jeff emerge whole from what he calls his plaster cocoon?[45] One answer is that he is due to be released, or delivered, a week from the time that the film opens. And Lisa says, "It's opening night of the last depressing week of *L. B. Jeffries in a Cast*."[46] It is as if Jeff is cast in a stage or screen play, but whether he will *ever* emerge from his cast plaster is its real subject. Another possible answer is that Jeff should already be out of the cast. This is the subject of one of the first definitely comprehensible conversations in the film (at 0.04.14—the preceding conversations having been barely audible):

> *Editor Gunnison (voice):* Congratulations, Jeff.
>
> *L. B. Jeffries (on phone):* For what?
>
> *Editor:* Getting rid of that cast.
>
> *Jeff:* Who said I was getting rid of it?

Far from getting rid of a cast, Jeff will actually gain another. Jeff ends up in *Rear Window* with a full lower body cast—as the result of that almost surreal and paralytic fall from his rear window. The new cast, of course, reveals no lie about broken bones.[47] It bears no inscription.

At the end of Cornell Woolrich's "Rear Window," Detective Boyne—on whom Hayes based Coyne and on whom Hitchcock modeled Doyle—hazards, "We can take that cast off your leg, now."[48] The detective seems to suppose that Jeff's leg was broken and that it has now healed. If, however, we hear the stress on the word *that* in his statement—"We can take *that* cast off your leg, now"—then we need wonder whether there will not be a cast to follow, whether a replacement (for the cast on the left leg) or a new cast (for the right leg). If we hear the stress on the word *now*—"We can take that cast off your leg, *now*"—then we should wonder why the cast was not removed in the past (as Gunnison supposes it has been) and so worry whether the cast might just as well not be removed in the future. But Lisa, it would seem, has already cast a spell that requires Jeff's being encased, at least until he behaves more like a woman's man.

Disability and Impotence

One of the common myths about polios is that poliomyelitic paralysis leaves them without sexual capacity. Most people believed that polios cannot feel physical pain or sexual sensation of any kind, including even the sort of itching that plagues Jeff under his cast. Jeff has a telltale "scratcher" for relieving his itch, which he slides down his cast. From scratching he derives a pleasure that betokens the possibility of a future cure from his disability understood as sexual impotence. Lisa pays heed to the scratching as if it were a sign of recovery from a severe disease. In her memoir *A Spring in My Step*, Joan McDonnell describes humorously the itch that many polios feel inside their necessary plaster casts. "Indeed, if [polios] could never move their leg, the itch would surely make them discover some way of moving it. Maybe that's how orthopaedic hospitals get people walking again. It's got nothing to do with medical skill— just a little itching powder down inside a plaster of paris and anyone will move."[49]

Do You Have Any Feelings?

Allen Lee reports the following incident in *My Soul More Bent:*

> There was Bill who was asked one day the question that I have found in numerous scar-counting sessions to be the most irritating of all. This time it came from a dignified, well-mannered woman.
>
> "But do you have any *feelings* in your legs, sir?"
>
> "Indeed I do," was Bill's answer.
>
> "But I can't believe that it doesn't feel different to the touch at least," she insisted. And then, after a moment's hesitation, she added bravely,
>
> "Sir, would you mind if I *touch* your leg?"
>
> "Not at all madam," Bill agreed affably, and then added quickly, "That is, if I can touch yours."[50]

Elaine Strauss writes, "A grave mistake—especially common in the 1950s— is the assumption that polio victims do not feel pain."[51] Many first-person polio books have tried to dispel the error. The chapter "The Male-Female Relationship" in Laurance Marx's *Keep Trying* (1974) tries to explode the myth. So too do the polio Robert Mauro's manual *Real Crip Sex* and his first-person narrative *Sucking Air, Doing Wheelies*. Sexual relationships for polios are likewise treated in Mark O'Brien's poetry and in J. G. Farrell's novels *The Lung* and *Girl in the Head* (1967).[52] In the Australian television mini-series *Shadows of the Heart*, a polio girl wears her brace in a lovemaking scene.[53] The chapter "Marriage" in Dixson's *My Way with Polio* also treats the subject.[54] The movie *Lucky Break,* as we have seen, addresses the relevant difficulty that polios are seen as unsexy and see themselves that way.

That their families perceived polios as not feeling sexual attraction and as being sexually impotent is one of the common reasons polios often left home after their discharge from the polio wards. This estrangement from family is the theme of the British movie *The Raging Moon* (1971; also known as *Long Ago Tomorrow*), based on the polio Peter Marshall's autobiographical book of the same name.[55] In *The Raging Moon,* Malcolm McDowell and his female counterpart are polio victims who refuse to accept their families' incomprehension and pity. Despite serious obstacles at the disability home, they fall in love—and have a sexual affair.[56]

Very few are the polios who do not experience sexual love because, like Richard Chaput as he describes his experience in *Not to Doubt* (1964), they are forever *encased* in an iron lung and choose to be chaste.[57] Such tales are the subject of books like Stehle's *Incurably Romantic,* which documents photographically the erotic life of patients in the Philadelphia Home for Incurables.[58]

Beyond the claim that polios have sex lives just like anyone else, certain telling reports have it that polios are actually *more* active than others. Elaine Strauss writes, "It is absolutely not true that a paralyzed person has lost all sexual feeling. Maybe we are even sexier! With so much time for thinking and 'phantasicizing,' along with an increased need for tender care, perhaps the urge for sexual relations and expressions of love and affection become stronger."[59] Strauss's view, that paralyzed persons are more highly sexed than other people, is an updated articulation of an ancient Greek view that the physical "compensation" for crippling of the legs and thighs is greater concupiscence. So Montaigne writes in his essay *Of Cripples.*[60]

Montaigne points out that the Amazons purposefully crippled their male infants in order to transform the boys into adult men who would thus be good for nothing but breeding! Crippled Oedipus had plenty of sex drive.[61] As for Jeff, only time will tell.

Shell Shock

Polio often presents itself in two ways at the same time. First, the physiological manifestation is "actual paralysis" lasting a few months or extending throughout a lifetime. Second, the psychological manifestation is often "hysterical paralysis," sometimes also associated with wartime shell shock. In Sholem Asch's Yiddish-American novel *East River* (1946), Nathan seems to suffer both from physical paralysis (polio) and from hysterical paralysis.[62]

In his "Aetiology of Hysteria" (1896), Sigmund Freud stresses that hysterical paraplegia is often the result of childhood sexual trauma.[63] Yet he fails to consider how the psychological trauma of having had a disease like infantile paralysis might have long-term psychological consequences that border on paralysis. Comparable here is Sigmund Freud's often myopic description of the presumably hysterical paralysis and "cure" of the orchestra conductor Bruno Walter. Although Freud had written brilliantly on infantile cerebral paralysis (1897), he failed to recognize that even hypochondriacal hysterical paralysis was sometimes based in neuromuscular paralytic diseases like polio, which affected so many children.[64]

In fact, patients who had paralytic polio often also had something like hysterical paralysis. Hugh Gallagher points out, regarding polios, in *FDR's Splendid Deception*: "Patients came to Warm Springs after the acute stage of their illness, sometimes years after . . . [They] were often in a state of mind bordering on shell shock."[65] At work here are both the psychological trauma of finding oneself unable to move some parts of the body, and physical effects (still not understood) of the polio virus on the biology of the brain.[66] Such aspects of the mind-body problem had been at the forefront of polio studies since Jean-Martin Charcot's work in the 1880s—as William James remarks in his *Varieties of Religious Experience*.[67] Sadly, they were dropped in the mid-twentieth century—although they surface brilliantly on the aesthetic plane in such works as *Rear Window*.

Some sort of more or less willful or unconscious hypochondriac dysfunction is always motivating the plot in *Rear Window*. This brings us back to the kind of paralysis that doctors of the period used to like to diagnose as hysterical. Originally, such diagnoses were restricted to women, for hysteria was thought to reside in the womb: in *Rear Window*, the woman sculptor works on a genderless figure with a gaping hole for its womb—an artwork she calls simply *Hunger*.

The almost unconsciously willed condition of hysterical paralysis resembles the condition of bodily immobility in Arthur Miller's play *Broken Glass*, which is set in New York in the 1930s. In this stage play, the heroine's discontent with being trapped in a loveless marriage to a now functionally impotent husband, together with her anxiety about the German anti-Semitism being reported on the radio, renders her paralyzed: her paralysis ceases when she confronts her marital problems.[68]

Hitchcock's *Vertigo* (1958) provides an analogy closer to home. This movie balances between life and death.[69] *Vertigo,* which opens with a hysterical rooftop flashback, involves a defective detective (the same Jimmy Stewart who plays Jeff in *Rear Window*). The female lead (Kim Novak) is a *corsetière,* and the detective appears in a corset. (See Frida Kahlo's brilliantly painted orthopedic corsets.)[70] The corset suggests the problem with the detective's personal involvements: he is paralyzed, as it were, by the maternal figure Midge, who tells him, "I will never leave you." More important, the corset is a reference to the speech in which Eleanor Roosevelt, wife of the corseted FDR, spoke of women's corsets. (The president was much bothered by his own need to wear a corset. In 1922, he wrote to his doctor Robert Lovett: "The corset I am getting on well with as far as walking goes . . . It almost cuts me in two, however, when I sit down. I am more glad than ever that I do not belong to the other sex!")[71]

The butcher knives and other cutting paraphernalia in Thorwald's apartment frighten Jeff, and not only because Jeff fears that Thorwald will use them on the corpse of Anna Thorwald. Nor is it only (as some interpreters have argued) because he fears castration, of the literal and figural sort from which Hemingway's nurse-loving Jack Barnes suffers in *The Sun Also Rises* (1926). It is also because Jeff fears that Thorwald might use his knives on him in some bizarre reenactment of the criminal leg amputation shown in *King's Row* (1942). Nurse Stella says that she would as soon lose her finger as the wedding band on it.[72] We do well to keep in mind, therefore, that amputation was an all-too-common treatment for polio when immobilization by means of a plaster cast failed. (In *The Care of the Invalid and Crippled Children in School* Dr. R. C. Emsllie had already written, "When a leg is completely useless—i.e., when it cannot be flung forward and backward—it is better to amputate it through the thigh.")[73] We should also remember here that Jeff in *Rear Window* is partly modeled on the wartime photographer Robert Capa, whose leg was blown off by a landmine in 1954.[74]

Depending on how you look at it, Jeff's physical condition is moreover the result either of a purposely inflicted wound, in the tradition of apoterpnophilia (self-amputation), or of an "accident."[75] Depending on one's viewpoint too, Jeff's condition may be real or feigned (and perhaps also hysterical). If it is real, then his condition might be temporary, like a broken leg on the mend, or it might be permanent, like a polio leg. If it is feigned, then Jeff might be faking it because he has a factitious disorder (is wearing braces or casts "for fun") or dysmorphophobia (fear about the appearance of one's body). Alternatively, Jeff might be hysterical, or suffering from survivor's guilt.[76]

Many people have suggested, in line with these speculations, that what is really wrong with Jeff is that he is impotent. As we have seen, his nurse, Stella, jokes about a possible hormone deficiency: Jeff's temperature does not go up when he sees partly naked women. Others note that Jeff is afraid of being brought to the sexual test. So scriptwriter Hayes remarks that "Jeff gives a sigh of relief, exhaling his breath, then looks down towards his legs in thought," later saying, "Lisa, I won't be able to give you any—pajamas."[77]

Just in Love

In certain situations fear of being impotent actually helps makes for impotence. In her first conversation with Jeff, Lisa asks him about his leg and stomach and then finally asks, "Anything else bothering you?" Irving Berlin wrote in his song "You're Just in Love," from *Call Me Madam* (1950), "You don't need analyzin' / It is not so surpisin' / . . . / You're not sick / You're just in love!"

Rear Window, with its superficially "macho" wartime photographer Jeff, recalls in this context two characters in the then celebrated fiction of Ernest Hemingway, who was himself a onetime war journalist. In *The Sun Also Rises* (1926) Jake Barnes falls in love with a nurse, but he cannot consummate a sexual relationship with her because his penis has been blown off.[78] In *A Farewell to Arms* (1929), Frederick Henry's war trauma recalls Hemingway's horrendous leg wound in World War I, when he fell in love with his nurse. It may be relevant that Hemingway's son Gregory (born in 1931) reports in *Papa: A Personal Memoir,* written before his surgical "gender transformation" into a woman (Gloria), that he was abandoned by his father on account of having had polio.[79] Depending on our viewpoint, of course, we might think of the masculine Jeff's physical situation as the cause of any sexual impotence or merely as the outward symbol of that impotence. ("Impotency" is the literal meaning of *disability.*)

In order to specify further the ambiguity about whether Jeff's broken leg does not actually render Jeff impotent (as opposed to merely symbolizing that impotency), let us consider parallel situations. The first situation informs Sholem Asch's influential novel *East River,* in which young Nathan's limbs have been "broken" partly by infantile paralysis and partly by an ensuing spiritual paralysis. His limbs remain paralyzed until Mary enters Nathan's tenement world. Playing the roles both of nurse (like Hitchcock's Stella in *Rear Window*) and of girlfriend (like Lisa), Mary massages the childlike Nathan as part of her attempt to cure him of his disability and his physical impotency. Eventually, Nathan becomes politically active, actually meeting Franklin Delano Roosevelt at a political rally. The second situation informs Christopher Reeve's made-for-television remake of *Rear Window* (1998). Here postrehabilitation patient Jason Kemp, a permanently paralyzed quadriplegic architect, hopes to walk one day, but in this case no vagueness remains about what is wrong with him: Reeve's movie shows both Kemp's disastrous accident and also the details of his recuperation. (This film is in the tradition of such documentarylike rehabilitation movies as Ida Lupino's *Never Fear.*) Likewise, we are left with no ambiguity about Kemp's past sexual capacity and present incapacity: Kemp was married and active sexually; now he is "damaged goods." However, he hopes for a medical miracle, along the lines anticipated by the optimistic Christopher Reeve Paralysis Foundation.[80]

In Hitchcock's *Rear Window,* Asch's *East River,* and Reeve's *Rear Window* we have three kinds of conditions relating to incapacity. In Hitchcock's *Rear Window,* the hero regards himself or is regarded by others as having a broken leg and perhaps also as being impotent. His broken leg, if that is what it is, should heal one day. In Asch's *East River,* the hero is physically able to make love, but he regards himself—and may be regarded by others—as sexually unattractive. His paralysis will not heal. In Reeve's *Rear Window,* the hero is sexually impotent but believes that he will heal.

A Work of Art

Jeff, the apparent exemplar of stasis in *Rear Window,* calls out for the status quo in his relationship with Lisa when Lisa is about to walk out on him. But is he really the only one who is sexually disabled? Let us here follow Jeff's advice to Detective Doyle, and not "jump to any conclusions." Is Lisa not an enabling part of the disabled couple in *Rear Window*? Is she especially attracted to Jeff because Jeff is disabled?

In considering the attractiveness of cripples to some people, the psychologist Richard Bruno argues that there are three types of "factitious disability disorders": devotees, pretenders, and wannabes. Preferring a handicapped person to be one's sexual partner is a well-documented fetish called apotemnophilia.[81] Paraphiliacs are people who prefer disabled sexual partners.[82] Especially in recent decades, the topic of attraction to people wearing orthopedic appliances and braces has left the specialized brothel or sculptor's studio and has gone mainstream. Consider artworks like John Currin's *The Cripple* and Jeff Koons's pieces that make use of leg braces.[83]

Is Lisa chaste, as Jeff is caught in a cast? Lisa's name is short for Elizabeth, meaning "consecrated to God," like a Sister. Is she nunlike? frigid? "Are you real, Mona Lisa? / Or just a cold and lonely lovely work of art?" So go Jay Livingston and Ray Evans's words to "Mona Lisa" (1949), which constitutes one of the songs on the sound track for *Rear Window*. In *Rear Window*, Jeff calls Lisa perfect; her counterpart exhibits relevant symptoms of sexual coldness in Woolrich's short story and Hayes's film script.[84] Some movie critics' nickname for the upper-class Grace Kelly was Ice Maiden.

Cold stone or statuary—many caretakers of polios see their wards as exactly that. Judith Rossner's *Looking for Mr. Goodbar* offers an example.[85] In the polio narrative *We Made Peace with Polio*, the parents think of their polio daughter as having turned to stone.[86] In his novel *The Lung*, J. G. Farrell's polio hero feels "as petrified as a stone" in his iron lung.[87]

Enchantments

Rear Window appears to be an enchanting comedy of remarriage, a romantic drama of restoration. In such comedies, the man or the woman or sometimes both come to marry the same person a second time; this second time, however he or she has been "cured," or both have, of their immaturity or merely fraternal, sororal, and usually also ambiguously nonsexual role in relationship toward the partner. For this transformation to take place in *Rear Window*, the frigid Lisa, for one, must murder her old self to become a new self. That self would be a look-alike to her old self in much the same way that Anna Thorwald (Thorwald's woman friend in Meritville) looks like the "real" Anna Thorwald (the bedridden counterpart to the disabled Jeff). The same might be said for Jeff, who, as we have seen practically dies when he falls from his rear window. This incident rather brings about the sort of rebirth that Lisa apparently wants: a greater hobbling. And Lisa, who generally knows what clothes to wear, now gets to wear the pants.

No wonder, then, that Lisa is so happy to get invalid Mrs. Thorwald's wedding ring. At this central point in *Rear Window*, moreover, Lisa has "stolen the case"—and the cast—from *Rear Window*'s male detective. Her retrieval of the ring is one of the few events where interaction occurs between the main plot and its various rearview subplots: Lisa now shows her rear end through Jeff's rear window. Other women, far less meaningfully, have bent over and revealed their rear ends—among them Miss Torso, the leg artist.[88]

The main informing song, or chant, in *Rear Window* is, of course, "Lisa," which Franz Waxman composed especially for the film. In *Rear Window*, Hitchcock has the divorcé songwriter (played by Ross Bagdasarian) compose the song at his piano.

> Lisa, with your daffodil April face,
> Lisa, full of starry-eyed laughing *grace*
> Hold me and whisper
> the sweet words I'm yearning for
> Drown me in kisses,
> Caresses I'm burning for.

Lisa (Grace Kelly) remarks to Jeff about the song: "It's enchanting. It's almost as if it were being written especially for us."[89] The songwriter says he gets his inspiration from his landlady. He means that he needs his songwriter's fee in order to pay her the rent. (Still, it is suggested in *Rear Window* that Lisa Fremont, who hails from a wealthy area, 63rd Street, "owns" these tenement buildings. She identifies with their various apartments as if they were her own—as in the case of Miss Lonelyhearts. Likewise, Lisa understands the tenants almost as if they were herself—as in the case of Miss Torso.)[90] If the songwriter is not composing his "Lisa" for this Lisa that Grace embodies, then he may as well be. (Soon after playing the part of the piano player who composes the song "Lisa" during the course of Hitchcock's *Rear Window*, Ross Bagdasarian—who was also known as David Seville—produced a bestselling song in 1958: "The Witchdoctor," as sung by Alvin and the Chipmunks; it has the memorable line "You've been keeping love from me just like you were a miser.")

In *Rear Window* Hitchcock makes his cameo appearance as the clock winder or clock repairman—as if he were measuring out the tempo in the musical score of "Lisa."[91] In this metonymic context, it is worth recalling that Hitchcock claimed, with some irony, that he did not really approve of composer Waxman's doing the score for *Rear Window*. He was suspicious of Waxman.[92] How come?

Perhaps it was partly because Hitchcock wanted and needed to play down the aspects of *Rear Window* that appeared to allude overtly to polio. Waxman was too close to the polio issue; for example, he had been involved in the theatrical productions for Roosevelt's funeral in 1945. In the 1950s, moreover, Waxman worked for years with Dore Schary on making *Sunrise at Campobello*. With his special interest in the temporary stops and starts of the polio experience and with corsets like the one Jeff wears in *Rear Window* (of the type FDR popularized), Waxman played up the paralytic aspects of Jeff's static condition, both by means of the lyrical content of the music he chose or wrote (about living beings becoming still) and by means of its musical form. This form, remarkable in cinematography, is suggested in Waxman's sequential stop-and-start "radio station" surfing sounds for *Rear Window*. They are sometimes barely audible as words, yet the static suggests the breaking of links between the various stations. The sounds compel the would-be listener to become an auditory spy. Francis Ford Coppola picks up on this kind of espionage in *The Conversation*: the former espionage agent and polio survivor Harry Caul uses electronic long-distance sound-recording equipment in much the same imperfect way that the war correspondent L. B. Jeffries uses long-distance photographic devices.

Waxman's jazzy start-and-stop musical sequences match Hitchcock's newspaper-cartoon visuals—those serial, window-framed, action sequences like Sunday funnies—which are sometimes barely visible. Nathanael West had conceived his influential novel *Miss Lonelyhearts* (1933) as "a novel in the form of a comic strip."[93] What Hitchcock probably disliked in the score for *Rear Window* was, after all, precisely its covert suitability for the task at hand.

The song "Lisa" is a response to the old favorite "Mona Lisa" that we hear coming from the rear windows of Jeff's neighbors in through Jeff's rear window. (Nat King Cole sang "Mona Lisa" in the 1950 movie *Captain Carey, USA;* it was a million copy bestseller.) Unusually in the history of cinema, the entire filming of *Rear Window* illustrates and gives content to the composition of "Lisa." "Lisa" is the song that transfixes Lisa.

Another song in *Rear Window* is Bing Crosby's version of "To See You Is to Love You," which we hear issuing from the radio as Miss Lonelyhearts is pouring out wine—for no one. ("To see you is to love you and I see you everywhere." "Every place I look you're there." "That same old dream tonight.") This song was used in the movie *Road to Bali* (1953)—which refers implicitly to the travel book by the polio William O. Douglas pictured near the end of *Rear Window.* "Lisa" is the song that saves Miss Lonelyhearts from suicide.

A Rear Window on the Iron Lung

> But it was only I trembling
> Waiting to be cut out
> Of my white cocoon
> Will I ever be a butterfly?
>
> —Robert Mauro, "White Cocoon," in *Landscape of My Disability* (1998)

In discussion with his editor Gunnison, Jeff calls his cast a cocoon.[94] This term *cocoon* had at least several interrelated meanings in this context in the 1950s.

First, *cocoon* means "temporary case for a chrysaloid." Such is the cast, or plaster case, from which Jeff may or may not emerge, thanks to some metamorphosis. If he does emerge, Jeff would be trading his now partly disabled, monopedal existence for one of two conditions. He might emerge in fully able-bodied possession of bipedal kinesis—as Gunnison assumes will happen. Or he might emerge with fully nonpedal status—as actually happens, thanks to his being cast out of his own rear window. (Virginia Acosta, in associating the iron lung from which she emerged with the cocoonlike incubator from which her children came forth into a polio-free world, touches on the same meaning of *cocoon.*)[95]

Second, *cocoon* means "submarine vehicle." Iron-lunger Bentz Plage-mann's novel *Steel Cocoon* (1958) provides a good example: it focuses on submariners' prisonlike air chambers. Third, *cocoon* often means "iron lung." Iron lungs, like submarines, suggest prison-like dependency and portend, for the hopeful, eventual delivery. In 1954, the polio Sharon Term wrote that the iron "lung became like a nice cocoon for me, because I could breathe in it and nothing hurt and I could get warm. I could sleep peacefully."[96] Robert Mauro, who wrote his book *Landscape of My Disability* from inside the cocoon home that was his iron lung, wonders in "White Cocoon" whether he will ever get out alive. The novelist J. G. Farrell captures this spirit in his often ironic novel *The Lung*: "After all, it was just a white metal box on wheels. Any similarity between this box and a coffin was purely coincidental, the result of morbid fantasies brought on by his normally depressive disposition."[97] Not surprisingly, the medical profession—and especially nurses—often preferred the term *steel cocoon* to *iron lung*, perhaps on account of the suggestion of temporary immobility and a promise of eventual delivery.[98]

Does Hitchcock's Jeff have in mind something like an iron lung when he talks about being in a cocoon? The iron lung plays a prominent role in several episodes of the television series *Alfred Hitchcock Presents*. In *No Pain*, for example, a young man in an iron lung has a beautiful, devoted wife, who has found a healthy young man. Who will murder whom?[99] Likewise, in *Cell 227*, the iron lung is associated with murder of or by an invalid.[100] Compare how, in Dick Francis's polio novel *Forfeit*, the main character's wife is dependent on a cuirass-type ventilator, and the plot involves a threat to turn off her life support.[101] Iron lungs as such still provide the motivating topos for Ray Turner's *Huston's Laws* and Arthur Hailey's *Overload*, which involves an iron-lung patient in a national electrical power blackout.[102]

Rear Window suggests the rearview mirrors that cinematographers actually attached to iron lungs. Jeff's overhead and rearview mirrors and various spyglasses function much as the rear windows for iron lung patients that the cinematographic industry often credited itself with inventing. Such windows were adjustable, reflective glasses that allowed the iron lung patient to see more than the ceiling of the room. Writes Omega Baker in her poetic meditation "Iron Lung" (1995): "Attached above my pale, ceiling-turned face is a large, rectangular mirror, considerately positioned to allow me to see the open doorway of my room and a small section of the hallway beyond. Bored and lonely, I watch the mirror for signs of life in the hall."[103] In the 1950s, this rearview mirror gave a view of the area behind, where one might see oneself as the other.[104] The man in the iron lung is thus already part of a photographic contraption.

One urban legend linking the origin of the iron lung's rearview mirror with the movie industry involves a well-publicized change made to the older Emerson lungs, which had had, instead of a glass mirror, only a small piece of stainless steel by means of which patients might see.[105] In the 1940s, a Hollywood movie crew thought of attaching rearview mirrors to the iron lungs at Rancho los Amigos.[106] J. G. Farrell in *The Lung* suggests parallels between the rearview mirror of an iron lung and the television screen or a neighbor's rear-window frame:

> A mirror had been placed in a slot above his head, angled to give him a view of that part of the room that lay behind him. Looking into it he saw the door open and Dr. Baker enter. For an instant he caught himself thinking that this was merely some television play he was watching, that some competent, professional scriptwriter was pulling the strings and that consequently everything would turn out fine in the end. A sad ending in this kind of programme was unthinkable. Donning a third dimension, however, the doctor's face appeared beside the mirror.[107]

The disabled narrator in Woolrich's "Rear Window," the literary source for Hayes's script for *Rear Window*, says that his spying on neighbors is not that of an ordinary Peeping Tom.[108]

> Sure, I suppose it *was* a little like prying, could even have been mistaken for the fevered concentration of a Peeping Tom. That wasn't my fault, that wasn't the idea if it. The idea was, my *movements* were strictly limited just around this time. I could get from the window to the bed, and from the bed to the window, and that was all. The bay window was about the best feature my rear bedroom had in the warm weather. . . . Well, what should I do, sit there with my *eyes tightly shuttered?*[109]

The goal here involves a windowed understanding of oneself as a nearly immobile photographic mechanism.

Cornell Woolrich's short story leaves unspoken until the very end what the "cause" is of the hero's incapacity to move, just as Hitchcock leaves somewhat ambiguous what Jeff's real problem is. Woolrich himself had problems with movement and stasis: the tradition has it that he lived all his adult life in a hotel room with his domineering mother. He never got out.

The Accidental Case of the Falling Cast

As we have seen, Jeff's invalidism raises diagnostic questions. How did it come about, etiologically, that his bones do not work? What might that indicate, symbolically, about his physical capacities and about his psychological, hysterical, or nervous condition? Prognostically speaking, will the condition of Jeff's bones *ever* improve? At the end of *Rear Window,* the invalid Jeff does not emerge from his cast or cocoon. (It is worth recalling here that, by contrast, we eventually see the apparently wheelchair-bound child in *Rear Window* actually standing while being groomed by her father.)[110] And in the last scene, Jeff is called El Bee. The prefix *El* is a jocular rhetorical put-down.[111] Lisa is now his even more powerful caretaker—his Queen Bee, as it were, the very nickname that the leg artist Jeff had given to Miss Torso.

Lisa, then, would seem to have won out in the battle between the presumed kinesis of travel and the apparent stasis of marriage. In the last scene, she appears at first to be reading a travel book, as if preparing to accompany Jeff on one of his wartime photography ventures into the mountains. After all, she has already demonstrated her prowess in that direction when, high heels and all, she climbed the exterior walls of the tenement to Jeff's courtyard (from which Jeff, by contrast, has fallen). When Lisa determines that Jeff is asleep, she puts down the book and takes up the fashion magazine *Harper's Bazaar.*

What book is it that she puts down? It is unnamed in Hayes's script, and most critics fail even to notice it.[112] Hitchcock, though, purposely chose Supreme Court Justice William O. Douglas's recently published *Beyond the High Himalayas.*[113] Why that particular travel book? On the one hand, it contains a reference to the June 1953 execution of the spies Ethel and Julius

Rosenberg, with which Douglas had a great deal to do. Spying, the offense of which the Rosenbergs had been convicted, resembles Jeff's voyeurism.[114] The punishment meted out to the Rosenbergs was execution—a far more severe penalty than that six months' imprisonment which Stella *seems* to promise Jeff for being a Peeping Tom (like Tom Doyle). Douglas stayed the executions and faced impeachment charges. On the other hand, though, the subject matter of the book is germane to the dialectic of stasis and kinesis at the heart of *Rear Window*. Douglas, who had been appointed in 1939 to the Supreme Court by FDR, was also a polio, one who "recovered" his mobility not by staying at home (as Lisa wants Jeff to do with her) but rather by freely climbing the high Himalayan mountains (as Jeff wants to do *without* Lisa Fremont, whose surname, of course, means "free mountain"). The July 13, 1953, issue of *Life* magazine featured two major cover stories: the first about Sir Edmund Hillary and Tenzing Norgay climbing Mt. Everest, and the second about thirty-three thousand children receiving gamma globulin during that year's polio epidemic. William O. Douglas insisted that partly paralyzed polios should take up mountain-climbing. (Besides Douglas, other members of the court had links with polio; for example, Governor Earl Warren, soon to be Chief Justice, had written an introduction to Charles H. Andrews's book *No Time for Tears*—described there as "the story of a ten-year old boy's desperate but successful battle to survive polio, and his family's role in guiding him back to a normal life.")[115]

His own infantile paralysis at an early age had made William O. Douglas weak, introspective, and much pampered by his mother. When a teenager, however, Douglas says that he read the work of Plato, who believed in "euthanizing" such human cripples as Douglas was—and we might infer, as Anna Thorwald was.[116] So, Douglas exercised hard in order to become able-bodied. (Douglas later got what he says was "a sort of Lown's syndrome"—though the symptoms he describes closely resemble those of what we now call post-polio syndrome.)[117] That "therapeutic" mountain hike that Douglas went on in 1951 is the subject of the book that Lisa puts down. Some years later, in his essay "Polio" in *Go East Young Man*, Douglas explained that "it was infantile paralysis that drove me to the outdoors," and to mountaineering.[118]

In the last scenes of *Rear Window*, it remains a moot issue how the immobile Jeff will travel to the Himalayas (by jeep? water buffalo?). Similarly suppressed now is the question whether he will see the war in Indochina (as planned in the script), or Kashmir (as planned with his editor), or Pakistan (as planned with Lisa).[119] The high-heeled mountaineer Lisa Fremont had wanted to go "all the way" in the sexual sense with Jeff.[120] Jeff, however, had wanted to go "around the world" (in the travel sense) without Lisa. Lisa has good reason to wonder how far in the sexual sense *she* has to go.

Lisa: How far does a girl have to go—before you notice her?

Jeff: If she's pretty enough, she doesn't have to *go* anywhere. She just has "to be."[121]

"To be" might also mean "to just stay put" like a good model, paralyzed for the still-photographer and by still photography. By the end, the question in *Rear Window* is no longer whether or when Jeff and Lisa will remove the corset from their relationship.[122] Jeff is now set, or cast. He will make no real exit from *L. B. Jeffries in a Cast*. The plaster cast spreading over his body is an intermediate stage in the symbolic production of a work of sculpture—static nature.[123] This wartime still photographer's predicament is like that reported by the war poet Rupert Brooke in "Paralysis": "Fast in my linen prison I press / On impassable bars."[124]

ⅠⅠⅠ POLITICS

This country needs, and unless I mistake its temper, the country demands bold persistent experimentation.

—Franklin Delano Roosevelt, commencement address at Oglethorpe University, Georgia, 1932

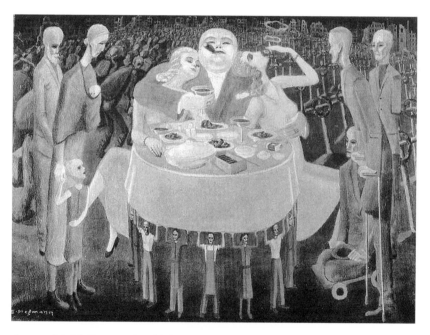

Arm und Reich (Poor and rich), by Arnulf Erich Stegmann.

7 POLIO AND THE GREAT WARS

One of the members of this Committee mentioned to me the other day, at the White House, that for the first time, so far as he knew, in all medical history, research into one definite known problem is adequately financed and every person, every scientist, who is engaged in this research work has been able to come to this Committee and the Warm Springs Foundation and be given sufficient funds to carry on the work that he is doing.

That is why I feel very happy about the contribution that the Foundation has made and is making to extending our work and fighting one of our most serious epidemic forms of disease in every part of the country.

—Franklin Delano Roosevelt, November 28, 1935

Reliance on the private sector for national health funding is, as we have seen in Chapter 5 on handi-capitalism, one influential legacy of the Roosevelt era's unusually successful NFIP. The foundation was an institution that originated both from the private needs of Roosevelt himself (and the concomitant insight into other people's desires and fears) and from the public exigencies of domestic and international crises, the Depression and World War II in particular. Public health institutions in the United States are still fraught with the contradictions attendant on the definitions of the private and public sectors.

National Health: Private and Public

Among the most important aspects of the American response to the world polio crisis was the phenomenal rise to prominence in the United States of the private National Foundation for Infantile Paralysis and its influence on the development of a definition of the public good in terms of private donations. (It is especially remarkable by comparison with the responses in Canada and European countries.)[1] One man here made a remarkable difference. Roosevelt, with his successful experiments with polio treatment and his triumphant political career, helped found the NFIP in 1937. It is partly thanks to him that the United States has its peculiar debates about public health policy and its particular way of defining the public and private sectors and the dialectic between them.

The NFIP owes its beginnings to FDR's experience with hydrotherapy in Warm Springs, Georgia. Roosevelt, who got polio in 1921, made his first therapeutic visit there in 1924. At that time he wrote to Eleanor from Warm Springs: "The walking and general exercising in the water is fine and I have worked out some special exercises also. This is really a discovery of a place and there is no doubt that I've got to do it some more."[2] At Warm Springs, claimed Roosevelt, he enjoyed life more than anywhere else. (Many photographs show him there with the withered leg that so many writers claim that he or his handlers tried to hide.) He worked at Warm Springs for the betterment of his own individual body, even as he worked on political papers for the weal of the body politic.

Roosevelt liked Warm Springs so much that he bought it in 1926. Over the next two decades—until his death at Warm Springs in 1945—Roosevelt made some fifty visits there. Some of these visits lasted for months. Warm Springs became, for Roosevelt, *the* site of "bold experimentation" in the twin realms of medical rehabilitation and political reform. Consider a few aspects of his work and thinking in these areas.

First, by 1925, FDR was known at Warm Springs as Dr. Roosevelt, so active a role was he taking in the direction of the rehabilitative and medical operations there.[3] Roosevelt jokingly told an audience at Warm Springs, "These . . . physiotherapists don't know anything about [water therapy]. I invented it first."[4]

Second, Roosevelt saw his work at Warm Springs as having a potential application to other people than polios. As he wrote to Eleanor from Warm Springs in the mid-1920s, "I feel that a great 'cure' for infantile paralysis and kindred diseases could well be established here."[5] Even before the official incorporation of Warm Springs, FDR wrote thus to Eleanor: "Most of the patients are suffering from infantile paralysis though we have two arthritis cases at the present time and expect several others, and also hope to have a good many people come there next winter for a few weeks of after-cure succeeding operations or serious illness."[6]

Third, he saw the wholesale attention paid to polio and its cure as a major experiment in medical finance. In his "informal remarks" at Thanksgiving dinner at Warm Springs in 1935, Roosevelt said: "One of the members . . . mentioned to me the other day, at the White House, that for the first time, so far as he knew, in all medical history, research into one definite known problem is adequately financed and every person, every scientist, who is engaged in this research work has been able to come to this Committee and the Warm Springs Foundation and be given sufficient funds to carry on the work that he is doing." What was being done for polios at Warm Springs should be done to help find a cure all diseases.

Fourth, at Thanksgiving dinner in Warm Springs in 1939 Roosevelt stressed the need for social inclusion: "And now—this is not the first dinner we have had here—it is going to be a question before most of us die as to whether this dining room is going to be big enough or not. However, we have all sorts of tricks up our sleeves; we can extend this dining room either this way or that way, behind me, or even out sideways."

A related problem was institutionalized and semiofficial racism, to which Roosevelt sometimes had to "kowtow" for electoral reasons.[7] When the governor of Georgia attacked Roosevelt for being a cripple—and hence supposedly unable to hold office—he was actually assailing Roosevelt's frequent endorsements of racial equality. It was relevant that Roosevelt alluded, in his speech on Thanksgiving in 1938, to European Jews and called on *all* American citizens to offer "prayers for the oppressed minorities in other lands."[8]

A onetime "American aristocrat," Roosevelt established a reliable and politically acceptable way to fund the war against polio by seeming to balance what we might now call the private and public spheres. On occasion in Georgia, for example, Roosevelt would speak to bankers about the needs of the country's crippled people, discuss the work going on at Warm Springs, and then stress how that should be extended to serve all: "No state government, no national government, can afford to embark on a program that would look after the needs of 350,000 crippled persons in this country. It has to be a development of private charity."[9] Bankers visited Warm Springs and donated.

When Roosevelt was elected governor of New York in 1928, Warm Springs became less of a one-man affair and was well on its way toward becoming a truly national foundation. The drive for national office and for the private national foundation went hand in hand, even when it came to FDR's articulation of policy. At the famous Oglethorpe University commencement address (1932), where he was photographed with his old-fashioned canes, Roosevelt declared the need "to inject life into our ailing economic order." He went on: "This country needs, and unless I mistake its temper, the country demands *bold persistent experimentation* [my emphasis]. It is common sense to take a method and try it. If it fails, admit it frankly and try another. But above all, try something." He had faced unpleasant facts about what had happened to his individual body; now he applied what he had learned to the state of the body politic. "We need enthusiasm, imagination, and the ability to face facts, even unpleasant ones, bravely." So "Bold persistent experimentation" became the rallying cry for the New Deal.[10]

For Roosevelt, then, two parallel worlds existed: the "little world" of Warm Springs and the larger world of American domestic and international intrigue. His informal remarks to patients at Warm Springs in 1937 typically allude to the dialectic. "The country is going along all right and that is true, too, of Warm Springs. In the past year I have been devoting much of my time to the country and I am inclined to think that in the future I shall be able to devote a little more of my time to Warm Springs."

Roosevelt established the National Foundation for Infantile Paralysis in order to coordinate all fund-raising efforts for the treatment and eradication of polio. The scope of the NFIP was much broader than that of the Warm Springs Foundation, and it proved to be a tremendous fundraiser, of epic proportions theretofore unheard of.

In fact, historians of public health care often suggest that the idiosyncratically private mechanisms in the United States for funding of public health care are those bequeathed to us by the NFIP. The NFIP's organizational structures and goals transposed to other levels seem to suffuse the present-day public health and medical systems. The contradictions between private and public inherent in the contemporary financing of health care and epidemiology suggest that the need still pertains for the bold experimentation that Roosevelt promised at Oglethorpe.

What happened to the NFIP itself? Beginning in the 1950s, the NFIP as Roosevelt conceived it—as a real instrument of national health policy and

practice—simply disappeared. It fought against even useful experimentation; for example, the NFIP argued for keeping the Sabin vaccine out of the
United States; and, instead of supporting the worldwide eradication of polio and the treatment of polio survivors, the foundation simply declared "a
complete victory" over polio and all its problems.[11] In 1967, the National
Foundation for Infantile Paralysis renamed itself the March of Dimes Birth
Defects Foundation. An analogy to such an organizational turning away
from the realm of politics informs the history of the National Society for
Crippled Children: founded in 1919, it engineered its transformation in the
1950s, taking on the lily (the symbol of resurrection) as its official logo and
renaming itself the Easter Seals Society in 1967. Some of the sociology of
the process is explained in David Sills's work *The Volunteers: Means and
Ends in a National Organization,* written when he was acting director of
the Bureau of Applied Social Research at Columbia University.[12]

The bold experiment in medicine and public health pioneered by Roosevelt, together with its peculiar mixture of private and public backing, was
all but forgotten, even as the victory over polio was reified into misleading
political ideologies and more voluntarism flourished, along with walkathons. The dual American reliance on the private and public sectors to
support public health institutions was now enlisted to combat Communism. The poliomyelitic rhetoric of the earlier war against National Socialism is captured in Elizabeth Cox's novel *Night Talk,* in which one brother
fights international foes in the U.S. Army and the other fights polio.[13] The
rhetoric of the war against Communism is clearer. During the McCarthy
period (1950–1954) it was often said that "world communism" was just like
polio, if not even worse. (So ran the argument already in W. F. Carroll's
Whence? Why? Whither?)[14] The confusion or tension between the private
and public sectors in American public health institutions continues to the
present day. The success of the National Foundation for Infantile Paralysis
in the United States—it "stood beyond all challenge as the most successful
voluntary health organization on earth"—ruled out the need to supply
substantial public assistance for polio.[15] Christopher Rutty is quite right to
point out that "the strong state-led response to polio was the clearest feature distinguishing the Canadian polio experience from the American."[16]

As we have seen, myriad interrelated politically charged questions come
into play when we ponder the history of the polio in the United States.
What should the role of expensive technology be when keeping a few peo-

ple alive? Is euthanasia a good idea? How should we think about medical quarantines in relation to political coexistence? What is the proper
political relationship between a domestic war on a particular epidemic
disease and an international war on a particular enemy army? What is
the long-term significance of the still-celebrated model: movie and radio
stars working to collect billions of dimes, with the March of Dimes, the
President's Ball Association, and movie chains in handi-capitalist lockstep?
What relevance has this quasi-philanthropic model to fund-raising and
aesthetics? How does it affect epidemic pathology and political sociopathology? How did the experience of infantile paralysis affect our understanding of individual childhoods and of political maturity? How did issues of race affect the problems of defining and treating epidemiological
disease?

One or two questions remain common to all these and many more:
How did the vaunted victory over polio encourage us to take for granted
the historically idiosyncratic combination of public and private philanthropy that we assumed had given rise to that victory? What have we
gained and lost by the consequential, partly happenstance definition of the
dialectic between public and private sectors in the public health arena?

The War against Polio

In her book *AIDS and Its Metaphors,* Susan Sontag is displeased whenever
diseases are treated "metaphorically"; by extension, she is pleased when
they are treated "un-metaphorically." The metaphorization she most ab-
hors involves the military sphere. "Not all metaphors applied to illness and
their treatment are equally unsavory and distorting. The ones I am most
eager to see retired—more than ever since the emergence of AIDS—is the
military metaphor."

Sontag has it that "military imagery on thinking about sickness and
health overmobilizes, it overdescribes, and it powerfully contributes to the
excommunicating and stigmatizing of the ill." Given Sontag's view that polio was treated appropriately "unmetaphorically," one would expect the
ideology of polio to have remained aloof from military metaphors.[17] In
fact, nothing could be further from the truth. Sontag got polio wrong—
and, I should think, also the broad dialectic of disease and politics.

Generally speaking, the military metaphor for dealing with disease came into widespread use during the 1880s. That decade coincides both with the appearance of the theory that bacteria are the agents of disease and also with the advent of the polio epidemics.[18] The older notion is one of "enemy germs" trying to infiltrate the castle that is the body politic in much the same way that a virus invades the organism that is the individual body.[19] In any case, from 1914 until the early 1960s, thousands of documents show that polio was looked upon as a national enemy, much like the Axis powers. The shadow of the "Crippler" polio, on the domestic front, matched that of Nazism, internationally—as suggested by the shadowy swastika that threatened healthy American children, as depicted by tens of thousands of American posters of the period. Infected polios were treated much like enemy infiltrators, and they were likewise assigned to militarily guarded areas and concentrated together in specialized "camps."

Crippled young polios, especially during the Cold War, were looked upon as "brave little soldiers." One of Roosevelt's informal Thanksgiving Day speeches at Warm Springs, in 1939, draws the parallel most clearly between the war on polio and international conflict: "You know, I am in favor of war. I am very much in favor of war, the kind of war that we are conducting here at Warm Springs, the kind of war that, aided and abetted by what we have been doing at Warm Springs now for fourteen or fifteen years, is spreading all over the country—the war against the crippling of men and women and, especially, of children."[20] (Compare this quotation with Roosevelt's "I Hate War" speech, delivered at Chautauqua, New York, on August 14, 1936.) The president went on to argue (against Sontag's view as expressed half a century later) for the *properness* of his use here of the word *war*.[21] The illustrator John Falter's well-known poster "This Fight Is Yours" for the March of Dimes is thus typical in its depiction of an American soldier liberating and protecting a young polio survivor in cowboy costume.

The popular film series *King of the Royal Mounted* likewise suggests that the struggle against polio in the 1940s was a counterpart to the war against the Nazis.[22] In this series a Canadian scientist discovers a substance (compound X) that will cure infantile paralysis but also contains magnetic properties that make enemy mines effective against the British fleet. Foreign agents open a sham polio sanitarium; although it ostensibly helps paralysis victims, its main purpose is to ship compound X to assist the enemy in its battle against Britain. Sergeant King discovers the fraud and exposes the deceit. Much other "literature" of the period promised and seemed to

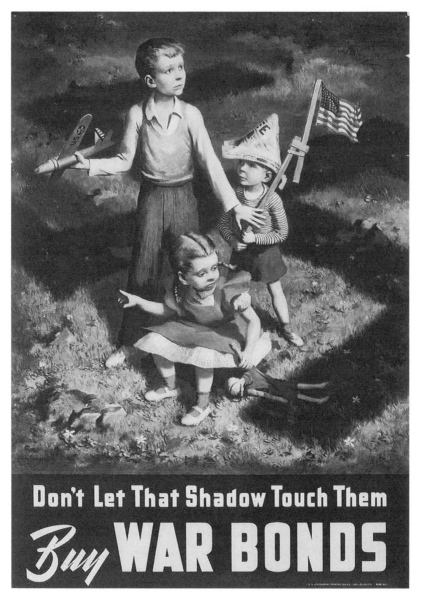

"Don't Let That Shadow Touch Them."

deliver a sort of definitive military victory over polio. Basil O'Connor—chairman of the National Foundation for Infantile Paralysis—gave hundreds of talks with titles like *The Conquest of Infantile Paralysis*.[23] Alton L. Blakeslee wrote pamphlets like *Polio Can Be Conquered,* and Robert Coughlan published influential booklets with names like *The Coming Victory over Polio*.[24] Especially in the late 1950s, this ideology of military triumph suffused almost all medical media. Such publications distracted us from certain ongoing problems facing medicine and especially public health.

Children in the polio ward often believed that their own struggle against polio was a sort of military war. In her memoir *Polio Tragedy of 1941,* Acosta reports the following dialogue with her doctor: "I said to Dr. Elzinga, 'I have something to say. Please tell me if I am wrong.' I said, 'There are a lot of people who are killed in the war.' I said, 'I think we have a polio war.' When, in a few days, the doctor's son was killed, he told the little girl, 'You can call it a polio war.' "[25] The posters of this period and others likewise suggest the parallel between polio and war. In line with Sister Kenny's recommendation, military towels were issued to the polio wards for hot towel treatments. Leonard Kriegel describes how one young polio viewed their distribution: even "the towels were the same greenish brown as the blankets issued to American GIs, and they reinforced a boy's sense of being at war."[26] Roosevelt himself often employed the analogy between the war against polio and the war against the Axis powers to get what he wanted in both cases. In a note of thanks to the Australian opera singer Marjorie Lawrence, who was seriously crippled by polio in 1941, Roosevelt wrote, "From an old veteran to a young recruit, my message to you is, *Carry on*." Several times President Roosevelt asked Lawrence to sing "for seriously wounded men—particularly men who knew they would never walk."[27] This was a request recorded in Lawrence's book *Interrupted Melody* (1949; movie version, 1955).

That Sontag and others pretend that all this military metaphorization of polio did not happen is merely another sign of the overall forgetting about polio that characterizes the paralysis of culture and the culture of paralysis at the time. The advent of the "designer vaccine" helped to trigger a relevant anti-intellectualism and politicization of elementary and general problems in public health—an unfortunate situation from which we are now, it is to be hoped, beginning to recover.

8 REMEMBERING ROOSEVELT

Never in history has a great leader been unable to walk.

—Turnley Walker, *Roosevelt and the Warm Springs Story* (1953)

Most young North American polios of the 1950s admired Franklin Delano Roosevelt for having been a "warrior" on several fronts. He had served as assistant secretary of the Navy during and after World War I (1913–1920) when he helped in the war effort against Germany and its allies. Later, during his presidency of the United States (1933–1945), Roosevelt waged both a domestic war against poverty (1933–1935, during the Great Depression) and an international war against the Axis powers (1941–1945, during World War II).

The Maimed King

As a child, I most admired Roosevelt's quarter-century-long personal struggle with polio (1921–1945), one that he waged both on the level of his own polio-racked body and on the level of a body politic in need of a new system of public health and research. Roosevelt, it seemed to me, was a wise and seasoned veteran. In earlier days, people had spoken of "seasoning the troops"—that is, letting soldiers live together long enough before going into combat to be exposed to one another's germs in such a way that the survivors would be stronger for the experience. In fact, much of the electorate during Roosevelt's campaign for the governorship of New York in 1928 believed that FDR's crippled condition was the ultimately fortifying result of some heroic event during the Great War. Such misperceptions about Roosevelt's polio were understandable: not only were many polios at the time regularly mistaken for wounded veterans, but participants in popular discussions about the "real origin" of Roosevelt's bodily incapacitation actually sometimes mistook it for other conditions (including syphilis).

FDR's disease and its aftermath must have been life-shaping for him. Nowadays making this abstract claim about Roosevelt's polio has become almost standard. Garry Wills, for example, says that FDR understood "the importance of psychology—the people have to have the courage to keep seeking a cure, no matter what the cure is. Those who wanted ideological consistency or even policy coherence were rightly exasperated with Roosevelt. He switched economic plans as often as he changed treatments for polio." Doris Kearns Goodwin, in *Character above All: Ten Presidents from FDR to George Bush,* sees the battle with polio as one explanation for Roosevelt's character.[1] Goodwin's memoir *Wait till Next Year* concerns the illness of her mother and polio, including that of a boyfriend.[2] Not always were the effects that polio had on FDR "taken for granted" in this way. In the period from the mid-1950s to until the early 1990s, for example, dozens of books were written about FDR—including many by his doctors, family, and friends. Only a few even speculated that FDR's polio was important to understanding his character and ambitions; still fewer attempted to say exactly how it was important.

It is worth rehearsing here, though, that people exhibited greater understanding of Roosevelt's polio in the period *before* the mid-1950s than has generally been supposed. Many fiction authors include Roosevelt's polio prominently in novels and novellas—among them, for the early period, is Sholem Asch in *East River* (1946). Daniel Kirk's treatment of the subject in his children's book *Breakfast at the Liberty Diner* is a typical example for the later period.[3] (It was Eleanor Roosevelt who said of FDR, "I think probably the thing that took most courage in his life was his mastery and his meeting of polio.")[4]

Most of those who, early on, made a serious attempt outside the realm of fiction to understand Roosevelt's polio were people with a professional interest or personal stake in the matter. One of these people was Frances Perkins (1880–1965). Perkins was author of such works as *A Plan for Maternity Care* (1918) and had done crucial research in the field of public and industrial hygiene when Roosevelt, as governor of New York State, appointed her in 1929 to be his state industrial commissioner. When, as president of the United States, Roosevelt tapped her to be his labor secretary (1933–1945), Perkins was the first woman to be appointed to a cabinet post in the United States. In Perkins's *The Roosevelt I Knew*, published soon after Roosevelt's death, she tells how she saw FDR shortly after his bout with polio in 1921 and felt that "he had a firmer grip on life and on himself than ever before. He was serious, not playing now."[5] Perkins goes on to say that "Franklin Roosevelt underwent a spiritual transformation during the years of his illness . . . The man emerged completely warm-hearted, with humility of spirit and a deeper philosophy, having been to the depths of trouble, he understood the problems of people in trouble."[6]

Another writer who took Roosevelt's polio seriously was John Gunther, in *Roosevelt in Retrospect*.[7] (Gunther wrote about Roosevelt a year after writing *Death Be Not Proud,* a narrative about how Gunther's sixteen-year-old son Johnny struggled with brain cancer and finally died from it.)[8]

The more modern period in understanding of FDR's polio begins slowly. Jim Bishop's *FDR's Last Year* includes information about how often FDR was away from the White House and in Warm Springs.[9] In *The Making of Franklin D. Roosevelt,* Richard Thayer Goldberg argues that polio and its effects—against which Roosevelt often struggled to the point of denial—prepared him for the presidency.[10] A large part of *FDR's Splendid Deception* by the polio Hugh Gregory Gallagher focuses more narrowly on what FDR did to hide the fact that he was a polio.[11] (Goldberg, who is careful to note the same "deception," calls it one of the ironies of FDR's life.) Geoffrey C. Ward, the author of two books on Roosevelt, mentions his own experience as a polio.[12]

Polio authors who are graduates of Warm Springs often took a particular interest in FDR. Their work is difficult to find—some are not listed in any of the major American libraries—but they are important sources of information about FDR and polio generally. Ruth Butts Stevens's *Hi-ya Neighbor* presents "intimate glimpses of Franklin Delano Roosevelt at Warm Springs, Georgia."[13] Turnley Walker's *Roosevelt and the Warm Springs Story* has been criticized because it lacks reference material, yet most of what Walker says is borne out by many Warm Springs polios.[14] Most of these authors emphasize that Warm Springs was FDR's second greatest commitment in life. For the first eight years of his presidency (1933 to 1941), after all, Roosevelt spent almost half his time at Warm Springs. Some political biographers point out that FDR met the poorer people in

Georgia then, and that he benefited in other ways from the democratiz-
ing experience of Warm Springs.[15] A few writers point out that Roosevelt,
who had a reputation for out-doctoring the doctors at Warm Springs,
transformed himself then from "Doctor New Deal" into "Doctor Win the
War."[16] According to FDR's adviser Thomas Corcoran, "the capacity to endure political upsets came from the polio."[17] No wonder that friendly
Georgians at Warm Springs were the first to hail Roosevelt as "our next
president"—four years before the fact, in 1929!

Against the view that polio was important in the life of Roosevelt stood
an opinion that was its polar opposite. Alice Roosevelt Longworth (1884–
1981), who had known FDR since his childhood, claimed that polio did not
change him: "What an absurd idea! He was what he always would be! He
took the polio in his stride. He overcame this horrid disease. He was perfectly splendid in the way he overcame 'infantile.'"[18] Gallagher claims in
Splendid Deception that most mainline biographers did accept the view
that FDR had been little affected by polio. "As the biographies and memoirs began to appear, the denial continued in a curious way. The memoirs
generally acknowledged the president's handicap; some even occasionally
mentioned his wheelchair. None, however, acknowledged that the handicap was of any importance."[19]

Gallagher is correct in saying that public consciousness of polio was
generally "repressed" in the wake of the Salk vaccine in the 1950s, but, as
the evidence shows, that was not the case for earlier in the century. The
current notion about Roosevelt and polio is still that he and his handlers
did everything they could to hide and unconsciously or consciously deny
his polio. This interpretation is a projection onto the Roosevelt era of later
generations' forgetting of polio. (Gallagher's first-person polio narrative,
Black Bird Fly Away, almost suggests as much.)[20] Yet many factors militate
against the still all-too-common idea that Roosevelt's polio was more or
less invisible.

1. In so public a place as Madison Square Garden, FDR allowed himself
to be lifted up to the rostrum when he put forward the name of Al Smith
("the Happy Warrior") as Democratic nominee for the presidency for the
first time, in 1924.

2. Roosevelt, when he successfully nominated Al Smith to run on the
Democratic ticket for the second time, in 1928, walked with canes to the
podium. This was FDR's often celebrated demonstration to the world,

which had not really seen much of him since 1921 when he got polio, that he was now both a very crippled and also a very capable man.

3. Photographs at FDR's famous Oglethorpe speech about "bold persistent experimentation" show Roosevelt with a cane. Despite claims to the contrary, many such photographs exist.

4. To his first presidential inauguration, in 1933, Roosevelt invited sixty patients and staff members from Warm Springs, as reported by Fred Botts in the official Warm Springs serial publication *Polio Chronicle*.[21] The obviously paralyzed Roosevelt's inaugural speech that day included one of the most famous sentences ever delivered by an American president: "So, first of all, let me assert my firm belief that the only thing we have to fear is fear itself—nameless, unreasoning, unjustified terror which paralyzes needed efforts to convert retreat into advance."[22] Roosevelt, clearly referring to his own stricken situation, went on to say: "I am prepared under my constitutional duty to recommend the measures that a stricken nation in the midst of a stricken world may require." Roosevelt delivered these words, about his constitutional duty, after walking to the podium with the aid of crutches; he spoke them in the context of his assertion that Americans were "stricken by no plague of locusts." This first inaugural address was the speech of a man seeking to reveal his polio within political and politic context.

5. Roosevelt kept his disability secret to a far lesser extent than did other crippled public figures of the time. Kaiser Wilhelm II of Germany (who ruled from 1888 to 1918) kept undisclosed the withered hand with which he was born, and Joseph Goebbels was obsessive about keeping his withered polio leg hidden. Goebbels's physical condition was the result of polio at the age of four. Rejected for military service, Goebbels remained pathologically ashamed of his leg, even as he institutionalized policies for eliminating disabled people. The psychologist Wilhelm Reich argued in 1933 that "the irrational fear of syphilis was one of the major sources of National Socialism's political views and its anti-Semitism"; Reich might have done just as well to consider poliomyelitic paralysis.[23]

6. One of several politically inspired American rumors had it that FDR "was not really crippled by polio but suffered from periods of insanity caused by 'syphilis of the brain.'"[24] FDR's paralysis was frequently the subject of magazine articles like Earle Looker's "Is FDR Physically Fit to Be President?" first published in *Liberty*.[25]

7. Many people argued in the 1930s that Roosevelt's physical condition disqualified FDR for office. Georgia governor Eugene Talmadge said frequently that cripples like FDR should not be president. In a *New York Times* interview from 1935, for example, he was reported to say, "The greatest calamity to this country is that President Roosevelt can't walk around and hunt up people to talk to. The only voices to reach his wheelchair were the cries of the 'gimme crowd.' "[26] On another occasion Talmadge said that people could not respect "a man who can't walk a two by four."[27] It was known wherever men or women could read that FDR had polio.

It is useful to take up here the old saw that, after all, a diseased man can be a good, effective leader or legislator. Roosevelt, doctor for the public weal, was just such a one. In fact, the idea of the "Maimed King" became popular, thanks to Frazer's *Golden Bough,* just at the time of the first polio epidemics.[28] By the time Jessie Weston had written *From Ritual to Romance,* and T. S. Eliot *The Waste Land,* the idea of the crippled ruler was commonplace. Roosevelt relied on it in his campaign literature.[29] Illustrations in Dorothy and Philip Sterling's book *Polio Pioneers* show a disabled king curing disease.[30] After Roosevelt's death, his polio became the subject of a best-selling play and movie about his illness and presumed recovery from it.

King's Row and *Sunrise at Campobello*

The traditional argument that virtually no one in the 1950s thought that polio had mattered much to President Franklin Delano Roosevelt ignores not only books but also movies. Among these is the much-watched movie *King's Row* (1942), in which Drake McHugh (Ronald Reagan, later president of the United States) awakes from surgery an amputee and delivers the celebrated line "Where's the rest of me?" For years after he playacted McHugh, Reagan dwelled on amputation and paralysis. During one of his "celebrity visits" to Rancho los Amigos Medical Center, Reagan crowned a young polio victim in an iron lung and named her Miss Breathless, then spoke about her legless condition. Drake McHugh's question even became the title of Ronald Reagan's autobiography, *Where's the Rest of Me?*[31]

President Franklin Delano Roosevelt—the commander-in-chief of the

United States during World War II—did not have the use of his legs. Reagan's playing a legless person during this period was certainly important to his film audience (as the reviews of the time show). Moreover, his utter identification with Drake McHugh was a key moment in the formation of Reagan's own character. Reagan reports that during his preparations—four decades before he would become chief executive of the United States—for playing the part of McHugh, he spent much time "in stiff confinement, contemplating my torso and the smooth undisturbed flat of the covers where my legs should have been." After this period of apparently self-imposed stasis, Reagan felt that something uncanny was happening. "Gradually the affair began to terrify me. In some weird way, I felt something horrible had happened to my body." Finally, Reagan felt as if he too really had no legs. "I can't describe even now my feeling as I tried to reach for where my legs should be. 'Randy!' I screamed . . . 'Where's the rest of me?'" Two years after writing these words—and twenty-five years after the traumatic experience they recount—Reagan told an audience at Eureka College in 1967 that "polio was more terrifying than even the threat of the bomb: We have defeated polio and tuberculosis and a host of plague diseases that held even more terror for mankind than the threat of the bomb." The World War I flyleaf message "'America must win this war,'" so important to President Reagan's first inaugural address, aimed to encapsulate these struggles of the twentieth century.

The most famous line comparable to Ronald Reagan's "Where's the rest of me?" in *King's Row* must be Franklin Delano Roosevelt's words on waking up from his "polio fever" in Dore Schary's stage play *Sunrise at Campobello* (1958). This work tells the story of Franklin Delano Roosevelt from the time he got polio in August 1921 until he gave the "Happy Warrior" speech nominating Al Smith in 1924. *Sunrise at Campobello* won Tony awards for outstanding play, outstanding supporting or featured actor, outstanding director, and outstanding dramatic actor. (Ralph Bellamy writes about the experience of playing Roosevelt in his memoir.)[32] The movie version (1960) won a Golden Globe for best actress in a drama and was nominated for best actress in a leading role. Greer Garson, who played Eleanor Roosevelt, had already had long involvement in polio work: in 1944, for example, she had narrated the documentary polio movie *Miracle at Hickory* for the National Foundation for Infantile Paralysis; and in preparation for *Sunrise at Campobello*, Garson renewed her friendship with Eleanor Roosevelt and researched her life. Among the people involved in making the movie was Franz Waxman, the composer for Hitchcock's *Rear Window.*

Remarkably, Gallagher claims that *Sunrise at Campobello* "did not touch upon Roosevelt's paralysis or its accompanying psychological effects."[33] The claim is not original. (Goldberg's *Making of Franklin D. Roosevelt* had already stated that *Sunrise at Campobello* did not portray FDR's depression following his polio.)[34] But the claim is mistaken. In *Sunrise at Campobello*, Franklin Delano Roosevelt says he is angry about the lack of medical knowledge and the plethora of quack cures. He proclaims himself "fed up with all those friendly hints that come in the mail—everything from ancient nostrums to brand new gadgets invented by people all the way from Keokuk to Zanzibar." Schary's Roosevelt also has "nightmares about being trapped and unable to move." Depressed, he thinks of himself as if he were "a crab lying on its back."[35] More important, an ongoing debate takes place within *Sunrise at Campobello*—the fundamental motivating narratological dialectic of the play—whether Roosevelt should keep moving in "politics" (as Roosevelt's friend and adviser Louie Howe says) or stay put "at home" (as Roosevelt's mother, Sara, says).[36]

Most biographers say that Sara Roosevelt had in fact never wanted FDR to enter politics—even before he got polio. In *Sunrise at Campobello*, this is Louie Howe's view of Sara. The real Louie McHenry Howe was, according to Lea Stiles, writing in 1954, "the man behind Roosevelt."[37] In *Sunrise at Campobello*, the character Howe—an asthmatic who is killing himself with cigarettes—is both Roosevelt's foil and his motivator.

In actuality, Franklin Delano Roosevelt met Howe in 1912, when Franklin was suffering from typhoid and running for re-election to the New York State Senate. Howe, who had serious asthma, helped FDR win his campaign, thereby overcoming FDR's inability to campaign on the public stage like the other candidates. Schary's character Howe is presented as a man whose first love is the theater.[38] In *Sunrise at Campobello*, then, Howe is staging Roosevelt throughout the play—for the purpose of making a "joint play," later on, for the presidency of the United States.

Sara Roosevelt and Louie Howe present antithetical views of FDR's fears about his abilities and his ambition after he has had polio. On the one hand, Sara does not want Roosevelt to make a play for the presidency: "If Franklin's to have any permanent injury, the best place for him is Hyde

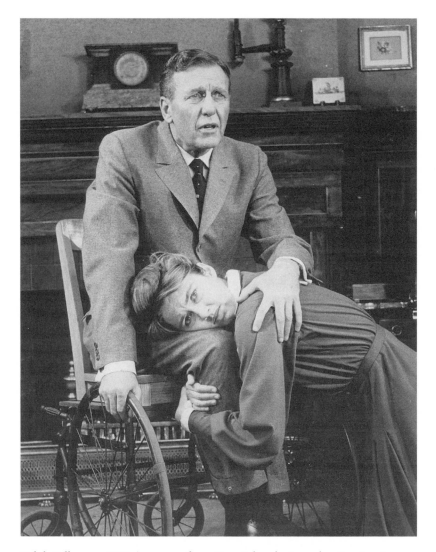

Ralph Bellamy as FDR, in a scene from Dore Schary's stage play *Sunrise at Campobello.*

Park. We can make a full life for him there. He can write, take care of the estate, raise his family as he was raised and there will be enough to keep him active without overtaxing him or spending his energy." Howe, on the other hand, presents FDR's hopes. Not to see this opposition between Sara and Howe—as Gallagher apparently does not—is to misunderstand the defining dialectic of *Sunrise at Campobello*. It is also to deny (as Gallagher does) the recognition that did exist in the 1950s of something like what we nowadays call post-polio syndrome. In *Sunrise at Campobello,* Roosevelt's mother, the fictional Sara, argues that Roosevelt should not "overextend" himself psychologically and physically. History eventually showed that, in some crucial respects, she may have been correct. Sara speaks directly to Roosevelt about going back to work in politics: "I only know that your stubbornness is not only your strength but your weakness." When she wants to install an elevator in their home in Hyde Park, he will not have it.[39] Her fears look forward to the eventual aggravation of the historical Roosevelt's paralysis.

Rights of the Handicapped

WE DON'T WANT TIN CUPS
WE WANT JOBS
—Inscription on hand-held placards at a disability rights demonstration

In a recent essay on civil rights, Tom Burke puts forward the thesis that "the politics of [civil rights] and disability was changed forever by the rise of a new generation of disabled people in the 1960s." He attributes the fact to "the polio epidemic of the 1950s" and "the Vietnam war." As Burke puts it, "the new generation [of disabled people] was larger, better educated, often less likely to be congenitally disabled . . . than its predecessors."[40] If Burke is correct about this matter, then we might conclude that polio veterans of the 1950s and disabled Vietnam veterans of the 1970s would have a good deal in common: little belief that their infection or any genetic risk might persist, say, and few traumatic memories of that sort. (Yet as Timothy Cook points out, polios were often discriminated against because people felt they were somehow contagious.)[41]

Moreover, polios identify themselves as handicapped persons more rarely than other apparently disabled persons. ("It's no use trying to get polio victims to enlist in handicapped causes, someone in the [disability rights] business once told me, because you guys don't think you are handicapped," writes Wilfrid Sheed in his polio memoir, *In Love with Daylight*.)[42] To put it another way, polios are more likely to struggle against such identification precisely on account of the culture of denial, compensation, and triumph in which they have persevered. Likewise, surviving polios are much less likely than victims of most disabling conditions and diseases—including especially the Vietnam war—to come from the economically less-advantaged social classes: polio tended to strike the "clean" neighborhoods at least as much as the "dirty" ones. Indeed, with acute cases of polio, survival often depended upon family wealth.

Burke is probably right enough, though, to posit a good number of disability rights activists among polios in the post–World War II era. Hundreds of polios are active in the civil rights arena. Dr. Linda Jane Laubenstein—the real-life model for Emma Brookner in Kramer's *The Normal Heart*—was among the first Americans to focus on the medical *and* political aspects of AIDS.[43] Henry Hampton produced and directed the 1987 PBS civil rights television series *Eyes on the Prize*. (It includes a section on the fate of the polio-stutterer Emmett Till.) Irving Zola helped to found the present-day academic field of disability studies.[44] Enid Foster became politically active in her hometown of Bulawayo, in present-day Zimbabwe.[45] Edward V. Roberts, left a quadriplegic after his bout with polio in 1953, became the first severely disabled student at the University of California at Berkeley in 1962. Judy Heuman, a quadriplegic after her bout with polio, entered high school in 1961; on graduating from college, she argued successfully that she should be allowed to teach in the New York City public schools; only then did she go to work at the Center for Independent Living and to hold other, higher offices. Justin Dart, Jr., a paraplegic after his bout with polio in 1948, became a successful disability rights activist with real influence on Presidents Ronald Reagan and George H. W. Bush. Hugh Gallagher, the subject of the movie *Coming to Terms* (1990), was an important figure in the passage of the 1968 Architectural Barriers Act. Gini Laurie was editor of the *Toomeyville Gazette* at the Toomey Pavilion Polio Rehabilitation Center in Cleveland, Ohio, and eventually transformed it, under the name *Rehabilitation Gazette*, into a key voice for disability rights.[46]

Given Burke's thesis about polios and veterans, one might expect a corresponding disability rights movement in other periods. After World War I and its great polio epidemic there was such a movement. (Burke overlooks it.) The early history of the disability rights movement in the United States includes the work of the polio Joseph F. Sullivan. He wrote *The Unheard Cry*, published the *Hospital School Journal*, and argued, against the tenor of the times (namely, that the handicapped were shameful and immoral) that cripples constituted "a noble class of humanity" and that all they needed was opportunity.[47] A reformer involved in the hospital-school movement (a precursor to polio schools), Sullivan put forward the thesis that the solution to "the problem of crippledom" was changing the society around the cripples.

The polios and veterans from the 1920s and 1930s did not succeed, whereas those from the 1950s and 1960s *apparently* have done so. Urgent financial and military conditions in the period between the two world wars help explain why. So too do conditions affecting the greater civil rights movement, the one about race. Another factor would be the sometimes "patronizing" influence of the NFIP. The National Foundation for Infantile Paralysis was in the business of taking dimes to find a cure; it was not in the business of giving rights. Such a slogan as *You've Given Us Your Dimes, Now Give Us Our Rights!* made good sense only in the post-Salk era of the 1960s.

In the United States, presidents often make efforts toward protecting rights. But apparently, President Franklin Delano Roosevelt, who founded NFIP, had too much else to do in the late 1930s to help out. The lesson is worth remarking in the case of the New York League of the Physically Handicapped, which was composed mainly of disabled (but not wheelchair-using) polios.[48] League members came together because they thought that FDR's New Deal policies would assist them in their quest for employment.[49] When in 1935 most polios were classified as unemployable under the New Deal, league members went to a New York City agency to demonstrate against the discriminatory policies. Later, the group conducted a three-week picket at the New York headquarters of the Works Progress Administration (WPA), with the result that the WPA hired about forty league members. The next year, in May 1936, league members met with WPA leader Harry Hopkins. Hopkins informed the league that he did not believe as many New Yorkers with disabilities were employable as the league contended, but he added that he would change his mind if he saw figures backing up the league's claim. The league eventually presented Hopkins with its *Thesis on Conditions of Physically Handicapped,* which described job discrimination in the private and public sectors, recommended that the Civil Service hire disabled veterans and handicapped civilians, and criticized public and private vocational rehabilitation for being under-

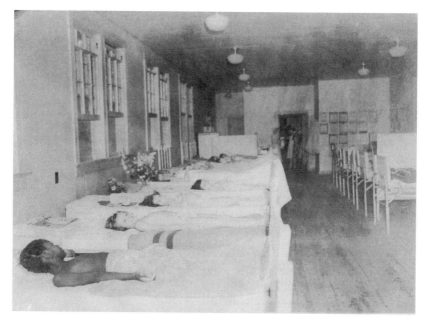

Integration of the races in the polio wards (1944): a first for the South.

funded and inadequate and for sending people into demeaning jobs. Hopkins ignored the *Thesis*. In the end, the league simply joined forces with the League for the Advancement of the Deaf in September 1936. The NFIP had won.[50]

Roosevelt's ignoring the league was hardly the only time FDR let civil rights down. Roosevelt even countenanced keeping African-Americans out of his beloved Warm Springs, with its tremendous backing from his various private foundations.[51] Some historians defend Roosevelt from the charge of racism by citing domestic political expediencies, including attacks by the governor of Georgia. (Roosevelt had to contend with charges that racial integration itself was the principal cause of polio.)[52] Racial integration at other polio hospitals was a landmark in American political history.[53]

Roosevelt's actual view was that the fight against polio, and against all disease, included the fight for the rights of all disabled persons. His informal remarks at Thanksgiving dinner, Warm Springs, Georgia, for November 23, 1939, include the following sentiments:

Even the older people here will be perhaps surprised a little when I tell them that fifty years ago, when some of us who are here tonight were alive, there was practically nothing being done in all of the United States to help crippled people to use their arms and legs again.

What did they do? Well, they were just sort of pushed off on the side; they were just unfortunate people. It was just what they used to call "an act of God" and there were a lot of very good religious people, people who belonged to churches, people who lived Christian lives, all over the United States who, when somebody in the family got infantile paralysis or something else in those days, would say that it was an act of God and they would do nothing more about it. The child or the grownup would be just sort of regarded as an unfortunate victim of something that no human being could do anything about. They were segregated; they were put up in the attic. It was one of the things you didn't talk about in the family or among the neighbors. And what is that? Half a century ago! And what a change there has been in those fifty years.[54]

The story of the "Miracle at Hickory," with its integrated polio wards and heartfelt backing from FDR, has yet to be fully disclosed. In the fifty years following his death, Roosevelt's Warm Springs graduates came out of the attic and went into the civil rights movements.

9 WHAT WE CAN LEARN, IF WE HURRY

Polio has taught me things I would never have known otherwise.
—Lorraine Beim, *Triumph Clear* (1946)

Where there is a will there is a way—as the very old proverb has it. A paralyzed person, certainly, will be skeptical about this proverb's rosy view of willpower. Yet even Franklin Delano Roosevelt said in his commencement address at Oglethorpe University in 1932, "It is common sense to take a method and try it. If it fails, admit it frankly and try another. But above all, try something."[1] Nevertheless, the question remains: What happened—continues to happen—to the *will* to deal with and understand polio and to comprehend the problems and opportunities that polio still presents? What can we (still) learn from polio?

An Orphan Disease?

In order to answer such questions, we need to draw up a short inventory of what we did *not* do, during the past half century—even though we had sufficient science, even at that time, to do it—and then we need to move on to the list of things to do about polio *now*, in the last days, we must hope, of its second mowing. Finally, we need to remember again what we have already forgotten. For all this we need to hurry up.

As we have seen, the fiction that "polio has been defeated" generally obscures the fact that many more people suffered and still suffer from polio than is generally understood. In the United States live 1.6 million people who had polio; polio is still the second-greatest cause of paralysis (after stroke).[2] Let me put this perspective into a global context: 24 million people worldwide are identified as having had polio.[3] Even at the point when no new incidences of polio occur on the planet, the direct medical effects of polio will continue to dog us for at least half a century beyond that. After all, polio should be understood not only in terms of its initial presentation and "early effects" but also with respect to its ongoing and debilitating aspects, which nowadays affect approximately 600 thousand Americans and about 7.5 million people worldwide. (I refer to its as yet little-understood sequelae, nowadays gathered under the rubric PPS.)

The conviction that most problems and opportunities involving polio had reached an end—that with the advent of the Salk and Sabin vaccines of the 1950s, polio had become what is called an orphan disease—tended to discourage us from attending to several important medical and public health issues involving the vaccine itself.[4] One such issue is our failure to eradicate polio completely by means of a universal vaccination, as we did with smallpox.[5] We seem to be doing that only now with polio. Procrastination over half a century has come at great cost in human suffering and imposed great financial burdens, and it deserves special study. A second such issue is our failure to investigate fully the ramifications of a disconcerting fact: that vaccines sometimes transmit the very disease they are meant to protect against.

A third issue, really a group of issues, is the failure to investigate faulty manufacturing methods, laboratory closures, preventable disasters like the Brazilian polio epidemic in the 1970s, and other forms of neglect that allow the disease to make comebacks in places where it seemed to have been eradicated.[6] A fourth issue involves the failure to consider Bernice Eddy's demonstration that Simian Virus 40 had infected some early polio vaccines.[7] This discovery was suppressed in a manner resembling the one Ibsen delineates in his *Enemy of the People* (1882). Only in the 1990s did interest in this issue come to the fore. In fact, the jury is still out on the not-unrelated question whether animal research during the period between 1950 and 1955 actually slowed down the development of a polio vaccine.[8]

Dr. Roland Berg, writing in 1948, had wished that *Polio and Its Problems*, which he called the "biography of a disease," could be polio's obituary. In recent years, many a book or film has purported to herald an obituary for polio. (The movie *The Last Word* is a typically well-meaning film still heralding this end of polio.)[9] Meanwhile, polio has already been manufactured from readily available raw materials. The possibility is there to terrorize any and all who want or allow it to do so. "As to whether we can ever stop using the polio vaccine"—or its equivalent—the unhappy answer is, No.[10]

After Polio

> There comes a time in the life of every such patient when the whole system—muscles, organs, bones, joints—begins to fall apart all at once, like the wonderful one hoss-shay. Every polio patient is warned to expect that time, every polio family lives with the foretold doom waiting for it at some unknown but expected time in the future. One learns to live with it by turning away from it, by not looking.
>
> —Wallace Stegner, *Crossing to Safety* (1987)

Post-polio syndrome is the contemporary term to describe the running together (the literal meaning of "syndrome") of two conditions that come along some decades after the onset of polio. The first of these is post-polio progressive muscular atrophy (PPPMA). One should distinguish PPPMA from "regular wear and tear" on the body—even though such normal wear and tear is usually quantitatively greater for polios than for other people. It is on just such a normally worn-out body that PPPMA gets to work, for years, often without the so-called polio survivor's knowing it. Eventually, physical symptoms appear. That is the moment when "the straw breaks the camel's back"—as Florence Nightingale put it in relation to other chronic medical problems.[11] At this moment when, they return, boomeranglike, the new symptoms compel many polios to experience some of the original trauma of the disease. The phenomenon inflicts on the consciousness both a haunting past experience (if the polio was old enough to remember) and a present reality. The person with PPS relives the polio on the ideal plane and also lives the post-polio condition in reality, as it is now. This situation is reminiscent of the diagnoses of hysterical paralysis delivered during the

1930s and 1940s. It also brings us to the second component of PPS, post-polio traumatic stress disorder (PPTSD).

The word *trauma* here refers to "a psychic injury, esp[ecially] one caused by an emotional or physical shock the memory of which is repressed and remains unhealed."[12] For the post-polio patient, the physical conse-quences of polio and PPPMA are aggravated psychologically by the origi-nal trauma.[13] I do *not* mean that the polio virus may have affected the brain. (However, that is an important matter for future researchers to con-sider.)[14] I *do* mean that recovery from the physical trauma often requires the patient to block out painful events and procedures psychologically, in much the same way that recovery, as understood in the 1940s and 1950s, re-quired patients to be distracted from physical weakness and difficulty. As we have seen, polio-children were often unable—or not allowed—to deal psychologically with what was happening to them at the time that they got polio. The consequent overcompensation for physical disability, or the ten-dency to ignore the body, for which polios were and are praised, is under-stood now as part of a socially constructed trauma. The problem is espe-cially poignant because what we would now call overexercise (such as that in which William O. Douglas engaged) stood polios in good stead when they were first recovering from the ravages of the disease; but now that they are post-polios, the habits of exercise inculcated in the past have be-come counterproductive of the good they once produced. Now, overexer-cise leads to or exacerbates further atrophy; underexercise, however, leads to further weakness and instability. Even the golden mean of Horace—the *aurea mediocritas*—is now become the merest illusion.[15]

The same cultural circumstances that led to the premature declaration that "paralytic" polio had been cured have also led to a consistent tendency to overlook PPS and, as Arthur Clarke emphasizes, often to declare that it doesn't even exist. About polio and post-polio syndrome, he says: "I speak with considerable feeling, for my own experience demonstrates the confu-sion surrounding this mysterious disease—the very existence of which is still denied by some physicians."[16] Yet a condition very like today's PPS has been repeatedly "discovered," forgotten, and then rediscovered, for a long time. Medical doctors who dealt with a similar problem in 1875 included Jean Charcot, M. Rayond, V. Cornil and R. Lepine, and M. Carrière. All such researchers showed that sequelae were to be expected for a large percentage of those polios who lived three or four decades beyond the time of the initial viral infection. In 1953, a few long-standing reviews or ongoing studies of PPS existed, like the one by W. Geiger, "Über progrediente postpoliomyelitische Zustandsbilder."[17] Yet people were very anxious to declare polio a short-lived disease. And from 1914 to 1950, most Canadian and American doctors seemed to go out of their way to neglect or even deny the reported clinical observations.[18]

The history of ignorance and denial of PPS is one reason some polios feel a certain relief when they are diagnosed with it. Thus William Phillips writes, "As strange as it may seem, I was comforted [*soulagé*] to learn that I was suffering from post-polio syndrome. 'Better a known devil than an unknown one.'"[19] What usually follows the elation of diagnosis is anxiety: What will happen to me—now and again? Fear of that anxiety helps explain why many polios draw little connection between their having had polio long ago and their developing "strange symptoms" a few decades later. Dixson, for example, writes in his autobiographical *My Way with Polio* that his first bout with polio was initially misdiagnosed as "rheumatic fever." Eventually, Dixson describes in his "Aftermath" how he is again diagnosed, decades later, with serious "rheumatic pains."[20] Dixson does not remark the similarity between his doctors' misdiagnoses. Another example involves the American therapist Milton Erickson. He writes that he had "a second attack of polio" decades after the first, but does not consider that what he calls "a second attack" was instead the "normal" long-term boomerang reaction from the first.

The long-range boomerang made polio's aftereffects especially difficult to study in its early years. It requires some four decades for PPS to manifest itself; but in the nineteenth century, when researchers were already trying to do such studies, life expectancy was only forty-nine years. Therefore, even if their statistical methods for studying disease and epidemics had been as sophisticated as ours (which they were not), PPS would not have shown itself in anything like a scientifically recognizable pattern.

Yet even today, statistical and diagnostic difficulties remain in dealing with PPS, partly because the usual figure cited for the number of polios worldwide (twenty-four million) is too low. Many people in addition had so-called abortive or nonparalytic polio without ever knowing it. And, as Charles Caverly argued in 1894, "It is impossible to estimate the number of abortive cases in an epidemic," owing to the nonappearance of polio symptoms in over 90 percent of cases.[21] In PPS the end fibers of motor nerves begin to lose function, but this condition is rarely properly diagnosed early on: the change does not reveal itself when the muscles are tested manually, and indeed, as Dr. Sharrard showed as early as 1953, more than half the anterior horn cells have to have been destroyed during the original polio infection in order for any weakness to show up in the early stages.[22] So the nonappearance of polio in the short run does not mean that PPS will not appear in the long run. A normally active lifestyle on the part of someone who has had polio unknowingly often leads to debilitation that is incompletely explained etiologically.

People often had polio without knowing it or were diagnosed with polio but didn't have it. The diagnosis of polio of the nonparalytic sort in the 1950s was often based merely on signs of aseptic meningitis (sometimes flulike symptoms) in patients from a neighborhood where polio cases had already occurred; and since a person can lose a great many motor units—the number reported varies between 20 percent and 60 percent—without giving any clinical evidence whatever of muscular weakness, many people who did have polio but had no observable muscle weakness would, without further tests—which were in any case expensive, invasive, and often unavailable—have been diagnosed (wrongly) as having had flu.[23]

Debilitation caused by an unacknowledged or unrecognized attack of polio decades earlier will often appear as "atypical" secondary injury or overuse, or as odd or premature gerontological conditions, or as "unusual" myalgic encephalomyelitis, fibromyalgia, multiple sclerosis (MS), chronic fatigue syndrome, or postviral syndrome.[24] The condition may erroneously be diagnosed as one of these—until a caring physician takes a careful case history, orders such tests as electroencephalographs, and makes detailed, comparative muscle-strength examinations over a period of years.

Many people misdiagnosed as having had flu often develop muscle weakness later on—owing to eventual neuronal damage—to the point that the motor nerves cannot support all their axonal sprouts.[25] The misdiagnosis is evident in statistical follow-up studies of people not diagnosed with polio who are siblings of twins who were diagnosed.[26] A Norwegian study includes anecdotal descriptions of a woman who had nonparalytic polio when she was six years old in 1952 but was diagnosed with post-polio in the late 1990s; in another case a woman complained of muscle weakness when she had polio in 1951, was diagnosed as having only nonparalytic polio, but developed symptoms of PPS in the late 1990s.[27]

Still Undone

Further mysteries await polio research. Consider the fact that we still do not know for sure how the poliovirus moves from the intestinal tract to the central nervous system. Does it move through the blood by means of a viremia?[28] It seems likely that knowing fully how the poliovirus makes this move would help us deal with similar viruses and several diseases.[29] A few medical scientists now hypothesize that even ALS (a disease of the gray anterior horn cells) has some viral component. Consider also that a newly defined intersection between genetics and poliovirology encourages research into the poliovirus as a "delivery system" for molecules that might support the regrowth of neurons.[30]

Orphan viruses are those viruses which are attached to no known symptoms—as far as we know. In some ways, therefore, they have represented a real opportunity for medical research. A few polio researchers recognized the opportunity early on. Dr. J. L. Melnick thus observed in 1954 that crucial to future medical research should be "the detection of new viruses, provisionally called 'orphan viruses'—as we know so little to what diseases they belong—from patients suspected of having non-paralytic poliomyelitis."[31] One might think here about numerous enteroviruses—Coxsackie A9, enteroviruses 70 and 71, and Japanese encephalitis virus—that apparently can cause poliolike paralysis and symptoms resembling those of PPS.[32] Some of these viruses—for example, Coxsackie virus RNA—have apparently been isolated from people with PPS symptoms, although it is not known whether such isolation is a common event.[33]

Many other areas of research remain to be tackled. Already in 1960, for example, Sven Gard had asked, "Exit poliomyelitis—What next?"[34] Just what has followed in polio's sociobiological and virological "niche" is not yet clear. The meaning of Gard's question, as regards environmental medicine, has become clearer. Beyond any such questions, we will never know what useful information we failed to collect by not having begun a study in the 1950s of polios along lines similar to the Framingham Heart Disease Epidemiological Study (ongoing since 1948) or to the Nurses' Health Study (at the Channing Laboratory of Harvard University).

Do physical accidents "set off" post-polio syndrome? Richard Bruno puts the question and answer as follows: "Can a traumatic event trigger post-polio sequelae? . . . Yes and No."[35] In fact, some experts in the field now believe that accidents, and falls like that in *Rear Window* in particular, are likely to trigger PPS. (Other experts say the same about falls triggering multiple sclerosis.)[36]

Many people suffer from symptoms that are possibly related to polio, and polios have been said to have a predisposition to contract various disorders (Creutzfeldt-Jakob disease, schizophrenia, and eye problems).[37] Not enough research has been done to determine what other predispositions may exist and what might be learned about them. About one such predisposition I am pretty clear: a disproportionately high number of polios stutter. The fact is not surprising from the merely etymological viewpoint. The cognate terms *stumble* and *stutter* mean the same thing, and nowhere does Jimmy Stewart's celebrated stutter work better than when he stumbles in *Rear Window*. ("I stumble in my speech and stutter in my legs" said one stuttering polio, the Roman emperor Claudius.)[38] Perhaps the psychological stress of having had polio exacerbates an underlying biological predisposition to stutter in some children.[39] Perhaps the physiological effects on mouth and tongue, and bulbar paralysis—often unnoticed at the time of the polio attack—may precipitate, or themselves constitute, a main "cause" of stuttering in this group. Whatever the link, so far we can only speculate. Only a few studies spanning the previous century—from Judson's *Influence of Growth on Acquired and Congenital Deformities* to the Pentagon's *Post-Polio Syndrome as a Model for Musculo-Tendinous Overuse Syndromes in Military and Civilian Populations*—are realistically exemplary.[40]

Nowhere is the paucity of research on polio more lamentable than in the political and sociological arenas. As we have seen, parallels can be drawn between the way private and public social institutions met the polio epidemics and the way we are meeting apparently similar health problems today. These latter include ALS (sometimes called slow polio), often initially

misdiagnosed as polio (as was the case with Lou Gehrig), and chronic fatigue syndrome (whose symptoms are sometimes much the same as those
of PPS, and it was already linked with polio in 1934).[41] In this tally, the great
epidemics should not be overlooked, such as influenza, which killed more
than twelve million people at the beginning of the twentieth century, or
HIV/AIDS, at the end of the twentieth century and into this one. Relevant
here, for understanding the sociologically sensitive link between xenopho-
bia and disease, is the New York City polio epidemic of 1916, which pro-
voked a massive quarantine (the largest in world history). The New York
City quarantine incited distrust among immigrant groups, especially Ital-
ians, who were singled out for singular discrimination because current statistics suggested that the number of polio cases was highest among that
group.[42] One nation almost always tends to blame another for an international epidemic! Thus, Americans called the post–World War I influenza
the Spanish influenza, and Englishmen called it Flanders grippe.[43] The
same phenomenon is apparent in the case of syphilis, which "was the
'French pox' to the English, *morbus Germanicus* to the Parisians, the 'Na-
ples sickness' to the Florentines, the 'Chinese disease' to the Japanese."[44]
How many newspapers in spring 2003 carried the headline "Chinese
SARS"?

Many people thought that the success of the polio vaccine portended
the end of *all* epidemics. The eminent historian William McNeill, author
of the influential book *Plagues and Peoples*, argued in 1983 that "one of the
things that separate us from our ancestors and make contemporary experience profoundly different from that of other ages is the disappearance of
epidemic disease as a serious factor in human life."[45] No wonder McNeill
failed to recognize AIDS for the epidemic that it was. (This is, of course,
not to claim that the poliovirus vaccine "caused" the HIV/AIDS epidemics—as some writers have asserted.)[46] McNeill seemed devoted to memorializing epidemics as events of the distant past, even as AIDS, which he ignored at the time, was making its triumphant entrance.

The AIDS activist Larry Kramer is troubled by such forgetfulness. "I
think one of the most disheartening things is everyone seems to have
forgotten the plague, and not just young people, but older people who
lived through it. It's almost like it didn't happen and everybody thinks it's
gone away."[47] Not surprisingly, Kramer's most influential work, *The Normal Heart*, attempts to show the parallel between the sociopathology of re-

pressing the facts and fictions about polio in the 1940s and 1950s (and, in-cidentally, also the facts and fictions about the Holocaust at the same period) and the sociopathology of denying the facts about AIDS or con-structing medically and politically dangerous mythologies about it.[48] The parallel here between polio and AIDS has a basis in the real history of American public health: Sandra Panem, in her book *AIDS Bureaucracy* (1988), goes some way toward showing how the repression and panic sur-rounding AIDS resemble those which surrounded polio: "As a public health emergency AIDS most closely resembles the polio epidemics of the 1940s and 1950s, notably in the public panic that accompanied both, their viral etiology, the attention paid to both by the media, and the fact that when each disease appeared in epidemic proportions, neither preventative or effective treatments were available."[49] The hero of Kramer's *Normal Heart* is a polio, Dr. Emma Brookner. Having had polio and become a medical doctor, Emma is apparently the first to bring to light the impor-tance of AIDS, to treat its victims with dignity, to try to protect society as a whole from its ravages, and to attempt to garner support for research into the biology of the disease. Emma notes how AIDS patients are treated in hospitals, as mere "objects," a reaction reminiscent of experience of treat-ment of polio patients during the epidemics. When an "examining doctor" tells Emma that she won't get the AIDS research grant for which she has applied, the rejection makes her feel much as if she were again in paralysis treatment. Too well she knows the political consequences for public health that "Nobody gets polio anymore."[50]

Kramer's Emma Brookner is based on the real-life personage of Dr. Linda Jane Laubenstein, whom polio likewise left confined to manual and electric wheelchairs, and who also suffered from severe respiratory dif-ficulties, usually diagnosed as asthma—as frequently happens in the case of polios.[51] Laubenstein was involved in the first work on AIDS. She was outspoken about neglect of the epidemic by government and society; her medical practice consisted predominantly of AIDS cases, and in 1983 she helped organize the Kaposi's Sarcoma Research Fund and the first full-scale medical conference on AIDS. Like me, Laubenstein was born in 1947 and had polio in the early 1950s. Her childhood immediately after polio is documented in her scrapbook, "My Life 1952–58," an example of the un-published literature by child-polios we have considered. Laubenstein died in 1993, of a heart attack—four decades after polio.[52]

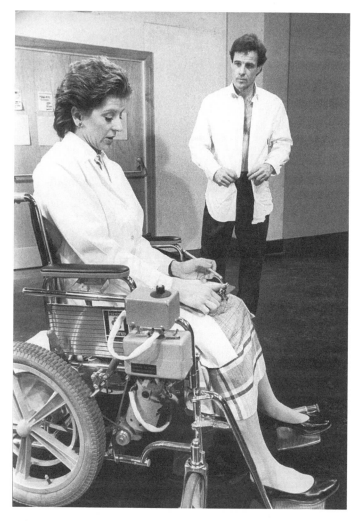

Polio and AIDS: scene from Larry Kramer's play *The Normal Heart*
(1985), starring Concetta Tomei and Brad Davis.

Medical Tolerance

Insofar as most doctors generally want to eradicate illness in their individual patients, their *art* of treatment usually sees as finally intolerable such
conditions as polio creates. Some doctors, understandably (if also irratio-

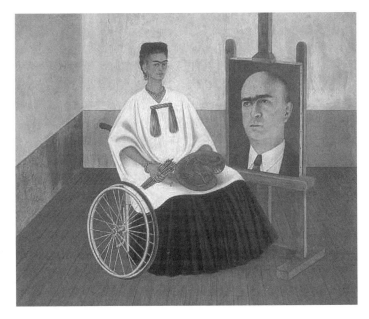

Self-Portrait with Portrait of Dr. Farill, by Frida Kahlo.

nally) thus become unable to bear up patients with chronic or disabling conditions and so, by their attitude, contribute toward those patients' spiritual and psychological difficulties. No wonder the polio activist Ed Roberts was proud *not* to go to a doctor. He wanted to come to terms with himself—to tolerate himself—as he was.[53]

There are, of course, exceptions to the caricatural view of the medical profession contained in the previous paragraph, when it comes both to individual doctors and to specific medical fields. One kind of exception can be seen in Frida Kahlo's great painting *Self-Portrait with Portrait of Dr. Farill* (1951), which she figuratively painted with her own blood. Dr. Juan Farill was Kahlo's own doctor. Himself able to walk only with crutches, he was Mexico's most distinguished orthopedist, and he organized the first Pan American Congress on Rehabilitation of the Handicapped.[54]

When it comes to the medical intolerance of specific "health specialties," it is often orthopedists, along with psychiatrists, who come in for special opprobrium in the case of polio treatment. It is as if orthopedists believe they might produce miracles in the style of Jesus when he told the paralytic to pick up his bed and walk.[55] The polio Mauro, in *The Landscape of My Disability,* writes in "On the Rack of Perfection" of suffering his orthopedic treatment.

> They put me on the rack and turned the crank
> crack tried to pull me back into perfect
> proportions a shade they wanted me
> straight not bent this is not the way
> to stand this is not the way to be
> this is not American
> the land of the free
> O say can you see you're hurting
> me they cast me in a plaster in their
> own image wrapped tight a snowy white
> Christmas gift waiting to be opened
> in the New Year where to them I'd
> finally blend right in and be more human
> again more like every man or woman again
> and no one would ever notice the scar
> they left unless I got undressed—
> at this they shook their heads
> but then nakedness is always
> the perfect test of every man
> who's ever been broken on the rack[56]

Orthopedic torture practiced toward the end of "perfect proportions"—as Mauro puts it, "they cast me in a plaster in their / own image"—is the pedagogic breaking on the rack about which polio singer Brother John Sellers also sang the blues in 1957.[57] It is the sort of treatment that gives rise to Frida Kahlo's near-desperate twin paintings, *Without Hope* (1945) and *Tree of Hope* (1946). (This is not to say that surgeries in general had no medical or social benefit. Without surgeries, many child polios—"frogs"—suffered those asymmetries in growth with which circus freak shows were once replete.)

The success of orthopedics, which generally seems to convey to polios the message "This is not the way to be," came in the wake of World War I

and the great polio epidemics of that time. A relatively more tolerant response set in at about the same time with a counterstatement from the
field of physiatry: "Learn to be the way you are." Orthopedics and physiatry have thus often been rivals for the same polio patients and disabled
veterans. As Dr. Julie Silver, in "Start with a Physiatrist," appropriately observes: "Both polio and physiatry came to the forefront during the first half
of the twentieth century. In fact, physiatrists who are doctors that special-
ize in physical medicine and rehabilitation largely entered the specialty due
to the polio epidemics when there was a large need for rehabilitation spe-
cialists."[58] In any case, views and practices about how to put up with—tolerate—disability varied widely between the poles of "cure" and "kill" during the decades following World War I.[59] Sometimes the argument for
sterilization of those with birth defects spilled over into urging polios to be
sterilized. In Germany, the Nazi spokesperson Joseph Goebbels promulgated in his newspaper *Der Angriff* (The attack) compulsory isolation
and mass euthanasia for most disabled people. Yet Goebbels was torn
about what to do with disabled war veterans and polios: Hitler had been
wounded in the leg by a grenade splinter during the Battle of the Somme
(1916), and Goebbels himself was a polio. The implications of these contradictions were brought out esoterically in the Goebbels character in G. W.
Pabst's wartime movie *Paracelsus.*

Most people with long-term disabilities learn none too soon that there is a
limit to what medical science can do to understand and to treat us. For the
smaller-spirited among doctors, moreover, we become their failures. Their
feeling of failure slips out in their secret emotional life; it reveals itself in
their dreams; it shows sometimes in memorably impolite, if also well-intentioned, words of advice. Even as we adult polios know enough to be
wary of doctors' feelings of guilt and inadequacy toward us, so we are often, in the last analysis, probably less dependent on doctors for the way we
"get along" than we are on other groups. Among these other groups are
architects, urban planners, and legislators—those who build the city and
interpret its books of justice—and engineers, who make devices like tele-
phones, stair-climbing wheelchairs, hearing aids, talking crosswalks, porta-
ble respirators, and voice recognition systems. In the last analysis, politics
and public health matter far more to us than medicine.

Athletics, Intellectual Gymnastics, and Overcompensation

> I no longer talk about how to seize a doctrine of compensation from disease. I don't talk about it, but it still haunts me.
>
> —Leonard Kriegel, *Falling into Life* (1991)

Some polios make up (compensate) for physical weakness by turning to intellectual endeavors—as painters, writers, and movie directors. Others turn to spiritual beliefs and good works—as do those who become missionaries (as suggested in works by Evelyn Bauer, Viola Pahl, Allen Lee, John Earl Lindell and Ethel Brooks, Keith A. Korstjens, Dorothy Pape, Lloyd C. Douglas, Alma Murdock, and others) and civil rights workers, like Enid Foster.[60] (In Dore Schary's play *Sunrise at Campobello,* Eleanor Roosevelt remarks that "God takes man into deep water not to drown him but to cleanse him.")[61] Still others take up physical exercise with such determination that they become stronger, to an extraordinary degree. Living at the time of the Superman comics, the polios become supermen. Already expert in physiotherapy, these polios build up the very muscle groups whose associated nerves polio damaged, along with other muscles groups that now serve the damaged ones in a compensatory or prosthetic manner. Some polios have excelled in certain kinds of sports. Over the long haul, unfortunately, these polio-athletes often suffer most from post-polio syndrome.

About *compensation* as such, Plagemann writes about his "teacher" at Warm Springs who would talk thus to her patient:

> "You have this muscle," the physical therapist would say, "or that muscle." And then she would point out his limitations. "You do not have these muscles," she would say, "and now you must learn to compensate for what you do not have by what you have."
>
> The word stirred memories in my mind. It had been a long time since I had read Emerson's essay, but it seemed to me that the secret lay in that word "compensation." I resisted this implication at first, saying that to give wider significance to this physical approach was naïve and humorless. I stood for a long time on the edge of these thoughts, hesitating, pushing away the help that I needed.
>
> At length I, too, learned to take myself to the mirror.[62]

Athletics

In the cases of hundreds of top polio athletes, the mind helped the remaining muscles strongly reconnect with the body. Among the baseball players was Bud Daley, the New York Yankees pitcher who made the All-Star team in 1959–60. (A natural right-hander whose right arm was shorter and weaker than the other, Daley taught himself to throw left-handed.) Among the runners was Olympics winner Wilma Rudolph, known as the world's fastest woman.[63] Her career is described in Krull's *Wilma Unlimited* and Coffey's *Wilma Rudolph*,[64] and the movie *Wilma* also tells her story. Other polio athletes include the golfer Jack Nicklaus, the bicyclist Conrad Dubé,[65] Tenley Albright, an Olympic gold medalist in figure skating, Ray "Human Frog" Ewry, who holds ten Olympic gold medals for jumping,[66] and Lis Hartel, the first woman to compete against men in Olympic equestrian sport, in which she won Olympic medals throughout the 1950s.

As we have seen, water provided many polios with a hydrotherapeutic medium and, in competition, the buoyancy of water tends to "level the playing field." Among famous polio swimmers have been Annette Kellerman (the subject of the movie *The Million Dollar Mermaid*), Barbara Hobelmann (who made "All-American" in 1951),[67] Nancy Merius, (the Olympic swimming champion who was the subject of a 1954 television program called *A Time for Courage*), Ethelda Bleibtrey, and Georgia Coleman (the diver).

Popular culture of the 1950s showed a fascination with polio water champions. One Olympic champion, Buster Crabbe (born Clarence Linden), founded a children's summer camp specifically for water sports. In the literature advertising the camp, which I myself attended, Crabbe emphasized his movie association with the Olympic swimmer Johnny Weissmuller—for example, in the *Jungle Jim* movie series.[68] *Mark of the Gorilla* (1950) starred Weissmuller, and *Captive Girl* (1950) starred Crabbe. Many such movies, like *The Ape* (1940), involved finding the cure for polio. *Jungle Jim* (1948), starring Weissmuller, starts out, as does *The Ape*, in documentary fashion. In *Jungle Jim*, a native killed by a leopard is carrying a golden vial containing a paralysis-inducing toxin from the jungle, which, when refined, cures polio.

Dozens of sports books were written explicitly for polio children: on baseball, Matt Christopher's *Catcher with a Glass Arm* (1964); on basket-

ball, C. H. Frick's *Five against the Odds* (1955) and, much later, Matt Christopher's *Shoot for the Hoop* (1995). Bill J. Carol's *Crazylegs Merrill* tells the
story of a polio who makes the school football team.[69] Most of the teenage
sports heroes in these books are praised for making up for their physical
weakness in certain muscles by developing physical strength in other muscles. American writing often thus features the polio triumphing over adversity in the competitive world of sport. (I am excluding here such venues
as the Paralympics, where polios like the swimmer Simon Åhlstad have always been successful contestants.)[70]

Many books about disabling disease are written from the viewpoint of
the sportswriter. Consider Albom Mitch's best-selling *Tuesdays with Morrie*
(1997), which concerns the paralysis and eventual death from ALS of Morrie Schwartz, who is portrayed as valiantly coming to terms with a terminal
paralytic disease. Mitch, a professional sportswriter at the time that he
wrote the book, had written an undergraduate thesis on sportswriting at
Brandeis University (where he had met Schwartz). Mitch, by his own account, wrote *Tuesdays with Morrie* as a sportswriter coming to terms with
his own brother's chronic illness. And *Tuesdays with Morrie* is framed by
two references to polio, which, like ALS, is a paralyzing disease of the gray
anterior horn cells. At the outset of the book, the author describes briefly
the funeral of Irving Zola, the polio and Brandeis disability rights activist.
It is when Schwartz attends Zola's funeral that this increasingly paralyzed
person gets the idea of staging a funeral for himself, while he is yet alive.
Next, then, we have the funeral of Morrie himself. When Mitch attends
Schwartz's living funeral, he learns that Schwartz's brother had paralytic polio. (In a series of public conversations in the mid-1990s with Ted
Koppel on ABC's *Nightline,* Schwartz said that he had always felt responsi-
ble for his brother's having gotten polio.)

For some polios, more than for most other people, performing music is
a supremely athletic challenge. We have already spoken of dancers who
have had polio. Violinist Itzhak Perlman and cellist Pierre Fournier, both
polios, certainly count among the great musicians.[71] The distinctive sound
of the jazz saxophonist David Sanborn is often linked to his having had
polio. Among the prominent polio-songwriters was Doc Pomus, whose
songs include "There Must Be a Better World Somewhere" and "I Count
the Tears."[72] Among singers one can mention Connie Boswell (of the Boswell Sisters), who usually performed sitting in a wheelchair and wearing
an evening dress. Others are Walter Jackson, Neil Young, Joni Mitchell,

Brother John Sellars, and Ian Dury ("I was . . . conceived at the back of the Ritz and born at the height of the Blitz!").[73] The three members of the Jamaican group Israel Vibrations—creators of "The Same Song"—were all crippled by polio in the 1950s. They first met as children at Mona Rehabilitation Centre in Kingston.[74] Earlier in the century Lois Catherine Marshall achieved fame, along with the opera diva Marjorie Lawrence, whom Franklin Delano Roosevelt counted "among my best soldiers" and whose story is told in the movie *Interrupted Melody*.

Does disability make for any difference in the performance? Consider the case of the brilliant jazz pianist Horace Purlan. Having lost the use of his fourth and fifth fingers to polio, Purlan compensated by using the thumb and first two fingers to complete those extended chords which are normally handled by the left hand, in the process developing a huge repertoire and a style all his own.

For polios, writing was often physically difficult and typewriting an athletic accomplishment, as perfected by the polio typist Ruth Ben'ari, from Warm Springs. Painting too must count as an athletic accomplishment for some polios, though not for all. Frida Kahlo, John Perceval, Alyce Frank, and Christine Pecket, for example, painted by hand in the "traditional" way. Yet other polios breach that tradition of painting in such a way as almost to define a polio school of painting.

Such polio painters can be divided into three groups. The first consists of those who have lost the use of their dominant hand. Nell Blaine (1922–1996) taught herself to paint with her left hand in 1959, when she got polio at the age of thirty-seven.[75] Similarly, Henriette Wyeth Hurd (1907–1997)—who was the sister of the Andrew Wyeth who painted *Christina's World*—got polio as a child and subsequently taught herself a unique technique of holding the brush between her first and second fingers. Her *Portrait of David* (1978) is a study of bodies at rest and in motion that bears on this discussion. Samuel L. Schmucker's dominant (right) arm was crippled by polio, so he holds the brush between his right index and second finger, with all the movement coming from the arm.[76]

The second group consists of foot painters. Paul Driver, a Briton who got polio in 1955, produces work concerned with the suspension of motion, as is the case with his *Tower Bridge*. Among the foot painters is the Dutchman Pieter Moleveld, who got polio in 1956, and the New Zealander Jim Duncan, who got polio in 1961.[77]

The third group consists of relatively well-known polio mouth painters.

From the time that Heather Strudwick, of Gibraltar and England, got polio in 1957 until her death in 1995, she was unable to leave her iron lung for more than a few hours a day.[78] She became a painter after reading about mouth and foot artists in J. H. Roesler's *God's Second Door* (1960), which tells about disabled artists painting with their mouths or feet. Among polio mouth painters are also the Australian Margaret Greig and the Canadian Earl Bailly. (I met Bailly at a gathering in Montreal in the late 1950s; at that time he gave me a copy of the booklet *His Trials and Triumphs,* which he had written with a pencil clenched in his teeth.) Two polio mouth painters merit special attention: the British ex-ballerina Elizabeth Twistington, whose work I described in the discussions on polios in photography and dance; and the anti-Nazi agitator Arnulf Erich Stegmann, who went on to found the Association of Foot and Mouth Painting Artists in 1956. Stegmann had lost the use of his hands and lower arms, and he was among the most brilliant of painters.[79]

Do the themes of kinesis and stasis in painting and, more important, the various kinetic painting techniques differ much, depending on whether they are practiced by polios or by other disabled persons? The Irishman Christy Brown, paralyzed with cerebral palsy, suggests in his first-person narrative *My Left Foot* (1954), that they do.[80] Studies of kinetic and non-kinetic techniques in the visual media bear him out.

Intellectual Gymnastics

Teenage polios often compensate by developing intellectual rather than physical skills. They take advantage of an enforced "quiet" lifestyle to read. Many first-person polio narratives thus include some moment such as the one that Betty Cavanna reports in *Joyride,* when the grandmother of the teenage polio assumes that her granddaughter simply must become a teacher:

Polio girl: Suppose I do not want to teach, Grandmother?

Grandmother: But of course you'll teach! What else can a girl like you do?[81]

In Luis and Millar's *Wheels for Ginny's Chariot,* a girl who does poorly in school depends on tutoring from her polio friend Ginny who "naturally" does well in school: "Mother said I ought to be ashamed to have to depend on a girl in a wheelchair for help, but I'm just not smart like you, Ginny."[82]

As for me, in the summer of 1956 I figured that I'd be making my way through life on intellectual merit rather than bodily strength. One afternoon, I met a beautiful young woman in a wheelchair playing a game called Hi-Q. Did I want to know how to play? You bet. That afternoon I learned to play.

A common hypothesis about compensation—that intellectual or physical accomplishment arises from suffering and spiritual sublimation—needs to be distinguished from the view that polio effectuates, in some corporeal or physiological way, an intellectual or moral superiority that was not there already. Dr. D. M. Greig, in his essay "The Cephalic Features of Sir Walter Scott" holds to this view when he argues that the great novelist's "poliomyelitis at 18 months turned to the central nervous system and increased blood-supply which his subsequent careful and prolonged treatment perpetuated . . . gradually approaching a matured anatomical perfection preparatory to fuller intellectual acquisitions, which in Scott's case passed on to genius."[83] A second view that can be distinguished explains the supposed intellectual superiority of polios by positing that physical paralysis occurs only in those who are already in some way intellectually or morally "superior." Some of the graduates of Warm Springs espouse this view in their polio autobiographies. After all, Alice Plaistridge, Roosevelt's physiotherapist, advocated this view.

Overcompensation

Not every disability has even the potential for a compensatory aspect. Much depends on the "biological facts" regarding the location and severity of the damage that poliomyelitis wrought. For those who cannot compensate, or who will soon die, the model of Horatio Alger–like "triumph over adversity" easily makes for cruel and unnecessary punishment. ("If Daley could do it, why can't I?") It is usually foolish to believe that "all is for the best in the best of all possible worlds"—the view of Dr. Pangloss in Voltaire's *Candide* (1759); it is just as silly to believe that for every bad thing that happens, an "equal and opposite" good thing happens.

It is also worth underscoring that just because you *can* do something does not mean you *should* do it. Early in my convalescence from polio, my parents encouraged me to listen repeatedly to Burl Ives's version of the song "The Little Engine That Could," which says, "All you have to do is really try. Then there's nothing you can't do."[84] (An alternative title was "Thinking One Can.") Polios were told—by well-intentioned guardians and medical professionals—that they *could* move if only they really tried.[85] Half a century later, Nancy Baldwin Carter critiqued such advice for polios in her book for polio survivors *Myths and Chicken Feet*.[86] Richard Bruno, too, criticizes this advice in *The Polio Paradox*.[87] The long-term effects that result when polios work their muscles to the point of experiencing fatigue or pain (following the triumphant old dictum, "No pain, no gain") tends to be devastating. The "disabled" polio, especially, needs to be wary of the high-sounding phrase "I am able." The encouragement to say "I can" and act as if you really could, without incurring damage, is everywhere for disabled people; iCan is even the name of a leading "disability community."[88] And POS'M—which mimics the Latin *possum* (meaning "I can") and stands for *patient operated selector mechanism*—is the "proprietary name for electronic devices that enable disabled persons to operate or control domestic fittings and machines."[89] Maybe you *can*, for a while. But if you are a polio, without a carefully chosen prosthetic POS'M, you probably *should* not. Almost every polio has been taunted with the charge of playing possum, meaning "feign[ing], dissembl[ing]; . . . pretend[ing] illness: in allusion to the opossum's habit of feigning death when threatened or attacked."[90] But the seeming play is, after all, the opossum's often successful way of staying alive. The famous can-do attitude of polios in the 1950s— the "triple-A personality" for which they were once celebrated—explains not only the extraordinary short-term successes of some polios but also the eventual long-term damage they suffer.[91] At the same time, the can-do rhetoric is probably an inevitable precondition for survival. In his essay "Whose Voice Is this Anyway?" the polio Irving Zola comments on this contradiction in the lives of many polios when he considers that "to a marked degree certain aspects of disabled people's lives have been inaccessible to themselves."[92]

One point of view shared by many polios is that their disease and its consequences have had *no* positive effect. (*If It Weren't for the Honor—I Would've Rather Walked* is Jan Little's telling title for *his* polio memoir.)[93] Many polios see unblinkingly the uncompensated aspect of their particular disabled lives without bitter despair. Thus Roxanne Frigon from Quebec writes, "For me, polio has had no positive effect—much to the con trary. My entire life has been very difficult, filled with obstacles, errors, and lack of comprehension."[94] At the same time, though, the negative view can render disabled people's lives inaccessible to themselves. Consider Charles Conley Ward's statement at the beginning of his as yet unpublished manuscript "Crippled Thunder" (1996).

> I have been in a wheelchair for 50 very long years [writes Ward] and I am here to tell you all of the quaint phrases regarding the world of crippledom are nothing more than politically correct, conscious soothing, sentimental clap-trap. Being crippled is a damnable way of experiencing the wonders of this world. Those that claim nature compensates for the deficiencies of a cripple's body are either deceiving themselves, trying to placate their conscience, or, have given the matter little thought. Of course, there is also the possibility that they are just plain stupid. The fact of the matter is there is absolutely nothing positive to say about being crippled.[95]

Ward bravely tries to write a polio survivor's narrative without redemptive aspects, but one has the feeling that he has chosen never really to live.[96]

The hypothesis that polio, and the attendant disabilities, offer no compensation does not necessarily mean that one would exchange the life that one has had, and has now, for another life that might have been. Every year or so now, in fact, an impersonal questionnaire or impolitic journalist asks me whether I would change my partly disabled life for a fully able-bodied one. But what does it really mean, I wonder, to ask a survivor (a person who lives on) whether he would like to revive (live again) his life—not from the beginning but rather starting from some apparently life-shaping event? (The Christian polio Buddy Robertson, who believed in resurrection of the body, looked for his "Mansion in the Sky"—but only *after* the death of the body.)[97] It is one thing to ask a man whether he would rather not have had an accident that left him injured. It is another to ask him—as many questionnaires sent to polios still do—whether he would not like to be rid of the continuing physical effects of that injury.

Few polios I know in Massachusetts, where I now live, would turn down becoming "whole-bodied." But most of the polios that I knew when I was growing up in Quebec *say* to me now, when I visit with them, that they would hesitate to change the lives they have led as crippled people. (Compare their reaction with the predicament of the blind man Virgil Adamson, hero of a medical case study in Oliver Sacks's *An Anthropologist on Mars* and of the 1999 movie *At First Sight*.[98] Adamson becomes desperately unhappy when, after four decades of blindness, he regains his sight.) The Quebec polio Eileen Gagnon writes, "If one were to say to me today that I could be rid of my polio on the condition that I would also be rid of everything ["à la condition de m'enlever aussi tout"] that I have learned during the course of this disease, I would hesitate."[99] Another Canadian, Georgina Bailey, wrote a not overly protesting little essay in 1950 for anglophone Canada's popular *MacLean's Magazine* that she entitled "I'm Glad I Had Polio."[100]

AFTERMATH

What makes a subject hard to understand—if it's something significant and important—is not that before you can understand it you need to be specially trained in abstruse matters, but the contrast between understanding the subject and what most people willfully want to see. Because of this the very things which are most obvious may become the hardest of all to understand. What has to be overcome is a difficulty having to do with the will, rather than with the intellect.

—Ludwig Wittgenstein, *Culture and Value* (1980)

Willful forgetfulness or denial of polio past—and the consequent failure to take up opportunities for the present—arises from what is called, with a certain grim irony, Post-Polio Traumatic Stress Disorder. This term applies not to the traumatic stress of individual polios but instead to the stress on a body politic celebrating a false triumph over an epidemic from which it is still too much in shock to see itself clearly. What has to be overcome on the political level is a difficulty having to do with the will as well as the intellect. The polios now alive are all more than forty-five years old—with very few exceptions, at least in the United States. If we want to study this group, we need to hurry. In a few decades, they—we—will be no more. Even the materials needed to conduct such a study in the future remain to be gathered, as this book helps show. Certainly, consideration of past experience with polio and knowledge of what medical doctors and others did *not* learn and do, in relation to what we might *yet* learn and do, will help prevent struggles with myriad future diseases and similarly terrifying conditions. With regard to whatever other fearful epidemic we may face one day and then essay to efface, we cannot afford politically to make once again the sort of mistakes we made with the polio epidemic. One day, perhaps, we will have effective vaccines and functional designer drugs. At that moment, though, let us not turn away from elementary problems of science, basic questions about treatment, fundamental issues in politics, and vital matters of culture and communication. Their study holds out the greatest promise for humankind. Let us therefore define the sociopathology of forgetting and set out the particular cases and local contexts where denial tends to be persistent. We want to remember how and why we forgot the aftermath of polio.

NOTES

Prologue

1. Roland H. Berg, *Polio and Its Problems* (Philadelphia: Lippincott, 1948).

2. Jane S. Smith, *Patenting the Sun: Polio and the Salk Vaccine* (New York: William Morrow, 1990).

3. Bentz Plagemann, *My Place to Stand* (New York: Farrar, Straus, 1949), vii.

4. *Oxford English Dictionary* (hereafter *OED*), s.v. *Biography,* n. 2.

5. *OED*, s.v. *Polio*, cites popular American sources: *Ladies' Home Journal,* February 1934, 1; *Guardian* 8 (September 26, 1962), 5.

6. Renate Rubenstein begins her book about her multiple sclerosis, *Take It and Leave It: Aspects of Being Ill* (London: Marlon Boyars, 1989), with: "The book is about being ill and about being me. / You can't separate the two." As cited in Judith Monks and Ronald Frankenberg, "Being Ill and Being Me: Self, Body, and Time in Multiple Sclerosis Narratives," 107–134, in Benedicte Ingstad and Susan Reynolds Whyte, *Disability and Culture* (Berkeley: University of California Press, 1995), 129.

7. For instance, *leprosy* and *leper.*

8. Peg Kehret, *Small Steps: The Year I Got Polio* (New York: Albert Whitman, 1996), 10.

9. Leonard Kriegel, *Falling into Life: Essays* (San Francisco: North Point, 1991), 87.

10. Mark Twain, *Three Thousand Years among the Microbes* (1905), in *Which Was the Dream? and Other Symbolic Writings of the Late Years,* ed. John Tuckey (Berkeley: University of California Press, 1967), 233. Twain's "germ" here is cholera. On paralysis, see Mark Twain, "The Damned Human Race" in *Letters from the Earth,* ed. Bernard DeVoto (New York: Harper & Row, 1962).

11. According to some histories, polio epidemics in the United States began with the 132 cases documented in Vermont in 1893–1894, which resulted in eighteen deaths

and thirty victims' being left with permanent paralysis. However, there had been several earlier outbreaks.

12. See Peter Graham, "Metapathography: Three Unruly Texts," *Literature and Medicine* 16 (1997): 70–87.

13. On *convivencia*, or conviviality—meaning "living together with conditions one dislikes but tolerates," see Marc Shell, *Children of the Earth: Literature, Politics, and Nationhood* (New York: Oxford University Press, 1994), 24–26.

14. *OED*, s.v. *Clinical*, 3a.

15. See Daniel J. Wilson, "Covenants of Work and Grace: Themes of Recovery and Redemption in Polio Narratives," *Literature and Medicine* 13 (1994): 22–41.

16. See, for example, Enid Foster, *It Can't Happen to Me* (Cape Town: Timmins, 1959). Foster was writing in Bulawayo, Southern Rhodesia (now Zimbabwe).

17. See, for example, Julie Silver, *Post-Polio Syndrome* (New Haven, Conn.: Yale University Press, 2001).

18. Sally Aitken, Pierette Caron, and Gilles Fournier, eds., *Histoire vécue de la polio au Québec* (Outremont, Canada: Carte Blanche, 2000); *Walking Fingers: The Story of Polio and Those Who Lived with It,* Sally Aitken, Helen D'Orazio, and Stewart Valin, eds. (Montreal: Véhicule, 2004); Janina Ochojska, *Niebo to inni: Z Janina Ochojska rozmawia Wojciech Bonowicz* (Kraków: Spoleczny Instytut Wydawniczy ZNAK, 2000); Barry North, comp., *Something to Lean On: The First Sixty Years of the British Polio Fellowship* (South Ruislip, England: British Polio Fellowship, 1999); Edmund Sass, with George Gottfried and Anthony Sorem, *Polio's Legacy: An Oral History* (Lanham, Md.: University Press of America, 1996).

19. Among manuscripts are those of Linda Jane Laubenstein (1950s, Schlesinger Library) and Charles Ward, "Crippled Thunder" (1999, Collection Selechonek); among the books, Elaine Strauss, *In My Heart I'm Still Dancing* (New Rochelle, N.Y.: Strauss, 1979).

20. See, for example, Monks and Frankenberg, "Being Ill and Being Me."

21. Russell F. Taylor, with Nelson Nix, J. F. Elliott, and Brian J. Sproule, *Polio '53: A Memorial for Russell Frederick Taylor* (Edmonton, Canada: University of Alberta Press, 1990).

22. Christopher James Rutty, "Do Something! . . . Do Anything! Poliomyelitis in Canada, 1927–1955," Ph.D. diss., University Toronto, 1995; A. K. Schanke, B. Lobben, and S. Oyhaugen, "The Norwegian Polio Study, 1994, Part 2: Early Experiences of Polio and Later Psychosocial Well-Being," *Spinal Cord* 37, no. 7 (July 1999): 515–521; T. Bache, "Andreas Christian Bull (1840–1920) and His Survey of Poliomyelitis," *Tidsskrift for Den Norske Laegeforening* 120, no. 27 (November 10, 2000): 3292–3293.

23. Anne Killalea, *Great Scourge: The Tasmanian Infantile Paralysis Epidemic, 1937–1938* (Tasmania, Australia: Tasmanian Historical Research Association, 1995); Robert Williamson Lovett and Herbert C. Emerson, *The Occurrence of Infantile Paralysis in Massachusetts in 1908,* reported for the Massachusetts State Board of Health (Boston: Wright & Potter, 1909).

24. E. A. Piszczek, H. J. Shaughnessy, J. Zichis, and S. O. Levinson, "Acute Anterior Poliomyelitis: Study of an Outbreak in West Suburban Cook County, Ill.: Preliminary Report," *Journal of the American Medical Association* 117 (1941): 1962–1965.

25. Walter S. Goodale, ed., *A Study of the Acute Anterior Poliomyelitis Epidemic which Occurred in the City of Buffalo, New York, U.S.A., during the Year 1912* (Buffalo, N.Y.: Department of Health [1912?]); Francis E. Fronczak, Frank R. Whelply, and Alfred E. Regan, *The Outbreak of Poliomyelitis: City of Buffalo, 1939* (Buffalo, N.Y.: Board of Health, 1940); Haven Emerson, *A Monograph on the Epidemic of Poliomyelitis (Infantile Paralysis): The Epidemic of Poliomyelitis in New York* (New York: Department of Health of New York City, 1917; rpr. New York: Arno, 1977); C. H. Lavinder, A. W. Freeman, and W. H. Frost, *Epidemiologic Studies of Poliomyelitis in New York City and the Northeastern United States during the Year 1916* (Washington, D.C.: U.S. Government Printing Office, 1918).

26. Angela Queste has written of Germany in the period from 1909 to 1970, and K. Eggers has written of Sweden in the period from 1880 to 1965. Both authors confirm the hypothesized connection between socioeconomic development and the incidence of polio-infections. See too Matts Bergmark, *Från pest till polio: Hur farsoterna ingripit i människornas öden* (1957; Avesta: Prisma, 1983).

27. On milk, see Duon H. Miller, "The Truth about Polio" (Coral Gables, Fl.: Polio Prevention, n.d.), four-page brochure; a more serious effort is A. C. Knapp, E. S. Godfrey Jr., and W. L. Aycock, "An Outbreak of Poliomyelitis Apparently Milk Borne" (Chicago: American Medical Association, 1926). On diet, see Benjamin Sandler, *Diet Prevents Polio* (Milwaukee, Wisc.: Lee Foundation for Nutritional Research, 1951).

28. William McNeill, *Plagues and Peoples* (Garden City, N.Y.: Anchor, 1976), esp. 254. See also Naomi Rogers, *Dirt and Disease: Polio before FDR* (New Brunswick, N.J.: Rutgers University Press, 1992).

29. Leonard Kriegel, *The Long Walk Home: An Adventure in Survival* (New York: Appleton-Century, 1964). See also Kriegel, *Falling into Life*, 85.

30. See, for example, Betty Banister, *Trapped: A Polio Victim's Fight for Life* (Saskatoon, Canada: Western Producer Prairie Books, 1975).

31. Charles Mee, *A Nearly Normal Life* (Boston: Little, Brown, 1999), 18–91; emphasis mine.

32. Dr. M. E. Knapp, "Observations on Infantile Paralysis: Symptoms and Treatment," *Lancet* 64 (May 1944): 164, argued that, for polios, mental alienation (as he calls it) is probably a "minor factor" and not "psychologic in origin."

33. Noreen Linduska, *My Polio Past* (Chicago: Pellegrini & Cudahy, 1947), 63, explains the meaning of a term originating with Kenny, *mental alienation,* as it applied to the theory and treatment of polio in the 1940s. "Once I heard of mental alienation," she writes, "I felt I had conquered polio."

34. See Rogers, *Dirt and Disease*; John Gliedman and William Roth, *The Unexpected Minority: Handicapped Children in America* (New York: Harcourt, Brace, Jovanovich, 1982), 1–51.

35. See Philip L. Safford and Elizabeth J. Safford, *A History of Childhood and Disability* (New York: Teachers College Press, 1995), 90–121; Dinah Maria Mulock Craik (Miss Mulock), *The Little Lame Prince and His Travelling Cloak* (London: Daldy, Isbister, 1875).

36. Sir Walter Scott, *Journal* (New York: Harper, 1890), 2:394, April 5, 1831, entry.

37. On narration, see Arthur Kleinman, *The Illness Narratives: Suffering, Healing, and the Human Condition* (New York: Basic, 1988); Howard Brody, *Stories of Sickness* (New Haven, Conn.: Yale University Press, 1987). On transformation, see Sharon R. Kaufman, "Illness, Biography, and the Interpretation of Self Following a Stroke," *Journal of Aging Studies* 213 (1988): 217–227.

38. Robert Murphy, *The Silent Body* (New York: Henry Holt, 1987).

39. See Graham, "Metapathography: Three Unruly Texts."

40. Murphy, *Silent Body*, 4; Monks and Frankenberg, "Being Ill and Being Me," 107–134 (second quotation).

41. Susan Sontag, *Illness as Metaphor* (New York: Farrar, Straus and Giroux, 1978), 5.

42. Susan Sontag, *AIDS and Its Metaphors* (New York: Farrar, Straus and Giroux, 1989), 15, 12.

43. Ibid., 39.

44. Foster recalls, "I had not realized, till then, that my face was so obviously affected. I tried to wink the right eye. It remained steadfastly open in an unwinking stare." Foster, *It Can't Happen*, 24.

45. See Rosemarie Garland Thomson, ed., *Freakery: Cultural Spectacles of the Extraordinary Body* (New York: New York University Press, 1996). For the polio known as Frog Boy, see papers in the Collection Selechonek. Relevant here too is the movie *The Goddess Bunny* (directed by Nick Bougas; VHS 1994), about the polio Johnnie Baima, who transformed himself into "Sandie Crisp."

46. Collection Selechonek.

47. See A. F. W. Peart, "An Outbreak of Poliomyelitis in Canadian Eskimos in Wintertime: Epidemiological Features," *Canadian Journal of Public Health* 40 (October 1949).

48. Consider, for instance, the title of Tony Gould's book, *A Summer Plague*.

49. Angola Press (ANGOP), in its report, "Le Président Dos Santos reçoit une prime pour la lutte contre la poliomyélite en Angola," August 17, 2000.

50. Franklin D. Roosevelt, first inaugural address, March 4, 1933.

51. My source for this figure is the Musée de l'Homme (Paris, France).

52. Peart, "Outbreak of Poliomyelitis."

53. *OED*, s.v. *Plague*, n. 2a. See Exodus 11.1.

54. For the Angel of Death, see Herb Keinon, "*The Prince of Egypt*—Moses and the Seven Dwarfs," (movie review), *Jerusalem Post*, April 2, 1999.

55. It would seem that most cases of polio went unreported.

56. National Office of Vital Statistics of the U.S. Public Health Service reports the figures as 5,072 and 38,153.

57. Sontag, *AIDS and Its Metaphors,* 93.

58. For a relevant study along the lines of literature and disease: Sander L. Gilman, *Franz Kafka: The Jewish Patient* (New York: Routledge, 1995). Examples of flu literature include Katherine Anne Porter, "Pale Horse, Pale Rider," in *Pale Horse, Pale Rider: Three Short Novels* (New York: Modern Library, 1939), and such works by Wallace Stegner as "Chip Off the Old Block," in *Collected Stories of Wallace Stegner* (New York: Random House, 1990).

59. See Robert S. Pynoos, Alan M. Steinberg, and Armen Goenjian, "Traumatic Stress in Childhood and Adolescence: Recent Developments and Current Controversies," in B. A. van der Kolk, Alexander C. McFarlane, and Lars Neisaeth, eds., *Traumatic Stress: The Effects of Overwhelming Experience on Mind, Body, and Society* (New York: Guildford, 1996).

60. Robert Dessaix, *Night Letters* (London: St. Martin's, 1997).

61. In 1959, there were 1,171 reported cases of polio in Quebec, where I grew up. Of these, 106 people died.

62. David Grubin, writer and producer, *The American Experience: FDR* (WGBH, 1994). Grubin relies on statistics gathered by Hugh Gallagher (see the interview with part 1 of Grubin's film). Concerning the medical statistics that in some times and places 25 percent of people who caught polio died within two weeks, see Hugh Gallagher's discussion in the published interview with David McCullough and Geoffrey Ward. Killalea's statistics for Tasmania in the 1930s are corroborating. Different medical traditions, however, have different tests for determining what is polio and what is not: in the 1950s doctors in the United States, for example, usually depended on a spinal tap; but doctors in Germany used other diagnostic tests.

63. Charles Dickens, *A Christmas Carol,* ed. Andrew Lang (London: Chapman and Hall, 1897 [1843]), 60.

64. Charles Schwab, *Man in a Wheelchair* (New York: Exposition, 1961), 13.

65. "One of the peculiarities of polio is that its victims, once they have recovered from the virus and settled down to whatever muscular control it has left them, live a sort of charmed life. Crippled as they are, they are rarely ill, they are surprisingly tough and durable, and they astonish their sound companions with their capacity to endure." Stegner goes on: "But that is not forever." Wallace Stegner, *Crossing to Safety* (New York: Random House, 1987), 273.

66. Piero della Francesca, *Resurrection* (1463), mural in fresco and tempera, 225 × 200 cm., Museo Civico, Sansepolcro. Stegner wrote about the influenza epidemic in "Chip off the Old Block," in his *Collected Stories.*

67. Such a leper colony was in operation on Massachusetts' Penikese Island from 1905 to 1921. See I. Thomas Buckley, *Penikese, Island of Hope: One of the Elizabeths—A Massachusetts Historical Site,* ed. Meg B. Springer (Brewster, Mass.: Stony Brook Publishing, 1997).

68. Sir Thomas Clouston, "A Case of General Paralysis at the Age of Sixteen," *Journal of Mental Science* 23 (1877).

69. *OED,* s.v. *Paresis.*

70. Montaigne, *The Essays* 3.11, "Of Cripples," trans. Charles Cotton, ed. William Carew Hazlitt (1877). "Le boiteux le faict le mieux."

71. On time and recovery after polio, see F. Davis, "Definitions of Time and Recovery in Paralytic Polio Convalescence," *American Journal of Sociology* 61 (1956): 582–587.

72. Shell, *Children of the Earth,* esp. 125, 208, n. 111.

73. See Joyce Ann Tepley, "Polio Memories from the Class of 1952 and Maturing with Polio," in "Appendix: Personal Stories," in Lauro Halstead and Naomi Naierman, eds., *Managing Post-Polio: A Guide to Living Well with Post Polio Syndrome* (Clearwater, Fla.: ABI Professional Publications, 1998), 191.

74. "Late effects of polio" is used in, for example, Frederick M Maynard and Joan L. Headley, eds., *Handbook on the Late Effects of Poliomyelitis for Physicians and Survivors,* 2nd ed. (Saint Louis, Mo.: Gazette International Networking Institute, 1999); see also Lauro S. Halstead and David O. Wiechers, eds., *Research and Clinical Aspects of the Late Effects of Poliomyelitis* (New York: March of Dimes Birth Defects Foundation, 1987). For the term *late sequelae of polio,* see M. C. Dalakas, "The Post-Polio Syndrome as an Evolved Clinical Entity: Definition and Clinical Description," *Annals of the New York Academy of Sciences* 753 (May 1995): 68–80.

75. See Theodore L. Munsat, *Post-Polio Syndrome* (Burlington, Mass.: Butterworth-Heinemann, 1991); and Halstead and Naierman, *Managing Post-Polio.*

76. David O. Wiechers, "Effects of Polio: Historical Perspectives," esp. 1–5, in Halstead and Wiechers, *Research and Clinical Aspects,* dates the first diagnoses or descriptions of what we now call PPS to the 1870s.

77. Albert B. Sabin argued that many cases of "summer grippe" or "sore throat" were actually polio.

78. See Albert. B. Sabin and A. J. Steigman, "Poliomyelitis Virus of Low Virulence in Patients with Epidemic 'Summer Grippe or Sore Throat,' " *American Journal Hygiene* 49 (1949): 176–193. The figure six million is cited by Dr. Richard L. Bruno of the International Post-Polio Task Force at Englewood Hospital and Medical Center, Englewood, New Jersey.

79. Again, the figure (65 percent) is cited by Dr. Richard L. Bruno of the International Post-Polio Task Force.

80. Helen Henderson, "Polio Still Stalks," *Toronto Star,* August 17, 2001, F-1. "Although North America was declared polio-free seven years ago, post-polio syndrome is in fact emerging as one of the hidden time bombs of the twenty-first century."

1. One Polio Story

1. On the military significance of poliomyelitis during World War II, see John Rodman Paul, *History of Poliomyelitis* (New Haven, Conn.: Yale University Press, 1971), 346 ff., 421. The Canadian representative was A. J. Rhodes, director, Research Institute, Hospital for Sick Children, Toronto, Canada. He was the *rapporteur* for the group.

2. See the polio pin (1954) illustrated in Dorothy and Philip Sterling, *Polio Pioneers: The Story of the Fight against Polio* (Garden City, N.J.: Doubleday, 1955).

3. Nina Gilden Seavey, Jane S. Smith, and Paul Wagner, *A Paralyzing Fear: The Triumph over Polio in America* (New York: TV Books, 1998), 174.

4. On Kahlo's nickname "Peg-leg," see Andrea Kettenmann, *Frida Kahlo: Pain and Passion, 1907–1954* (Cologne: Benedikt Taschen,1993), 10.

5. Tony Gould, *A Summer Plague: Polio and Its Survivors* (New Haven, Conn.: Yale University Press, 1995). B. Davies, "Death Walks in Summer," *Canadian Magazine* 82 (July 1932): 7.

6. Dr. Joseph P. Moody, with W. de Groot van Embden, *Arctic Doctor* (New York: Dodd, Mead, 1955). See also A. F. W. Peart, "An Outbreak of Poliomyelitis in Canadian Eskimos in Wintertime," *Canadian Journal Public Health* 40 (1949), esp. 405; and Paul, *History of Poliomyelitis,* and other studies mentioned there, 360–361.

7. Saint-Augustine Saguenay is on the coast in Quebec, not far from the border with Labrador. See V. Pavilanis and A. Frappier, "A Winter Epidemic of Poliomyelitis in Saint-Augustine, Que.," *Canadian Medical Association Journal* 79 (July 1, 1958): 11–14.

8. Charles Solomon Caverly, *Infantile Paralysis in Vermont, 1894–1922: A Memorial to Charles S. Caverly, M.D.* (Burlington: Vermont State Department of Publication; Burlington, Vt.: State Department of Public Health, 1924).

9. Dominion Bureau of Statistics. See Christopher J. Rutty, " 'Do Something! . . . Do Anything!': Poliomyelitis in Canada, 1927–1962," Ph.D. diss., University of Toronto, 1995, 397.

10. Ibid., 399.

11. Roosevelt's family did not report FDR's polio to the Canadian authorities. See the correspondence sent by Dr. E. H. Bennet to Dr. Robert Lovett on August 27, 1921, and also Lovett's response to Bennet on August 31, 1921. Both letters are contained in the Robert W. Lovett Collection of the Francis A. Countway Library of Medicine, Harvard University, Boston; see Richard Thayer Goldberg, *The Making of Franklin D. Roosevelt: Triumph over Adversity* (Cambridge, Mass.: Abt, 1981), 43.

12. Mia Farrow, *What Falls Away: A Memoir* (New York: Doubleday, 1997), 1.

13. "Well said, old mole! canst work i' the earth so fast? / A worthy pioner!" William Shakespeare, *Hamlet,* 1.5.

14. Garth Drabinsky, *Closer to the Sun: An Autobiography* (Toronto: McClelland and Stewart, 1995), 13.

15. Earl Bailly, *His Trials and Triumphs* (n.p., 1957), 3. Vivienne Overheu, *It Helps to Be Stubborn* (Perth, Australia: Saint Georges, 1984), 7.

16. Betty Cavanna, *Joyride* (New York: Morrow, 1974), 24.

17. Writes Jenny Danielson in an e-mail message of December 16, 2000: "I can not remember much of anything prior to my polio days in 1955 at the age of 14. I've been told that the high temperature during polio and the body trying to regulate the disease of polio and trying to survive that polio probably wiped out any earlier memories as a child. I have missed much of my earlier life and no memory whatsoever.—Jenny"

18. Judith Rossner, *Looking for Mr. Goodbar* (New York: Simon and Shuster, 1975), 13: "When she was four her limbs had been briefly paralyzed by polio. She remembered none of it. Not the hospital, not the sisters who took care of her, not the respirator she'd needed to breathe. The illness was said to have altered her personality, and maybe that was why she couldn't remember; she'd become another person."

19. Owen Dixson, a Briton, begins his polio autobiography as follows: "Some people claim they can well remember personal and historical happenings that occurred when they were still at a very early age. For myself, I can only recall a very few incidents during the five years of my pre-polio existence." Owen Dixson, *My Way with Polio: An Autobiography by Owen Dixson* (London: Merritt and Hatcher, n.d. [1960]), 3.

20. Peter Brooks, "Freud's Masterplot," in *Reading for the Plot: Designs and Intention in Narrative* (Oxford: Clarendon 1984), 90–112.

21. Cathy Caruth, *Trauma: Explorations in Memory* (Baltimore, Md.: Johns Hopkins University Press, 1995), 4–5.

22. Martha Ramsey, *Where I Stopped: Remembering Rape at Thirteen* (New York: Putnam's Sons, 1995). Susan J. Brison, "Trauma Narratives and the Remaking of the Self," in M. Bal, J. Crewe, and L. Spitzer, eds., *Acts of Memory: Cultural Recall in the Present* (Hanover, N.H.: University Press of New England, 1999), 40.

23. Leonard Kriegel, *Falling into Life: Essays* (San Francisco: North Point, 1991), 88.

24. Gen. 2:24 (I cite the King James version throughout).

25. The Collection Selechonek includes official Public Health Board quarantine signs from the 1950s.

26. See Howard Markel, *Quarantine! East European Jewish Immigrants and the New York City Epidemics of 1892* (Baltimore, Md.: Johns Hopkins University Press, 1997).

27. On the earlier American controversy between those who argued for sanitary measures, as being more important than quarantine in dealing with epidemics, see J. H. Powell, *Bring Out Your Dead: The Great Plague of Yellow Fever in Philadelphia in 1793* (New York: Time, 1949), 14.

28. Paul, *History of Poliomyelitis,* 148.

29. Concerning this subject in Lange's oeuvre, see "Interview with Photographer Dorothea Lange by Suzanne B. Riess, 1960–1961," sponsored by the Regional Oral History Office of the Bancroft Library, University of California, Berkeley," in a transcript, *Dorothea Lange: The Making of a Documentary Photographer,* at the Schlesinger Library, Harvard University. See also Roger Daniels, "Dorothea Lange and the War Relocation Authority: Photographing Japanese Americans," in Elizabeth Partridge, ed., *Dorothea Lange: A Visual Life* (Washington, D.C.: Smithsonian Institution Press, 1994).

30. Tom Atkins, *One Door Closes, Another Opens: Personal Experiences of Polio* (London: Waltham Forest Oral History Workshop—Vestry House Museum, 1994).

31. Nancy M. Frick, "The Contribution of Childhood Physical and Emotional Trauma to the Development of the Post-Polio Personality," *Proceedings of the Ontario March of Dimes Conference on Post-Polio Sequelae* (Toronto: Ontario March of Dimes, 1995). Revised April 2000.

32. See Fred Davis, *Passage through Crisis: Polio Victims and Their Families* (New

Brunswick, N.J.: Transaction, 1991 [1963]), ix–x. The 1991 version has a new introduction. Davis cites Peter Conrad, "Classics Revisited," *Disabilities and Chronic Disease Quarterly* 4, no. 3 (July 1984): 20–21.

33. Robert Lovering (who had polio in 1946) offers discussions of self-image, social acceptance, and architectural barriers in *Out of the Ordinary: A Digest on Disability* (Phoenix, Ariz.: ARCS, 1985). See also Irving Kenneth Zola, *Missing Pieces: A Chronicle of Living With a Disability* (Philadelphia: Temple University Press, 1982). See also Irving Kenneth Zola, ed., *Ordinary Lives: Voices of Disability and Disease* (Cambridge, Mass.: Apple-wood Books, 1982).

34. Emily Dickinson, *The Complete Poems of Emily Dickinson*, ed. T. H. Johnson (Boston: Little, Brown), 162.

35. Camille Savard, "Témoignage," in Sally Aitken, Pierette Caron, and Gilles Fournier, eds., *Histoire vécue de la polio au Québec* (Outremont, Canada: Carte Blanche, 2000), 205. "Je constate combien c'est terrible d'avoir tant souffert et tant travaillé pour me retrouver, aujourd'hui, au point de départ."

36. Peg Kehret, "Epilogue," in *Small Steps: The Year I Got Polio* (New York: Albert Whitman, 1996), 173–174.

37. Robert Mauro, *The Landscape of My Disability* (Berkeley, Calif.: Lemonade Factory, 1998), 4.

38. For examples of "almost complete" recoveries, see Edmund Sass, with George Gottfried and Anthony Sorem, *Polio's Legacy: An Oral History* (Lanham, Md.: University Press of America, 1996), 193–224.

39. Georgina Bailey, "I'm Glad I Had Polio," *Maclean's*, October 1, 1950.

40. "Doctor Says 3/4 of Victims Recover Fully from Polio," *Winnipeg Free Press*, September 1, 1953. See also Rutty," 'Do Something!' " 190.

41. See especially Frederick M. Maynard and Sunny Roller, "Recognizing Typical Coping Styles of Polio Survivors Can Improve Rehabilitation," undated paper, Department of Physical Rehabilitation, University of Michigan; Karen P. Butterfield and Jean Ross, eds., *Mind over Muscle: Surviving Polio in New Zealand* (Palmerston North, New Zealand: Dunsmore, 1994): 115–117. See also Brenda Jo Brueggemann, "On (Almost) Passing," *College English* 59 (Octoer 1997): 647–660.

42. For the term *passers*, see Nancy Baldwin Carter, *Myths and Chicken Feet: A Polio Survivor Looks at Survival* (Omaha: Nebraska Polio Survivors Association Press, 1992), 1.

43. Ibid., 11.

44. Kriegel comes to recognize this notion that the body rules the mind when, after years of successfully negotiating walking, he falls and, for the first time, discovers that he can no longer get up on his own. "My body had decided—and decided on its own, autonomously—that the moment had come for me to face the question of endings. It was the body that chose its time of recognition." Kriegel, *Falling into Life*, 17.

45. "Recognition, as the name indicates," says Aristotle, "is a change from ignorance to knowledge, producing love or hate between the persons destined by the poet for good or bad fortune. The best form of recognition," claims Aristotle, "is coincident

with a reversal, as in the *Oedipus*." Aristotle, *Poetics*, trans. S. H. Butcher (New York: Hill and Wang, 1961), pt. 11. In Oedipus' case the reversal, triggered by a Corinthian drunkard's outrageous statement about Oedipus' familial origin (that he is a *plastos*) or by an obscure statement by the Oracle at Delphi about his progenitors (that he will kill his father and marry his mother), is an apparent return to childhood or even to the womb *(delphos)*. For the polio, the actual boomerang of recognition is triggered at the moment that PPS strikes.

46. Adapted from Apollodorus, *Bibliotheca* 3.5.8; 348–349, in *Apollodorus: The Library*, trans. James George Frazer, 2 vols. (Cambridge, Mass.: Harvard University Press, 1921).

47. On punning meanings of *Oedipous* in Sophocles' play, see Marc Shell, *The End of Kinship* (Palo Alto, Calif.: Stanford University Press, 1988).

48. In Judith Rossner's novel *Looking for Mr. Goodbar,* the scar keeps coming up as an important thing, for example, near the end (202).

49. The full history of surgery for infant polios still remains to be written; however, various standard manuals used by surgeons during the period of 1930 to 1960 lay out the options.

50. J. Krol, ed., *Rehabilitation Surgery for Deformities Due to Poliomyelitis,* illustrated by Patrick Virolle (Geneva: World Health Organization, February 1994).

51. For an analysis of this term, *plastos,* in Sophocles' *Oedipous tyrannous* (l. 780), see my *The Economy of Literature* (Baltimore, Md.: Johns Hopkins University Press, 1978), esp. 98.

52. Many polios, looking back on their treatment, use the language of torture when describing the application of hot branding irons to the backs of patients until the blood shows and congeals. See Paul, *History of Poliomyelitis.* Plagemann refers to the torture of being upside-down for a week on a Bradford frame in Warm Springs, Bentz Plagemann, *My Place to Stand* (London: Gollancz, 1950), 148, 166.

53. "Many individuals have difficulties adjusting to new disabilities. For some people with PPS, reliving their childhood experiences with polio can be a traumatic and even terrifying experience." Source: Post-Polio Health International (PHI), formerly Gazette International Networking (GINI), http://www.geocities.com/HotSprings/4760/GINIfaq.html.

54. Constantine P. Cavafy's poem, "Body, Remember" (1918), is included in *Cavafy Collected Poems,* trans. Edmund Keeley and Philip Sherrard (Princeton, N.J.: Princeton University Press, 1980).

55. When I tried to obtain records from Quebec, I learned that none were extant. And when, in 1998, I contacted the Ottawa offices of Dr. Alton Goldbloom's son, he told me that his father's records had been destroyed about a decade earlier.

56. Caroline Eyring Miner and Edward L. Kimball, *Camilla: A Biography of Camilla Eyring Kimball* (Salt Lake City, Utah: Deseret Books, 1980).

57. Comments by Basil C. McLean of Strong Memorial Hospital, Rochester, New York, commenting on John A. Anderson, "Diagnosis and Treatment of Poliomyelitis in the Early Stage," in International Poliomyelitis Congress, ed., *Poliomyelitis: Papers and*

Discussions Presented at the First International Poliomyelitis Conference (Philadelphia: Lippincott, 1949), 120.

58. Thus, Paul Decoste kept his children away from the Hôtel-Dieu de Chicoutimi. See his "Témoignage," in Aitken, Caron, and Fournier, *Histoire vécue*, 242. Eventually Decoste's children were seen at Hôpital Pasteur in Montréal.

59. Dore Schary, *Sunrise at Campobello: A Play in Three Acts* (New York: Random House, 1958), 19.

60. On blowing straws, see Daniel J. Wilson, "Covenants of Work and Grace: Themes of Recovery and Redemption in Polio Narratives," *Literature and Medicine* 13 (1994): 22–41. On Perceval, see *Fifty Years of Perceval Drawings*, comp. Ken McGregor (Sydney: Bay Books, 1989). See also John Perceval, *Boys' Ward, Stonnington* (1938), pencil on paper, 30 × 24 cm., private collection, in *Fifty Years of Perceval Drawings*, 51.

61. Turnley Walker, *Rise Up and Walk* (New York: Dutton, 1950). Walker's book is from the series of articles "I Am a Polio" syndicated by the North American Newspaper Alliance. John Gunther wrote about this book: "A tender and discerning book about the kind of faith and courage that overcomes a tragedy. Anyone who has suffered the ravages of illness, particularly those crippled by infantile paralysis, will find an inspiring message in this book."

62. Edward Said, *Out of Place: A Memoir* (New York: Knopf, 1999).

63. As reported in Anne Killalea, *The Great Scourge: The Tasmanian Infantile Paralysis Epidemic, 1937–38* (Sandy Bay, Australia: Tasmanian Historical Research Association, 1995), 101. See also Richard Chaput, *Not to Doubt* (New York: Pageant, 1960); Richard Chaput, *All I Can Give* (Canfield, Ohio: Alba House Communications, 1972).

64. On relative per capita sizes of polio epidemics, see "Major World Infantile Paralysis Epidemics (Non-Virgin Soil)," in Killalea, *Great Scourge*, 135–136. The only known epidemic that might well have been worse than that of Tasmania (421 per 100,000) would be the one in Iceland in 1924 (sometimes said to be 480 per 100,000). By comparison, the New York City epidemic in 1916—usually taken to be the worst—was only 28.5 per 100,000.

65. Said Albright in interview: "I don't remember fear about being sick. The fear I had was staying in the—hospital overnight. I couldn't imagine anything worse. But no one—told me how serious it was. In fact, they took the sign *POLIO* off my door."

66. Marie Morgart, *Abandoned Child* (Virginia Beach, Va.: Cornerstone, 1995), n.p.

67. Suzanne Martel, "Témoignage," in Aitken, Caron, and Fournier, *Histoire vécue*.

68. Rossner, *Looking for Mr. Goodbar*, 155. Consider also the heroine's dream of being strapped down and bound, 210.

69. Morgart, *Abandoned*, writes that "the physical difference between my legs did bother me." That is why she asked this question.

70. Davis, *Passage through Crisis*, 21.

71. In Antonioni's *Il Deserto rosso* (*The Red Desert*, 1964) the heroine comes to fear that her son has polio. Eventually she discovers that the boy is faking. Her fear that her son has polio is replaced by a fear that she is not needed.

72. For other children in this situation, see Davis, *Passage through Crisis*, 25. In the

movie *Where the Money Is* (2000), starring Paul Newman and Linda Fiorentino and directed by Marek Kanievska, a nurse discovers that one of her catatonic patients actually faked his paralytic stroke to get out of prison.

73. Garth Drabinsky, *Closer to the Sun: An Autobiography* (Toronto: McClelland and Stewart, 1995), 14.

74. Davis, *Passage through Crisis,* 36, 27.

75. See Garrett Oppenheim, *The Golden Handicap: A Spiritual Quest* (Virginia Beach, Va.: A. R. E. Press, 1993). See also Garrett Oppenheim, "A Karmic Case of Polio," *Journal of Regression Therapy* 2, no. 1 (Spring 1987): 58–60, in which he attributes the onset of his polio to problems in former lives.

76. Luke 17:32.

77. The words *infantile* and *ineffable* are two sides of the same coin, the first meaning "that which cannot speak" and the second "that which cannot be spoken or expressed."

78. Pat Cunningham Devoto, *My Last Days as Roy Rogers* (New York: Time Warner, 1999), 285. The man who says this turns out to be a crook.

79. William Russel MacAusland, *Poliomyelitis, with Especial Reference to the Treatment* (Philadelphia: Lea & Febiger, 1927), 85, citing the New York City poliomyelitis epidemic (1916).

80. Miner and Kimball, *Camilla.*

81. In *The Epidemiology of Rheumatic Fever* (New York, 1957 [1930]), John R. Paul writes, "There is little evidence to support the removal of tonsils which are diseased as a means of preventing rheumatic fever" (140). He writes elsewhere about problems that tonsillectomies actually cause. Associated with rheumatic fever is *scarlatina*, another word for scarlet fever.

82. See M. Talmey, "Reflections on Predisposing Factors in Infantile Paralysis," *New York Medical Journal* 104 (1916): 202. See also W. L. Aycock and E. H. Luther, "The Occurrence of Poliomyelitis Following Tonsillectomy," *New England Journal of Medicine* 200 (1929): 164.

83. See Paul, *History of Poliomyelitis,* 189.

84. "The Sum of Our Knowledge" is the title of the last chapter of Berg's 1948 book, *Polio and Its Problems.* For the Akron history, see 90–96. Writes Berg of the studies done at Akron (95–96): "These findings were important, for they showed that a person can harbor the virus in his body and indeed spread it to others without suffering any ill effect himself. However, when an additional factor is added, such as a tonsil operation or tooth extraction, it may render the subject more susceptible to a serious type of the disease. The study emphasizes the dangers of tonsil operations during the months when poliomyelitis is prevalent, even though cases of the disease have not been reported in the community. It showed that a tonsillectomy may transform a mild, sub-clinical infection of infantile paralysis into a sever, paralyzing and fatal disease. This was the lesson learned from the Tragedy at Akron."

85. L. Jessner and S. Kaplan, "Children's Emotional Reactions to Tonsillectomy," in

J. E. Milton, ed., *Problems of Infancy and Childhood: Transactions of the Third Conference* (New York: Josiah Macy, Jr., Foundation, 1949). This work is referenced in Anna Freud, "The Role of Bodily Illness in the Mental Life of Children," *Psychoanalytic Study of the Child* 7 (1952): 69–81. Anna Freud discusses "a recent symposium on the Emotional Reactions of Children to Tonsillectomy and Adenoidectomy."

86. See Sass, *Polio's Legacy,* 266. For the Boines method, see George J. Boines, "The Use of Curare in a Repository Medium in the Management of Acute Poliomyelitis," *American Practice* (November 1952): 879–880. Dr. George J. Boines was in contact with Elizabeth Kenny between 1941 and 1946; see item 143.E.10.6F, box 4, Minnesota Historical Institute. On the curare cure, see Elaine Strauss, *In My Heart I'm Still Dancing* (New Rochelle, N.Y.: Strauss, 1979), 124. Curare as a treatment was recommended by Evelynne G. Knouf; see "Medical Management of the Patient with Acute Poliomyelitis: General Considerations," in Albert G. Bower, *Diagnosis and Treatment of the Acute Phase of Poliomyelitis and Its Complications* (Baltimore, Md.: Williams and Wilkins, 1954), 44.

87. Enid Foster, *It Can't Happen to Me* (Cape Town: Timmins, 1959), 37.

88. For Haast's case, see Mark R. Glasberg, "Amyotrophic Lateral Sclerosis: Unorthodox Treatments," in *Amyotrophic Lateral Sclerosis: A Comprehensive Guide to Management* (New York: Demos, 1994), 53–61; quotation on 54. See also Harry Kursh, *Cobras in His Garden* (Irvington-on-Hudson, N.Y.: Harvey House, 1965). Lorenzo Wilson Milam, *The Cripple Liberation Front Marching Band Blues* (San Diego, Calif.: Mho & Mho Works, 1984).

89. Wrote Rudyard Kipling, in "Our Fathers of Old": "Bleed and blister as much as you will, / Blister and bleed him as oft as you please." Rudyard Kipling, *The Collected Works of Rudyard Kipling,* 28 vols. (Garden City, N.Y.: Doubleday, 1941), vol. 13.

90. Thanks to the fact that so many surgeons were out of work after the World War I, many new surgeries developed, some merely cosmetic and others harmful in the end.

91. The 1951 photograph of Mary Guy, one of the Tasmanians who suffered this treatment, shows the rigid positioning of all body parts except the head: Anne Killalea, *Great Scourge,* 103. Killalea notes that this photograph is included in a photo album at Wingfield House, a Tasmanian "polio after-care home" of the period (151).

92. See Victor Cohn, *Sister Kenny: The Woman Who Challenged the Doctors* (Minneapolis: University of Minnesota Press, 1975).

93. Elizabeth Kenny, with Martha Otenso, *And They Shall Walk: The Life Story of Sister Elizabeth Kenny* (New York: Dodd & Mead, 1943).

94. John Florian M. Pohl, *The Kenny Concept of Infantile Paralysis and Its Treatment* (Minneapolis: Bruce, 1943). See also Wallace Hasbrouk Cole, *The Kenny Method of Treatment for Infantile Paralysis* (New York: National Foundation for Infantile Paralysis, 1942). On guidelines for nurses, see A *Guide for Nurses in the Nursing Care of Patients with Infantile Paralysis: Including Nursing Aspects of the Kenny Method* (New York: National Foundation for Infantile Paralysis, 1943). On parents, see Joint Orthopedic Nursing Advisory Service of the National Organization for Public Health Nursing and

the National League of Nursing Education, *A Guide for Parents in the Nursing Care of Patients with Infantile Paralysis in the Home,* 2d ed. (New York: National Foundation for Infantile Paralysis, 1944).

95. In January 1952, the annual Gallup survey showed that Kenny was the most admired woman in America. For the previous twenty years, it had been Eleanor Roosevelt.

96. Milam, *Cripple,* 48.

97. Turnley Walker, *Roosevelt and the Warm Springs Story* (New York: A. A. Wyn, 1953).

98. Joseph S. Barr, "The Management of Poliomyelitis: The Late Stage," in *Poliomyelitis: Papers and Discussions Presented at the First International Poliomyelitis Conference* (Philadelphia: Lippincott, 1949), 201.

99. R. W. Lovett, "Fatigue and Exercise in the Treatment of Infantile Paralysis: A Study of 1,836 Cases," *Journal of the American Medical Association* 69 (1917): 168; see also Lovett and W. P. Lucas, "Infantile Paralysis: A Study of 635 Cases from the Children's Hospital, Boston, with Especial Reference to Treatment," *Journal of the American Medical Association* 51 (1908): 1,677.

100. W. J. W. Sharrard, "The Distribution of the Permanent Paralysis in the Lower Limb in Poliomyelitis: A Clinical and Pathological Study," *Journal of Bone and Joint Surgery* 37, no. B.4 (November 1955): 540–558. The reference here is to J. J. Sedden's work in England on testing polio-affected muscles: J. J. Sedden, "Poliomyelitis: Part 2—Treatment of Poliomyelitis," in E. Rock Carling and Sir J. Paterson Ross, eds., *British Surgical Practice, Surgical Progress: 1954* (London: Butterworth, 1955), 162.

101. William P. Frank, "Diagnosis and Differential Diagnosis of Poliomyelitis," in Bower, *Diagnosis and Treatment of the Acute Phase,* 15, 39.

102. Charles L. Lowman, "Orthopedic Treatment, Including Bracing," ibid., 210.

103. Kipling, "Our Fathers of Old," *Collected Works.*

104. *National Review* 1 (Melbourne), August 31, 1973, 1455; emphasis mine.

105. Schary, *Sunrise at Campobello,* 19.

106. On vaccination and the iron lung, Sharon Stern says: "When I was still in the acute hospital, in the lung, I remember seeing on the news that the vaccine was being tried in spot areas around the country. Most of the news stories reported cases where the children actually came down with polio from the vaccine. There was a lot of controversy then. Nobody really trusted the vaccine and so they did emphasize, at least in my memory, those cases where the kids got polio from the vaccine. I don't remember thinking or feeling much about it either way. My mother wept about it, she actually wept. She said to me, 'Couldn't you have waited for seven months?' but there was no answer . . . I couldn't answer." http://www.pbs.org/wgbh/peoplescentury/episodes.

107. Edward Le Comte, *Long Road Back: The Story of My Encounter with Polio* (New York: Philosophical Library, 1958). In the case of Le Comte, an associate professor of English at Columbia University who got polio in 1954, there had been some question whether to have the vaccine in 1955–56 or not (40–41, 116). Wilfrid Sheed, *In Love With Daylight: A Memory of a Recovery* (New York: Simon and Shuster, 1995), 54: "They

never did learn very much about polio, if you'll recall, except how to prevent it, and I was surprised at the force of my irritation the day I first read about Dr. Jonas Salk and his famous vaccine." He adds, "We were *last* year's cover story now" (56). In fiction for adolescents, too, the difficulties surrounding the introduction of the vaccine play a key role. Consider the beginning of one, set in the summer of 1955: Susan Terris, *Wings and Roots* (New York: Farrar, Straus and Giroux, 1982), 8. Jeannie is a young girl who has been vaccinated against polio and has volunteered to do work in a polio ward. She meets Kit, a young polio who contracted polio just before the Salk vaccine was introduced. They have this conversation: " 'I'm going to be a doctor,' " Jeannie said. 'Wonderful! Marvelous! You'll be a *doctor,* and I'll be the crip making potholders at the Goodwill workshop. And you've had the vaccine, so you'll never get what I got. Nor will anyone else after this lousy year. How's that for lousy, stinking timing? Dr. Jonas Salk's going to wipe out polio, and I'm going to be left like this forever. Why me?' " Like such real-life polios as William Douglas, Kit goes on to become something of a mountain climber; Jeannie and Kit become the closest of friends.

108. This was one of the general controversies surrounding the vaccine. See Aaron E. Klein, *Trial by Fury: The Polio Vaccine Controversy* (New York: Charles Scribner's Sons, 1972).

109. Jerome Brooks, *Big Dipper Marathon* (New York: Dutton, 1979), 8. The boy's having contracted polio, presumably from the vaccine, is considered a "freakish" fact (55): "a statistic maybe in *The Guinness Book of World Records.*"

110. See Eleanor McBean, "The Hidden Dangers in the Polio Vaccine," chap. 4 of *The Poisoned Needle* (self-published, 1960); Mira Louise, *Protection from Polio and Animal Research* (1956); in Collection Selechonek. There were much earlier printings. This one featured eighty pages of newspaper clippings. McBean worked with other anti-vaccine crackpots, such as Herbert M. Shelton and Morris A. Beale.

111. Virginia Lee Counterman Acosta, *Polio Tragedy of 1941* (n.p., 1999), 85. The post-polio Acosta returns to the subject of childhood polio precisely in order to explain the vaccine to children: "I have written this book so first graders and up can read and understand it. I have seen children get their polio vaccinations. They say that it hurts. I tell them they will never know the pain of polio. When you read this book, you will understand." These words appear on the back cover of the book.

112. Bubbie is Yiddish for "grandmother." Zeyde (later) is "grandfather."

113. See Davis, *Passage through Crisis,* 41.

114. Cavanna, *Joyride,* 41.

115. Roxane Frigon, "Témoignage," in Aitken, Caron, and Fournier, *Histoire vécue,* 62. "Ce témoignage me permet, pour la première fois de ma vie, de réellement parler de mon handicap."

116. Lewis Carroll [Charles Lutwidge Dodgson], chap. 5, "Advice from a Caterpillar," in *Alice's Adventures in Wonderland,* illus. Sir John Tenniel (London: Macmillan, 1865).

117. William Shakespeare, *Romeo and Juliet,* 2.2.

118. A relatively recent version of the *Captain America* story (the movie of 1989–

1990) goes as follows: In the 1940s, the U.S. government recruits a scientist from Germany, from behind the Nazi lines, to help create a fighter to take on the "Red Skull." This fighter is a young polio victim, Steve Rogers, who becomes Captain America, after having been frozen in Alaska for forty years and then taking a special serum that changes him into a superman. See the cover of *Captain America* comics, no. 39 (June 1944). Joel Matus, *Leroy and the Caveman* (New York: Atheneum, 1993), has a similar plot; its story intertwines these elements: a caveman, World War II German spies, an orphan, and a boy recovering from polio.

119. *The Wizard of Oz* (film, 1939).

120. Old Hickory makes this complaint near the beginning of the movie, while working on the wind machine in the barn in Kansas.

121. L. Frank Baum, *The Wonderful Wizard of Oz* (Chicago: G. M. Hill, 1900), chap. 5.

122. The Tin Man later tells us he was frozen one day while "chopping that tree—minding my own business."

123. See *A Decade of Doing*, a twenty-page pamphlet on the history of the medical treatment of polio in the United States, published in 1948 by the National Foundation for Infantile Paralysis. A grant was given to Dr. George Washington Carver to develop a combined massage and peanut oil therapy for the treatment of polio. (The oil is still available today—Curtis Rubbing Oil, named after Carver's assistant, Dr. A. W. Curtis.)

124. For leg amputation and restoration, see L. Frank Baum, *The Tin Woodman of Oz: A Faithful Story of the Astonishing Adventure Undertaken by the Tin Woodman,* illustrated by John Rae Neill (Chicago: Reilly and Britton, 1918). Chapter 1 already promises a story of limb removal and restoration. For voice reparation, see Baum, *Tin Woodman,* chap. 2, which begins thus: "The Emperor of the Winkies paused in his story to reach for an oil-can, with which he carefully oiled the joints in his tin throat, for his voice had begun to squeak a little."

2. In the Family

1. See *Life,* July 1944, cited in Patricia M. Sarchet, "Archeology of Deadly Meanings: Polio and HIV Photographs," M.A. thesis, State University of New York, Buffalo, 1968. Eisenstadt was also involved in the movie *Sunrise at Campobello.*

2. According to several sources, some 250,000 disabled persons died in the gas chambers.

3. The Young Men's / Young Women's Hebrew Association at the corner of Côte Sainte Catherine Road and Westbury Avenue, in Snowdon, Montreal, Quebec.

4. With regard to the theme song, "Hi Lili Hilo," complementary aspects of *Lili* (1953, words and music by Branislau Kaper and Helen Deutsch; starring Leslie Caron and Mel Ferrer) encouraged this sort of identification.

5. Tony Kemeny, with Roy Hayes, *A Puppet No More* (n.p.: Thomas Litho & Printing, 1963). Kemeny was not a Jewish child but an escaped orphan with polio and conse-

quent paralysis of the legs. Out of loneliness, he taught himself puppetry (starting with puppets made from dirty socks!) and adopted his personal creed: "No one should make the children pay to see puppets." In the streets of wartime Budapest, an inmate of Dachau concentration camp, the official mascot of the 103d American Infantry Division, and an accused spy.

6. This book, in the Collection Selechonek, was purchased in 2000 from Center Ministry, P.O. Box 158933, Nashville, Tenn. 37215.

7. Ilona Karmel, *Stephania* (New York: Houghton Mifflin, 1953).

8. Karmel's later work, *An Estate of Memory* (Boston: Houghton Mifflin, 1969), re-creates the daily lives of four Jewish women in a Nazi concentration camp in Poland. See Ann Shapiro, Sara Horowitz, Ellen Schiff, and Miriyam Glazer, eds., *Jewish American Women Writers: A Bio-Bibliographical and Critical Sourcebook* (Westport, Conn.: Greenwood, 1994), and Lilian Kremer, *Women's Holocaust Writing: Memory and Imagination* (Lincoln: University of Nebraska Press, 1999).

9. During her bout with polio, Elaine Strauss imagines that she is being tortured by Nazis. Elaine Strauss, *In My Heart I'm Still Dancing* (New Rochelle, N.Y.: Strauss, 1979), 20.

10. *Captain America* comics, created by Jacky Kirby and Joe Simon, were commonly issued from 1941 to 1954.

11. Larry Kramer, *The Normal Heart*, foreword by Joseph Papp (New York: Dutton, 1985). Franklin Bialystok, *Delayed Impact: The Holocaust and the Canadian Jewish Community* (Montreal: McGill–Queen's University Press, 2000), 68. The second quotation is from Cyril Levitt, of Toronto, a third-generation Jewish Canadian who lived in the 1950s (Bialystok's interview with Levitt in Toronto in May 1995); emphasis added by Bialystok.

12. On the Tin Woodman's accident, see also Marc Shell, *Stutter* (Cambridge, Mass.: Harvard University Press, forthcoming).

13. Leviticus treats such matters as tattooing: "You shall not cut into your flesh for the dead, nor cut any marks on yourselves; I am the Lord." Lev. 19:28.

14. 1 Sam. 31:4.

15. See *OED*, s.v. *Shush, Sh*, etc.

16. Dorothy Edwards Shuttlesworth, *Exploring Nature with Your Child: An Introduction to the Enjoyment and Understanding of Nature* (New York: Greystone, 1952).

17. Matt. 23:5. One scholarly view is that magical amulets were the original phylacteries. See Joshua Trachtenberg's controversial *Jewish Magic and Superstition* (Cleveland: Meridian, 1961), esp. 145–146.

18. Exod. 13:16; Deut. 6:4–9, 11:13–21.

19. Jerome Brooks, *The Big Dipper Marathon* (New York: Dutton, 1979), 12, 14, 17, 21.

20. See Danièle LeBlanc, "Témoignage," in Sally Aitken, Pierette Caron, and Gilles Fournier, eds., *Histoire vécue de la polio au Québec* (Outremont, Canada: Carte Blanche, 2000), 249. "On ne parlait jamais de polio dans la famille, surtout pas! J'ai essayé d'en parler dans les dernières années, mais c'était un sujet délicat, presque tabou."

21. A. Barnett, *The Iron Cradle* (New York: Crowell, 1954). Mara does not acknowledge Barnett's book as the source of her title.

22. Carol Mara, *Iron Cradles* (St. Leonards, Australia: Allen and Unwin, 1999), 279–280.

23. When Arvid Wallgren in 1921 described the epidemic of the poliolike acute aseptic meningitis (or "serous meningitis"), many doctors figured wrongly that what had been thought of as nonparalytic poliomyelitis was actually Wallgren's disease. For parents who wanted to tell their children (or for doctors who wanted to tell their patients' parents) that what seemed to be polio was not polio, Wallgren's disease was a perfect cover. See Arvid Wallgren, "Une nouvelle maladie infectieuse du système nerveux central," *Acta pediatrica, Upsala* 4 (1925): 4.

24. The Irish physician Henry Kennedy believed that there was a paralysis to be classified as "the temporary paralysis of early life." Henry Kennedy, "Observations on Paralytic Affections Met with in Children," *Dublin Medical Press: Journal of Medicine and Medical Affairs* 6 (1841): 201–204; Kennedy, "On Some of the Forms of Paralysis which Occur in Early Life," *Dublin Quarterly Journal of Medical Science* 9 (1850): 85. Other doctors, including Richard de Nancy and F. Rilliet, took a similar point of view, against that of Jacob von Heine, who argued (correctly) for a "spinal origin" of the disease. See John R. Paul, *A History of Poliomyelitis* (New Haven, Conn.: Yale University Press, 1971), 33.

25. This quotation is taken from Eddie Bollenbach and Marcia Falconer, "Non-Paralytic Polio and PPS," on the Lincolnshire PPS Web page. They refer to H. A. Howe and D. Bodian, *Neural Mechanisms of Poliomyelitis* (New York: Commonwealth Fund, 1942). See also R. L. Bruno, R. Sapolsky, J. R. Zimmerman, and N. M. Frick, "Pathophysiology of a Central Cause of Post-Polio Fatigue," in M. C. Dalakas, H. Bartfeld, and L. T. Kurland, eds., *The Post-Polio Syndrome: Advances in the Pathogenesis and Treatment* (New York: New York Academy of Sciences, 1995), 257–275.

26. See W. J. Sharrard, "The Distribution of the Permanent Paralysis in the Lower Limb in Poliomyelitis," *Journal of Bone and Joint Surgery* 37B (1955): 540–558.

27. Many people with nonparalytic polio probably were paralytic cases with diffuse weakness who recovered quickly. See M. C. Dalakas, "The Post-Polio Syndrome as an Evolved Clinical Entity: Definition and Clinical Description," in Dalakas, Bartfeld, and Kurland, *The Post-Polio Syndrome*, 68–80.

28. Edward J. Doherty, *The Saint of Paralytics,* 2nd ed. (Los Angeles: Times-Mirror, 1925); this book concerns Milton H. Berry of Hollywood, California.

29. Letter of 1665 from Marie de l'Incarnation, in Léo Gagné and Jean-Pierre Asselin, *Sainte-Anne-de-Beaupré: Trois cents ans de pèlerinage* (Sainte-Anne-de-Beaupré, Quebec: 1984), 14. Anne was the patron saint both of Brittany (uncomfortably part of France) and of Quebec (uncomfortably part of Canada).

30. Brother John Sellars with Guy Lafitte (tenor sax), Georges Arvanitis (piano), Pierre Michelot (bass), and Kenny Clarke (drums), recorded in Paris on May 13, 1957 (teal and silver Columbia label #SEG 7740).

31. In a letter of 1906 to his publisher Grant Richards, Joyce states, "My intention was to write a chapter of the moral history of my country and I chose Dublin for the scene because that city seemed to me the centre of paralysis." James Joyce, *Selected Letters of James Joyce*, ed. Richard Ellman (New York: Viking, 1975), 2:134. In Joyce's story "The Sisters," in *Dubliners* (1914), a young boy is faced with a case of actual paralysis.

32. Father André was born Alfred Bessette.

33. *Poliomyelitis: Papers and Discussions Presented at the Third International Poliomyelitis Conference,* ed. International Poliomyelitis Congress (Philadelphia: Lippincott, 1955), 555.

34. Mary Grimley Mason, *Life Prints: A Memoir of Healing and Discovery* (New York: Feminist Press of the City University of New York, 2000), 30. Her family moved to Montreal in 1936, when she was eight years old.

35. In the polio ward, Acosta witnesses the deaths of iron-lung patients and wonders whether she herself will be one. She believes that there is "a polio heaven for polios who die." Virginia Lee Counterman Acosta, *Polio Tragedy of 1941* (n.p., 1999), 9, 10.

36. *Cripple's Reward,* record album cover artist, Buddy Robertson; label, K-Town Records. Robertson sings "Cripple's Reward," a song about being handicapped and how God is going to give him a mansion someday.

37. For the comparison with the *Decameron,* see Bentz Plagemann, *My Place to Stand* (London: Gollancz, 1950), 136.

38. Ibid., 179.

39. Alton Goldbloom, *The Care of the Child* (Toronto, 1945), esp. 279–280. In July of 1946, my parents' friends Harriet and Sharkey gave this book to my parents. Goldbloom is depicted together with Sister Kenny in Aitken, Caron, and Fournier, *Histoire vécue,* 28.

40. Hyman left off trying to get into medical school after being rejected for two years running.

41. Diana B. Kidd, *The Physical Treatment of Anterior Poliomyelitis together with an Outline of Treatment of Other Nervous Conditions* (London: Faber and Faber, 1943), 101.

42. H. M. Visotsky, D. A. Hamburg, M. E. Goss, and B. Z. Lebovits, "Coping Behavior under Extreme Stress: Observations of Patients with Severe Poliomyelitis," *Archives of General Psychiatry* 5 (1961): 27–53, cited in Mary T. Westbrook, "Early Memories of Having Polio: Survivors' Memories versus the Official Myths," paper presented at the First Australian International Post-Polio conference, Sydney, Australia, November 1996.

43. See, for example, David A. Hamburg's eventual contribution to Joy G. Dryfoos, *Full-Service Schools: A Revolution in Health and Social Services for Children, Youth, and Families* (San Francisco: Jossey-Bass, 1994).

44. Late in the epidemics, several articles discussed the severe stress experienced by polio patients who required respiratory support. Some patients were reported to be experiencing hallucinations when placed in an iron lung. Being weaned away from respiratory support was described as particularly frightening. I. Mendelson, P. Solomon, and E. Lindemann, "Hallucinations of Poliomyelitis Patients during Treatment in a Respi-

rator," *Journal of Nervous and Mental Diseases* 126 (1958): 421–428; D. G. Prugh and C. K. Tagiuri, "Emotional Aspects of the Respirator Care of Patients with Poliomyelitis," *Psychosomatic Medicine* 16 (1954): 104–128; M. A. Seidenfeld, "Psychological Implications of Breathing Difficulties in Poliomyelitis," *American Journal of Orthopsychiatry* 25 (1955): 788–801.

45. H. W. Newell, "Differences in Personality in the Surviving Pair of Identical Triplets." *American Journal of Orthopsychiatry* 1 (1930): 61–80. Other references include E. H. Barbour, "Adjustment during Four Years of Patients Handicapped by Poliomyelitis," *New England Journal of Medicine* 213 (1935): 563–565; W. W. Barraclough, "Mental Reactions of Normal Children to Physical Illness," *American Journal of Psychiatry* 93 (1937): 865–877; F. S. Copellman, "Follow-up of One Hundred Children with Poliomyelitis," *The Family* 25 (1944): 289–297; L. M. Fairchild, "Some Psychological Factors Observed in Poliomyelitis Patients," *American Journal of Physical Medicine* 31 (1952): 275–281; M. Seidenfeld, "The Psychological Sequelae of Poliomyelitis in Children," 14–28.

46. Roland Berg, *Polio and Its Problems* (Philadelphia: Lippincott, 1948), 149.

47. "Nous avons rêvé de beaux et forts garçons." Paul Decoste wrote this some forty years after his children contracted polio. See his "Témoignage," in Aitken, Caron, and Fournier, *Histoire vécue*, 241. He continues (245): "Comment décrire à quel point cette épreuve a pu meurtrir nos coeurs de jeunes mariés?"

48. Garrett Oppenheim and Gwen Oppenheim, *The Golden Handicap, A Spiritual Quest: A Polio Victim Asks "Why" and Turns His Life Around* (Virginia Beach, Va.: ARE Press, 1993). James Oppenheim, *Mystic Warrior* (New York: Knopf, 1921).

49. Dinah Maria Mulock Craik (Miss Mulock), *The Little Lame Prince and His Travelling Cloak* (London: Daldy, Isbister, 1875).

50. "Polio and Your Pocket Book: In the Rare Case, It Can Be a Financial Crippler," *Financial Post*, August 28, 1954, cited in Christopher J. Rutty, " 'Do Something! . . . Do Anything!' Poliomyelitis in Canada, 1927–1962," Ph.D. diss., University of Toronto, 1995, 436.

51. "Rich Young was so fascinated by these almost ritualized meetings that he made a study of the behavior of parents and closely associated relatives and friends of polio patients, which he published in *Mental Hygiene*. He discovered that, far more than [with] any other illnesses, families suffered anxiety over polio and the fear of the unknown." Robert F. Hall, who wrote these words and was himself a polio, continues: "How often we wished [close relatives] would just pounce and ask us if we were afraid or if it hurt. But they didn't. They were only anxious to help, to share our feelings which we usually found difficult to express. But, because they didn't know what we have been through, they could only imagine what it was like. Their imagined specters created worry and tension, which showed in their anxious faces. It was their silent looks that so often raised barriers between us." Robert F. Hall, *Through the Storm: A Polio Story* (St. Cloud, Minn.: North Star Press of St. Cloud, 1990), 22, 23.

52. J. D. M. Griffin, W. A. Hawke, and W. W. Barraclough, "Mental Hygiene in an Orthopaedic Hospital," *Journal of Pediatrics* 13 (1938): 75–85.

53. They also prescribed a program of "wholesome" activities for the children; good music, books (not comics), movies (excellent nature movies, rather than cartoons, which were "too exciting and stimulating"), and various creative activities. Westbrook, "Early Memories."

54. William Green, "The Management of Poliomyelitis: The Convalescent State," in *Poliomyelitis: Papers and Discussions Presented at the First International Poliomyelitis Conference* (Philadelphia: Lippincott, 1949), 189.

55. Seidenfeld, "The Psychological Sequelae of Poliomyelitis in Children."

56. Fairchild, "Some Psychological Factors Observed"; Westbrook, "Early Memories."

57. Victor Cohn, *Four Billion Dimes* (Minneapolis: Star and Tribune, [1955]), 88, 91 (illustration).

58. See Phyllis York, D. A. York, and Ted Wachtel, *Toughlove Solution* (New York: Doubleday, 1988); Stanley L. Lipshultz, "Tough Love in the 50s: Mainstreaming and Support Groups," 210 ff., cited in Lauro S. Halstead and Naomi Naierman, eds., *Managing Post-Polio: A Guide to Living Well with Post-Polio Syndrome* (Clearwater, Fla.: Vandamere, 1998).

59. See, for one overview, J. A. Kessler, *Psychopathology of Childhood* (Englewood Cliffs, N.J.: Prentice Hall, 1966).

60. Joan Hunter, "A Child of a Lesser God," *Psychoanalytic Psychotherapy* 7, no. 1 (1993): 39–51, presents a case history of psychotherapy with a thirty-five-year-old man whose legs were paralyzed as a result of polio when he was eighteen months old and who presented with chronic depression. Thanks to therapy, he began to use his polio less as a defense, and the picture of himself as a "child of a lesser god" began to disappear.

61. Oleh G. Tkaczenko, "Tiefenpsychologische Aspekte des Stotterns" (The depth-psychological aspects of stuttering), *Zeitschrift für Individualpsychologie* 15, no. 4 (1990): 298–306. From an individual psychological perspective, stuttering represents a symptom of the Adlerian "organ inferiority." An originally mild lack of speech fluency can be compounded by the attitudes of parents and siblings. For a discussion of this view, see Shell, *Stutter*.

62. Some doctors say that Christina Olson suffered from Still's Disease. With regard to sidling, it is the woman as much as the painting that interests me in the present context. See Jean Olson Brooks and Deborah Dalfonso, *Christina Olson: Her World beyond the Canvas* (Rockport, Me.: Down East Books, 1998).

63. Elizabeth du Preez, *Elizabeth Sings: The Collected Writings of Elizabeth du Preez*, ed. J. J. and E. I. du Preez (Cape Town: Maskew Miller, 1957). Jacob E. Finesinger, "A Depression in a Six-Year-Old Boy with Acute Poliomyelitis," in Ruth Eissler et al., eds., *The Psychoanalytic Study of the Child*, vol. 13 (New York: International Universities Press, 1958). See also Celiker R. Kutsal et al., "Depression in Children with Hemophilic Arthropathy and Poliomyelitis: A Preliminary Report," *Turkish Journal of Pediatrics* 42, no. 1 (January–March 2000)): 27–30.

64. J. G. Farrell, *The Lung* (London: Hutchinson, 1965), 110.

65. *OED*, s.v. *Pestilent.* Cf. Susan Sontag, *Illness as Metaphor* (New York City: Farrar, Straus and Giroux, 1978), 58, for the play on "pest."

66. Christopher James Rutty, " 'A Grim Terror More Menacing, More Sinister, than Death Itself': Physicians, Poliomyelitis, and the Popular Press in Early Twentieth-Century Ontario," M.A. thesis, Department of History, University of Western Ontario, 1990.

67. Jane Boyle Needham, *Looking Up*, as told to Rosemary Taylor (New York: Putnam, 1958), 69.

68. Jerry Bledsoe, *The Angel Doll* (Asheboro, N.C.: Down Home Press, 1966). See also the movie version—*Angel Doll*, directed by Alexander Johnston, starring Keith Carradine, Diana Scarwide, Betsy Brantley, and Pat Hingle.

69. See Judith G. Zalesne (Bryn Mawr, Pa.), Letter to Editor, *Wall Street Journal,* August 21, 2000: "In 1942, when I was five, parents lived in dire fear of polio, the summer scourge. Parents were desperate to keep their kids off the streets, out of movie theaters, and away from the crowds."

70. According to my camp counselor: interview with Lenny Wisse, July 1999.

71. Suzanne Martel likewise reports her experience: "Après cette polio, j'ai dû porter des lunettes très épaisses parce que ma vue avait également beaucoup baissé" (After this polio I had to wear very thick glasses because my eyesight was weakened as well). "Témoignage," in Aitken, Caron, and Fournier, *Histoire vécue,* 139. Elaine Strauss has double vision after her bout with polio, in Strauss, *In My Heart,* 22, 35, 43.

72. See, for example, William Russel MacAusland, *Poliomyelitis, with Especial Reference to the Treatment* (Philadelphia: Lea & Febiger, 1927), 83.

73. Ibid., 85.

74. I was not able to get a proper diagnosis until 1969, however, when I consulted doctors in Cambridge, England, following a concussion from an automobile accident.

75. Mary Vermillion, "Re-embodying the Self: Representations of Rape in *Incidents in the Life of a Slave Girl* and *I Know Why the Caged Bird Sings,*" in *Maya Angelou's "I Know Why the Caged Bird Sings,"* ed. Harold Bloom (Philadelphia: Chelsea House, 1998), 153–166, esp. 162.

76. Mara Alper, *Stories No One Wants to Hear* (1993), twenty-seven minutes, distributed by Fanlight Productions.

77. " 'I don't think there's much love lost between us,' " the polio says to her hospitalized father. Judith Rossner, *Looking for Mr. Goodbar* (New York: Simon and Shuster, 1975), 64; see also 108, 188. When she learns that her father has a tumor, she doesn't even ask whether it is terminal (109).

78. *Good Times with Our Friends* (Boston: Houghton Mifflin, 1948). This was one of the first grade readers used in the English-language component of the classes arranged by the Protestant School Board of Montreal in the 1950s.

79. Owen Dixson, *My Way with Polio: An Autobiography by Owen Dixson* (London: Merritt and Hatcher, n.d. [1960]), 18.

80. Margery Williams, *The Velveteen Rabbit, or How Toys Become Real* (Garden City, N.Y.: Doubleday, n.d. [1922]).

81. Ruth Sawyer, *Old Con and Patrick,* illustrated by Cathal O'Toole (New York: Viking, 1946). Patrick, the lame young hero of this book, also has another pet: a blue jay with a shriveled leg.

82. See the photograph of FDR and Fala in Frances Cavannah, *Triumphant Adventure: The Story of Franklin Delano Roosevelt,* illustrated by Jo Polseno (New York: Rand McNally, 1964).

83. See the illustration by John Leech, "He had been Tim's blood horse all the way from church," in Charles Dickens, *A Christmas Carol,* ed. Andrew Lang, Gadshill edition (London: Chapman and Hall, 1897).

84. See Louis and Dorothy Sternburg, with Monica Dickens, *View from the Seesaw* (New York: Dodd, Mead, 1986). This book tells the story of a man who came down with polio during the summer of 1955 and of the rocking bed that enabled him to breathe.

85. Sawyer, *Old Con and Patrick.*

86. See Michael B. A. Oldstone, *Viruses, Plagues, and History* (Oxford: Oxford University Press, 1998).

87. Compare this situation with the arguments supporting Daniel Hudson Burnham's 1909 plan for the city of Chicago, in view of the Chicago fire of 1871.

88. See Robert Fishman, *Urban Utopias in the Twentieth Century: Ebenezer Howard, Frank Lloyd Wright, and Le Corbusier* (New York: Basic, 1977).

89. The smallpox epidemic ("le grand fléau") of 1885 killed 3,000 people out of a population of 157,000. More than 95 percent of those who died were Catholic. Two doctors associated with Quebec were involved: William Osler and William Hales Hingston. See Michael Bliss, *Montréal au temps du grand fléau: L'histoire de l'épidemie de 1885* (Montreal: Libre Expression, 1993), translated as *Plague: A Story of Smallpox in Montreal* (Toronto: HarperCollins, 1991).

90. Millie Teders's account is in Edmund J. Sass, *Polio's Legacy: An Oral History* (Lanham, Md.: University Press of America, 1996), 195.

91. The record is a 45-rpm single: "We Gotta Get out of This Place," written by Barry Mann and Cynthia Weil, with "I Can't Believe It" on the other side (July 1965; Columbia DB 7639 UK MGM K 13382 US).

92. At Concordia University Neil Compton, a wheelchair-bound polio, was chairperson of the Department of English. Together with Mr. Worrell, the director of the library, also a polio, he played an important role in the life of at least one student there who was, like them, a polio, and, like me, a resident of the Town of Mount Royal—Daphne Dale-Bentley. See her "Témoignage," in Aitken, Caron, and Fournier, *Histoire vécue,* esp. 165.

93. On the doctrine of *contagio carnalis,* see Marc Shell, *The End of Kinship* (Stanford, Calif.: Stanford University Press, 1988).

94. Mary Dorothy Sheridan, *The Handicapped Child and His Home* (London: National Children's Home, 1965). I read Dr. Sheridan's book in 1965, just as I was leaving

for college at Stanford. Joseph Laurance Marx quotes this passage in his *Keep Trying: A Practical Guide for the Handicapped Written by a Polio Victim* (New York: Harper and Row, 1974).

95. Edward Le Comte talks of *Sans Regret et sans honte,* by Heny Dory, in which a woman leaves her man after he gets "myélite." Edward Le Comte, *Long Road Back: The Story of My Encounter with Polio* (Boston: Beacon, 1957), 171.

96. Vivienne Overheu, *It Helps to Be Stubborn* (Perth, Australia: St. Georges, 1984), 103.

97. For the concerns when a pregnant woman gets polio, see Viola Pahl, *Gold in Life's Hourglass* (Surrey, Canada: Maple Lane, 1993), esp. 81. See also Pahl's first book, *Through the Iron Lung* (Thorold, Canada: Dryden Sinclair, 1955). An important example of the genre is the somewhat autobiographical work by Anne Finger, *Past Due: A Story of Disability, Pregnancy, and Birth* (Seattle: Seal Press, 1990), which was "done over" as a novel in Anne Finger, *Bone Truth* (Minneapolis, Minn.: Coffee House, 1994). On Finger, see Sharon Greytak's film *Weirded Out and Blown Away* (Cinema Guild, 1986). The medical literature on the subject includes M. Blair and C. E. Robertson, "Anterior Poliomyelitis in Pregnancy," *Canadian Medical Association Journal* 51 (December 1944): 552–553.

98. "Have I conceived all this people? Have I begotten them, that thou shouldest say unto me, Carry them in thy bosom, as a nursing father beareth the sucking child, unto the land which thou swarest unto their fathers?" (Num. 11:12). See Marc Shell, *Children of the Earth* (New York: Oxford University Press, 1994), 94.

99. *Ottawa Journal,* May 12, 1953. This particular item came from the Associated Press (Milwaukee).

100. For the Tepleys, see Halstead and Naierman, *Managing Post-Polio,* 191 ff., which includes a first-person polio narrative involving a brother and sister who both get polio. See also Luther Robinson, *We Made Peace with Polio* (Nashville, Tenn.: Broadman, 1960), which concerns polio in their family.

101. C. N. Herndon and R. G. Jennings, "A Twin-Family Study of Susceptibility to Poliomyelitis," *American Journal of Human Genetics* 3 (1951): 17–46; L. Nee, J. Dambrosia, E. Bern, R. Eldridge, and M. C. Alaska, "Post-Polio Syndrome in Twins and Their Siblings, Evidence That Post-Polio Syndrome Can Develop in Patients with Non-paralytic Polio," in Dalakas, Bartfeld, and Kurland, *The Post-Polio Syndrome,* 378–380.

102. Of a polio survivor, Helen Henderson reports, "She also worries about her brother, who had 'flu' about three weeks before she was paralyzed with polio." Helen Henderson, "Polio Still Stalks," *Toronto Star,* August 17, 2001, F-4.

103. For similar speculation about whether she got polio from a brother, see Overheu, *It Helps to Be Stubborn,* 27.

104. Here is a typical example of an e-mail on the subject: "Hello, LaVelda: . . . I just assumed my back problem was from a car accident when I was 18. Then I got to thinking how polio would have affected me by my father's genes. Do you know of any study that was done on children of parent/s that had polio? I haven't heard of any in Canada."

105. Jaana Suvisaari, Jari Haukka, Antti Tanskanen, Tapani Hovi, and Jouko Loenn-

qvist, "Association between Prenatal Exposure to Poliovirus Infection and Adult Schiz-ophrenia," *American Journal of Psychiatry* 156, no. 7 (July 1999): 1100–1102.

106. Diane Zemke Hawksford, *Polio: A Special Ride—One Nurse's Real Life Story of Her Experiences with Polio and Its Life-Long Ramifications in and through Her Brother* (Minnetonka, Minn.: Diagnostic Center of Learning Patterns, 1997). Julie Johnston, *Hero of Lesser Causes* (Toronto: Lester Publishing, 1992). Johnston wrote a screenplay, *Hero of Lesser Causes,* based on the novel, for Roy Krost Productions.

107. See Sass, *Polio's Legacy.* For similar problems in Tasmania, see Anne Killalea, *The Great Scourge: The Tasmanian Infantile Paralysis Epidemic, 1937–38* (Sandy Bay, Australia: Tasmanian Historical Research Association, 1995), 115.

108. Mara, *Iron Cradles,* 286–287. Mara's son William died at the age of thirteen, just five years before the book was published.

109. Jane Goodall, pt. 23, "Figan's Rise," in *Through a Window: My Thirty Years with the Chimpanzees of Gombe* (Boston: Houghton Mifflin, 1990).

110. For the name Jacob, see Gen. 25:26. For the wrestling match, see Gen. 32.

111. This stricture does not apply to birds. Because of the blow inflicted on Jacob by the mysterious "man," "therefore the children of Israel eat not the sinew of the thigh vein which is upon the hollow of the thigh to this day" (Gen. 32:33). The Torah refers to the incident at Gen. 32:24–30.

112. Ewald Mengel writes, in "Authority and Experience in the English Drama of the Sixteenth Century: *The History of Jacob and Esau,*" *Erfurt Electronic Studies in English* 5 (1995): 91, of Rebecca's hatred for her elder son.

113. Ishmael is the son of Hagar, Abraham's "concubine."

114. M. M. Mannon, *Here Lies the Blood* (Indianapolis: Bobbs-Merrill, 1942).

115. Moses leans on two people as if they were crutches, as I discuss in Shell, *Stutter.* Exod. 17:14: "Write this for a memorial in a book, and rehearse it in the ears of Joshua: for I will utterly put out the remembrance of Amalek from under heaven."

116. 1 Sam. 15:8–9,32–33.

117. Goodall, *Through a Window,* pt. 23.

118. Needham, *Looking Up,* 74.

119. *Long Day Tomorrow* (1971), directed by Bryan Forbes, with Malcolm McDowell, Nanette Newman, Georgia Brown; shot in the United Kingdom. Two paralyzed individuals, one an ex-athlete, find romance and love in a home for the disabled.

120. Peter Marshall, *The Raging Moon* (London: Hutchinson, 1964).

121. Allan V. Lee, *My Soul More Bent* (Minneapolis, Minn.: Augsburg, 1948), 58. Lee was stricken with polio prior to entering his senior year at Luther Theological Seminary, St. Paul, Minnesota.

122. *A Fight to the Finish: Stories of Polio* (1999), directed by Ken Mandel, was created and produced by Texas Scottish Rite Hospital for Children (TSRHC).

123. Strauss, *In My Heart,* 23.

124. For a son writing, see ibid., 38, where the son, Peter L. Strauss, has now become the Betts Professor of Law at Columbia University Law School. For a daughter writing, see ibid., 38, 135.

125. Kathryn Black, *In the Shadow of Polio: A Personal and Social History* (Reading, Mass.: Addison-Wesley, 1996). The author, whose mother died of polio in 1956 at the age of thirty-one, gives a detailed history of the polio years in the United States and recounts the disease's devastating effect on her family.

126. Sass, *Polio's Legacy,* 269.

127. Brooks, *Big Dipper Marathon,* 129.

128. "Honor thy father and thy mother" (Exod. 20:12).

129. In *A Muriel Rukeyser Reader,* ed. Jan Heller Levi, introduction by Adrienne Rich (New York: W. W. Norton, 1995).

130. Charles Ward, "Crippled Thunder," unpublished manuscript, copyright 1995, Collection Selechonek.

131. The succeeding sentences read as follows: "Stepfather and mother, later, had a fierce argument over the incident. Mother ensured in plain English that he was never to strike me again. She emphasized that I was not his child. She made sure stepfather understood he had no right to hit me and that it would never again happen. It didn't happen again, ever. Mother looked out for my well being and seemed to continue that role for the rest of her life. Even in death, I find she still guides me. My actions are, to a great extent influenced by mother. This all happened during a typically scorching, muggy, south side summer. South side of Chicago that is." Ibid.

132. Of Glynda, who had had polio in 1952 at the age of eighteen months, Amy Gardner writes in "Glynda's Bout with Polio as a Child": "We had to have an understanding. She was going to have to obey, settle down and let us all have some peace and joy again. I picked her up. She began kicking and screaming but I held her and carried her to her bedroom. I sat down on Scooter's bed and laid her across my knees. I thought I could never spank her because of her paralysis, but I turned her across my knees, 'bottom-side-up' and I spanked her hard enough for her to get my message and she got it. Just that one spanking and she was really home again. She never threw another tantrum and she was again playful and easy to live with." Amy Gardner, "Glynda's Bout with Polio as a Child," http://glynda's.com/story.asp.

133. Howells wrote *Hymnus Paradisi* after the death of his son, Michael, from polio at the age of nine. The *New Grove Dictionary of Music and Musicians,* Stanley Sadie, ed. (London: Macmillan, 1980), though, cites the cause as meningitis.

134. "Es ist genug," from Johann Sebastian Bach, Cantata no. 60 (fifth movement).

3. A Polio School

1. Walter Scott, *Waverly; or, 'Tis Sixty Years Since* (Edinburgh: Adam and Charles Black, 1892 [1814]). William Shakespeare, *Hamlet,* 3.2.

2. N. H. Rachlin, "Roller Skates as an Aid to Active Motion and Muscle Training in Cases of Poliomyelitis," *Journal of Bone and Joint Surgery* 14 (July 1932): 723; A. Windorfer, "Der Rollschuh zur Frühbehandlung der poliomyelitischen Beinlähmung" [Roller-skating in early therapy for poliomyelitic paralysis of the leg], *Kinderärztliche Praxis* no. 12 (March 1941): 76–79.

3. The book was a favorite first-person polio sports narrative for young peo-

ple. *Screwball*'s main character is Mike, twelve-year-old boy who had polio at age three. Rarely called upon to participate in sports at school, Mike decides to start playing hooky. Eventually, the town truant officer, who happens also to be the school gym teacher, leads the boy back onto "the right track" and Mike finds solace—and social acceptance—in wheel sports. First there is roller-skating, then soapbox car racing, and finally automobile driving. When Mike and his Dad buy a car, with all its prosthetic possibilities, the novel's successful conclusion is assured. Alberta Armer, *Screwball* (Cleveland: World Publishing, 1963), 12, 32, 74; 55; 57; 79, 80; 69, 59, 70. 72, 82, 93.

4. *OED*, s.v. "Trojan," 1b.

5. My parents never asked me why I kept failing gym, almost as if they feared to hear (yet again) the answer.

6. Killalea reports on shame caused by teachers. Anne Killalea, *The Great Scourge: The Tasmanian Infantile Paralysis Epidemic, 1937–38* (Sandy Bay, Australia: Tasmanian Historical Research Association, 1995), 130; see also Virginia Lee Counterman Acosta, *Polio Tragedy of 1941* (n.p., 1999), 44.

7. *OED*, s.v. "Horse-block."

8. Before Walter was two years old, he had an illness that left him lame for the rest of his life. Scott called the illness a "teething fever," but it was probably infantile paralysis. When he was six years old, an uncle gave him a small Shetland pony, no bigger than a Newfoundland dog, on which he could gallop over the countryside.

9. For a photograph of the author as Gene Autry, see Marc Shell, *Stutter* (Cambridge, Mass.: Harvard University Press, forthcoming).

10. Johann Wolfgang von Goethe, *Faust, Part 1*, Scene 4.

11. Richard Thayer Goldberg, *The Making of Franklin D. Roosevelt: Triumph over Disability* (Cambridge, Mass.: Abt, 1981), 73, 101, 135.

12. William O. Douglas, "Infantile Paralysis," chap. 3 in *Of Men and Mountains* (New York: Harper & Brothers, 1950).

13. See Edward Le Comte, *Long Road Back: The Story of My Encounter with Polio* (New York: Philosophical Library, 1958), 136.

14. Arthur C. Bartlett, *Game-Legs: The Biography of a Horse with a Heart*, illustrated by Harold C. Cue (New York: Cupples & Leon, 1928), 18.

15. At Eph. 5:31 the woman is a wife; at 1 Cor. 6:16 the woman is a prostitute. Matthew uses the same formulation.

16. Quotation is from the North American Riding for the Handicapped Association (NARHA). The method is also known as equine-assisted therapy.

17. See also "The Family Pet," in Marc Shell, *Children of the Earth* (New York: Oxford University Press, 1994).

18. Earlene W. Luis and Barbara F. Millar, *Wheels for Ginny's Chariot* (New York: Dodd, Mead, 1966). Ginny changes from a bitter teenager into a vibrant person who forgets herself and her own problems.

19. In *Tomboy and the Champ* (1961) the calf Champ gets stuck in mud and so does Tomboy—the orphan—who gets polio while trying to save it. Everyone has to save Champ, or Tomboy will die from pneumonia.

20. Acosta, *Polio Tragedy of 1941,* 42, 47.

21. Carolyn Stonnell Baber, *Little Billy,* illustrated by Luke T. Fleischman (Hollidaysburg, Pa.: Jason and Nordic, 1995). Danny is recovering from polio on a ranch in the 1940s and wants to train a mustang.

22. Dorothy Lyons, *Dark Sunshine,* illustrated by Wesley Dennis (New York: Harcourt, Brace, and World, 1968 [1951]).

23. Lois Johnson, *God's Green Liniment,* with Avis Johnson Thomas and Lois J. Rew (Alhambra, Calif.: Green Leaf, 1981). Vian Smith, *Tall and Proud* (Garden City, N.Y.: Doubleday, 1966).

24. Emily Crofford, *Healing Warrior: A Story about Sister Elizabeth Kenny,* illustated by Steve Michaels (Minneapolis, Minn.: Carolrhoda, 1989). Julie Johnston, *Hero of Lesser Causes* (Toronto: Lester, 1992), 33.

25. Arthur Tarnowski, *The Unbeaten Track* (London: Harvill, 1971). *Hammers over the Anvil* (1992, directed by Anna Turner) is an award-winning movie about a boy's coming of age in a small Australian town. Alan, crippled with polio, yearns to be a great horseback rider like his hero, East Driscoll, a horse-breaker.

26. Bartlett, *Game-Legs,* 17, 21, 56 ("Why don't you have me shot, too?"), 33, 62, 121 ("He felt that Sister was akin to him"), 122, 261, 256.

27. For balneology, see *Balneologie und Balneotherapie: Vortragszyklus, veranstaltet unter der Forderung des Internationalen Komitees für das ärztliche Fortbildungswesen* (Jena, Germany: Fischer, 1914). For hydropathy, see *The Water Doctor or Hydropathist* (Philadelphia: Carey & Hart, n.d. [ca. 1845]), with caricatures; Joel Shew, *Hydropathy; or, The Water Cure: Its Principles, Modes of Treatment* (New York: Wiley & Putnam, 1844). For hydrotherapy, see Thomas Smethurst, *Hydrotherapia; or, The Water Cure. Being a Practical View of the Cure in All Its Bearings, Exhibiting the Great Utility of Water As a Preservative of Health and Remedy for Disease, Founded On Observations and Experience Made at Grafenberg* (London: J. Snow, 1843). See also Durham Dunlop, *The Philosophy of the Bath; or, Air and Water in Health and Disease* (London: Simpkin, Marshall [Belfast, Archer and Sons, printers], 1868).

28. John Summers, *A Short Account of the Success of Warm Bathing in Paralytic Disorders,* 2d ed. (Bath: James Leake; C. Hitch and L. Hawes, 1751).

29. These include osteoarthritis, fibromyalgia, stroke, rheumatoid arthritis, low back pain, head injury, joint replacement surgery, tendinitis, spinal cord injury, arthroscopic surgery, bursitis, Parkinson's, joint reconstruction surgery, idiopathic joint pain, multiple sclerosis, scoliosis, balance disorders, and sprains and strains, rheumatology disorders, and spinal stabilization.

30. Charles Leroy Lowman, "Orthopedic Treatment, Including Bracing," in Albert G. Bower, *Diagnosis and Treatment of the Acute Phase of Poliomyelitis and Its Complications* (Baltimore, Md.: Williams and Wilkins, 1954), 208–209.

31. FDR began using the pool seriously at Vincent Astor's home in Rhinebeck, New York, in summer 1922. Goldberg, *Making of Franklin Delano Roosevelt,* 51.

32. William Russell MacAusland, *Poliomyelitis: With Especial Reference to the Treat-*

ment (Philadelphia: Lea & Febiger, 1927), 227. Warm Springs annual reports contain a good deal of information about the hydrotherapy practiced there.

33. Among the relevant works by Simon Baruch are *An Epitome of Hydrotherapy for Physicians, Architects and Nurses* (Philadelphia: Saunders, 1920); *The Principles and Practice of Hydrotherapy*, 3rd ed. (New York: Wood, 1908); and *The Uses of Water in Modern Medicine* (Detroit: George S. Davis, 1892). The committee, which served from 1943 to 1952, was appointed by Bernard Baruch in memory of his father, Simon Baruch, who had been a faculty member at Columbia University's College of Physicians and Surgeons. Wilhelm Winternitz, *Die Hydrotherapie auf physiologischer und klinischer Grundlage* (Vienna: Urban & Schwarzenberg, 1877–1880).

34. Charles Leroy Lowman, "Orthopedic Treatment, Including Bracing," in Bower, *Diagnosis and Treatment of the Acute Phase*, 208.

35. Carl Munde, *Dr. Charles Munde's Water-cure Establishment, at Florence, Mass.* (Florence, Mass.: n.p., 1856); *Willow Park Water Cure, and Hygienic Institute, at Westboro', Mass.* (Westboro, Mass.: n.p., n.d. [184–?]); *Dr. Wesselhoeft's Water-Cure Establishment (Brattleboro, Vt.). Report of over Two Hundred Interesting Cases from May 22d, 1851, to January 1st* (New York: E. O. Jenkins, 1853). See also *A Second Report of the Brattleboro Hydropathic Establishment* (Brattleboro, Vt.: J. B. Miner, 1849).

36. In 1909, a facility similar to Boston's was opened in Philadelphia.

37. See Anne Hardy, "Poliomyelitis and the Neurologists: The View from England, 1896–1966," *Journal of the History of Medicine* (Summer 1997).

38. For the anthropology of bathing, see especially *Uomo, Acqua e paesaggio: Atti dell'incontro di studio sul tema Irreggimentazione delle acque e trasformazione del paesaggio antico*, S. Maria Capua Vetere, November 22–23, 1996, eds. Alessandra Coen and Stefania Quilici Gigli (Rome: L'Erma di Bretschneider, 1997). See also Hellmut Stoffer, *Die Magie des Wassers: Eine Tiefenpsychologie und Anthropologie des Waschens, Badens und Schwimmens* (Meisenheim am Glan, Germany: Hain, 1966); Bernhard Maximilian Lersch, *Geschichte der Balneologie, Hydroposie und Pegologie, oder, Des Gebrauches des Wassers zu religiösen, diätetischen und medicinischen Zwecken: Ein Beitrag zur Geschichte des Cultus und der Medicin* (Würzburg, Germany: Verlag der Stahel'schen Buch- und Kunsthandlung, 1863).

39. The politics of bathing becomes clearer with regard to Roman baths. See *Les vertus médicinales de l'eau commune; ou, Recueil des meilleures pièces qui ont été écrites sur cette matière, traduit du Latin* (Paris: Cavelier, 1730).

40. For the Methodist view, see John Wesley, *Primitive Remedies* (Beverly Hills, Calif., Woodbridge, 1973); originally published in 1751 under title *Primitive Physick*. Harry Bischoff Weiss and Howard R. Kemble, *The Great American Water-Cure Craze: A History of Hydropathy in the United States* (Trenton, N.J.: Past Times Press, 1967). John Wesley, *Wesley's Family Physician, Revised, and [T. E.] Ware's Medical Adviser. A book of receipts, with directions for the use of Dr. Samuel Thomson's medicine and bath* (Salem, N.J.: Piror, 1839).

41. Bentz Plagemann, *My Place to Stand* (London: Gollancz, 1950), 145, 146.

42. Roosevelt, Extemporaneous Remarks to Patients at Warm Springs, Ga., March 24, 1937.

43. On Kellerman, see especially "Annette Kellerman," in Jeannine Dobbs, ed., "Class Essays, 1977," manuscript at the Schlesinger Library, Radcliffe College/Harvard University.

44. Rebekah Wright, *Hydrotherapy in Hospitals for Mental Diseases* (Boston: Tudor, 1932). Wright followed it up in 1940 with *Hydrotherapy in Psychiatric Hospitals.*

45. Lakeville State Sanatorium in Rutland, Massachusetts, was one of three additional state institutions authorized around 1907. Dozens of polios who survived the first months were institutionalized there for the rest of their lives.

46. Beginning in 1957, the mental patients at Rancho were moved elsewhere. Collen Adair Fliedner and G. Maureen Rodgers, *Rancho los Amigos Medical Center: Centennial, 1888–1988* (Downey, Calif.: Rancho los Amigos Medical Center, 1990), 127, 295.

47. C. Kling, A. Pettersson, and W. Wernsteidt, "The Presence of the Microbe of Infantile Paralysis in Human Beings," trans. A. V. Rosen, a report from the State Medical Institute of Sweden to the 15th International Congress on Hygiene and Demography, Washington, D.C., September–October 1912, reported the virus in human feces, but this work was unfortunately not much credited for decades. For the later period, see J. R. Paul, J. D. Trask, and C. S. Culotta, "Poliomyelitic Virus in Sewage," *Science* 90 (1939), esp. 258–259; and J. R. Paul, J. D. Trask, and S. Gard, "Poliomyelitic Virus in Urban Sewage," *Journal of Experimental Medicine* 71 (1940): 765–777; and J. R. Paul and J. D. Trask, "The Virus of Poliomyelitis in Stools and Sewage," *Journal of the American Medical Association* 116 (1941): 493–497.

48. Guidelines to the effect that children should not go swimming were available to parents. Among these was the series of "family pamphlets" published by Hearst's *Good Housekeeping* with the financial backing of the Lysol Corporation, as well as pamphlets distributed by the National Foundation for Infantile Paralysis.

49. A polio scare in the 1950s almost put Sunlite Pool (in Coney Island) out of business. Pat Cunningham Devoto, *My Last Days as Roy Rogers* (New York: Time Warner, 1999), 4.

50. That was also the name of a movie, *Polio Water: A Gothic Tale about a Little Girl's Secret* (short directed by Caroline Kava, United States, 1995 New York Film Festival).

51. Wesley, *Sermon 88, On Dress* (1838 [1791]), 3:15.

52. Ian Dury (1942–2000), the rock-and-roller, says in interview: "I was . . . conceived at the back of the Ritz and born at the height of the Blitz! . . . [I got polio] when I was seven . . . there were nine cases reported in Southend in August, during the heat wave. I'd been at the open air pool in Southend . . . they said I was going to die, but I rallied round after six months in the Royal Cornish Infirmary. They took me back to Essex on a stretcher." See www.nigeldick.com/guide.html.

53. Owen Dixson, *My Way with Polio: An Autobiography by Owen Dixson* (London: Merritt and Hatcher, n.d. [1960]), 4.

54. Elaine Strauss, *In My Heart I'm Still Dancing* (New Rochelle, N.Y.: Strauss, 1979), 158; see also 80.

55. J. G. Farrell, *The Lung* (London: Hutchinson, 1965), 134.

56. Johann Wolfgang von Goethe, *Wilhelm Meister's Apprenticeship*, translated by T. Carlyle (New York: Collier & Son, 1917 [1796]), bk. 4, chap. 12.

57. Erick Berry, *Green Door to the Sea* (New York: Viking, 1955), 56.

58. Arnold Beisser, *Flying without Wings: Personal Reflections on Being Disabled* (New York: Doubleday, 1989).

59. Stephen W. Meader, *Topsail Island Treasure*, illustrated by Marbury Brown (New York: Harcourt, Brace, and World, 1966); set in New Jersey's Topsail Island Park. The young polio combines his bird watching with exercising his leg, weakened by polio, and with searching for Captain Kidd's treasure.

60. Jerome Brooks, *The Big Dipper Marathon* (New York: Dutton, 1979), 100. Brooks quotes "The Daring Young Man on the Flying Trapeze," a well-known musical-hall favorite of the period: "He floats thro' the air / With the greatest of ease / The daring young man / On the Flying Trapeze."

61. Says Yu: "I see a lot of myself in Ryan. We are the crippled boys who fantasize about being a *ninja* warrior."

62. Enid Foster, *It Can't Happen to Me* (Cape Town: Timmins, 1959), 48–49. On the use and purpose of this apparatus, see Olive Frances Guthrie Smith, *Rehabilitation, Reeducation and Remedial Exercises* (Baltimore, Md.: Williams and Wilkins, 1943).

63. William Shakespeare, *Antony and Cleopatra*, 5.2. *Dolphinate* usually means "like a dauphin" (according to *OED*, s.v. "Dolphinate"), but I use it here to mean "like a dolphin."

64. In July 1951 Barbara Hobelmann, who had overcome polio to become an All-American swimmer, was on the cover of *Life Magazine*. Ethelda Bleibtrey of Waterford, New York, was the first woman to receive a medal in swimming for the United States (in the 1920s). She was also the first woman in the world to win three gold medals. *The DuPont Cavalcade Theater* included an episode, titled "A Time for Courage" (September 13, 1955), that starred Gloria Talbott and Hugh Beaumont in the "true story" of Olympic swimming champion Nancy Merius's battle to overcome polio.

65. See Digby Diehl's "authorized biography" of Williams, called *Million Dollar Mermaid* (New York: Simon and Schuster, 1999). In 1907 Annette Kellerman attracted national attention by performing water ballet at the New York Hippodrome as the first underwater ballerina. Kellerman also starred in several silent movies, including *Neptune's Daughter, Queen of the Sea,* and *A Daughter of the Gods.* In the last, Kellerman played a goddess so full of charm that when she fell into a pool of gnashing alligators, they were instantly transformed into swans.

66. George Gordon, Lord Byron, *The Island* (1823), in *the Works of Lord Byron*, vol. 5, ed. Ernest Harley Coleridge (London: Murray, 1904).

67. Berry, *Green Door to the Sea,* 56; emphasis mine.

68. Igor Burdenko and Scott Biehler, *Overcoming Paralysis: Into the Water and out*

of the Wheelchair (Garden City Park, N.Y.: Avery, 1999); the edition with this inscription is in the Collection Selechonek.

69. See Berry, *Green Door to the Sea,* dust jacket.

70. Ibid., 116.

71. See, for example, the cover of *Life Magazine,* February 22, 1954. Underwater breathing apparatus for human beings was explored in Jules Verne's novel *20,000 Leagues under the Sea* (Paris: Hetzel, 1870). The equipment was introduced as common technology in 1942 by Jacques Cousteau.

72. See Aman P. Schröter and Arjana C. Brunschwiler, *Wassertanzen, Aquatische Körperarbeit* [Waterdance, Aquatic Body Work] (Braunschweig, Germany: Aurum Verlag, n.d.).

73. The story *Waldo* is included in Heinlein, *Three by Heinlein* (Garden City, N.Y.: Doubleday, 1951). The movie *2001: A Space Odyssey* (1968), co-written with Stanley Kubrick, is based on Clarke's story "The Sentinel," in Arthur C. Clarke, *The Nine Billion Names of God: The Best Short Stories of Arthur C. Clarke* (New York: Harcourt, Brace, and World, 1967). Writes Clarke in the screenplay: "It is quite soft, and it stops them in their tracks, so that they stand *paralyzed* on the trail with their jaws hanging. A simple, maddeningly repetitious rhythm pulses out of the crystal cube and hypnotises all who come within its spell. For the first time—and the last, for two million years—the sound of drumming is heard in Africa"; emphasis mine. For the quotation on zero gravity, see Arthur C. Clarke, "Painful Memory of a Silent Stalker," *Times Higher Education Supplement,* History of Science, June 29, 2001, 34.

74. Inscrutable Films and Pacific News Service produced the movie *Breathing Lessons: The Life and Work of Mark O'Brien* (1996) by Jessica Yu.

75. Mark O'Brien, "Breathing," *Breathing,* 2nd ed. (Berkeley, Calif.: Lemonade Factory, 1998), 1. Concerning these sounds like breathing, compare the lyrics in Weird Al Yankovic, "Mr. Frump in the Iron Lung," in *Weird Al Yankovic,* Scotti Brothers, 1983. The song "Insect Kin"—by Bush—begins thus: "Iron lung I know you well / Deal with you like a bad spell." See also Radiohead's "My Iron Lung." First released September 1994.

76. *Star Wars* (1977), dir. George Lucas, with James Earl Jones as the voice of Darth Vader (Lucasfilm/20th Century Fox). See also Martin F. Norden, *The Cinema of Isolation: A History of Physical Disability in the Movies* (New Brunswick, N.J.: Rutgers University Press, 1994), esp. 293.

77. In Collection Selechonek.

78. Mark O'Brien, "The Man in the Iron Lung" (1988), in *The Man in the Iron Lung* (Berkeley, Calif.: Lemonade Factory, 1997), 1.

79. Walt Whitman, "A Carol Closing Sixty-Nine" (ca. 1888), in Walt Whitman, *Complete Poetry and Collected Prose,* ed. Justin Kaplan (New York: Viking, 1982).

80. Naomi Rogers, *Dirt and Disease: Polio before FDR* (New Brunswick, N.J.: Rutgers University Press, 1992), 168, citing Frank Freidel, *Franklin Delano Roosevelt: The Ordeal* (Boston: Little, Brown, 1954), 113.

81. *OED,* s.v. "Dance," n. 1.

82. S. A. Lee, "Is It the Last Dance? Ballet Dancers at Age 30," *Medical Problems of Performing Artists* 3, no. 1 (March 1988): 27–32.

83. W. Schweisheimer, "Look Out for Your Hands! Neuritis, Neuralgia, and Temporary Paralysis Must Be Watched," *Etude* 67 (1949): 85, 120–121.

84. A. G. Ryan, "Early History of Dance Medicine," *Journal of Dance Medicine and Science* 1, no. 1 (1997): 30–34; C. G. Shell, ed., *The Dancer as Athlete* (Champaign, Ill.: Human Kinetics, 1986).

85. "Human robots," on the other hand, move jerkily, in the fashion of early cinema.

86. The translation is by Sarah M. Lowe, in *The Diary of Frida Kahlo: An Intimate Self-Portrait,* introduction by Carlos Fuentes (Mexico City: Abrams and La Vaca Independiente, 1995), 233.

87. On Midas, see Shell, "Portia's Portrait: Representation as Exchange," in *Common Knowledge* 7, no. 1 (Spring 1998): 94–144. On Lot's wife, see Genesis 19:26.

88. A. G. Brandfonbrener, "Music of the Heart" (editorial), in *Medical Problems of Musicians and Dancers* 12, no. 4 (December 1997): 95–96. Strauss, *In My Heart,* 96.

89. Born Frances "Fanny" Rose Shore, Dinah Shore contracted polio when she was a year and a half old. She was left with a crippled right leg that was eventually strengthened by massage, swimming, and tennis.

90. *Moto* (Italian for "motion, movement") is found in the direction *con moto,* "with movement, fast." A *moto perpetuo* is a rapid piece that gives the impression of perpetual motion, such as Paganini's *Allegro de concert* and or the last movement of Ravel's Violin Sonata.

91. Richard Burton, *Anatomy of Melancholy* (London: George Bell and Sons, 1926), I.i.I.iv.

92. Carolyn Bereznak Kenny is the polio who cofounded Capilano College's music therapy program and helped design Canada's first master's program in music therapy.

93. Dore Schary, *Sunrise at Campobello: A Play in Three Acts* (New York: Random House, 1958), 57; emphasis mine.

94. Sarah M. Lowe, *Frida Kahlo* (New York: Universe, 1991), 233.

95. Marc Alexander, *The Dance Goes On: The Life and Art of Elizabeth Twistington Higgins,* photographs by Graham and Jacqui Sergeant, foreword by Prince Phillip, Duke of Edinburgh (Churt, England: Leader Books, 1980); Elizabeth Twistington Higgins, *Still Life* (London: Mowbray, 1969). Quotation from Alexander, *Dance,* 38.

96. Photographs showing Twistington's paintings are to be found in Higgins, *Still Life,* 66.

97. On Twistington's work, see "Past Masters," in Marc Alexander, *Canvases of Courage: A Gallery of Art Inspired by Triumph over Adversity* (Churt, England: Leader Books, 1991).

98. Alexander, *Dance,* 109–110; Alexander, *Canvases,* 23–27.

99. Balanchine's *Valse* was based on Maurice Ravel's ballet *Valses nobles et sentimentales* (composed 1911, orchestrated 1912, and completed in 1920).

100. *Treasures from American Film Archives* (program 3) includes part of *La Valse*

(1951, six minutes), with George Balanchine's choreography performed by the dancers for whom he created it.

101. In 1932, Balanchine had used Emmanuel Chabrier's music for *Cotillon,* a thematic predecessor of *La Valse,* with its devilish circle of dancers.

102. James Burnett, *Ravel: His Life and Times* (New York: Hippocrene, 1983).

103. See Holly Brubach, "Muse, Interrupted," *New York Times Magazine,* November 22, 1998, 60. See also Arlene Croce, "Tanny," *New Yorker,* January 15, 2001, 64–65.

104. Tanaquil Le Clercq, with Martha Swope, *Mourka: The Autobiography of a Cat* (New York: Stein and Day, 1964).

105. The book includes writing by the physicist and dancer Kenneth Laws and a foreword by Francia Russell, who worked with Balanchine in the 1950s.

106. Joan Clarke, *All on One Good Dancing Leg* (Sydney: Hale & Iremonger, 1994).

107. Ana Castillo, *Peel My Love Like an Onion* (New York: Doubleday, 1999), 4.

108. *Brace Yourself* played in San Francisco in September 2001. Liebe Wetzel, *Lunatique Fantastique* featured her mime puppetry.

109. Shannon has used crutches since the age of five, when he was diagnosed with a rare form of arthritis that prevents him from putting weight on his legs for any extended length of time.

110. I was struck, too, by the apparent resurrection of the acrobats, who Lili fears have died in a fall.

111. Ida Lupino, "My Fight for Life," in *Photoplay* (New York: Macfadden, 1946).

112. Franco went on to become an influential Hollywood script consultant.

113. An eighty-two-minute drama starring Sally Forrest, Keefe Brasselle, Hugh O'Brian, Lawrence Dobkin, and Eve Miller.

114. Quoted in John R. Paul, *A History of Poliomyelitis* (New Haven, Conn.: Yale University Press), 305.

115. For his novel *Arrowsmith* (New York: Grosset & Dunlap, 1932 [1925]), Sinclair Lewis collaborated with Dr. Paul De Kruif.

116. See Leonard Kriegel, *Falling into Life: Essays* (San Francisco: North Point, 1991), 66.

117. See the journal *Moving Picture World,* and Norden, *Cinema of Isolation,* 19.

118. Included in *The Complete Glenn Miller,* 13 CDs, RC Bluebird, no. 228.

119. *The Leather Saint* (1956, directed by Alvin Ganzer), with a cast that includes Paul Douglas, John Derek, Jody Lawrance, Cesar Romero, Richard Hannon, and Ernest Truex.

120. *This Is Your Life.* For a photograph of this episode, see Higgins, *Still Life,* 51. "With my parents and Eamonn Andrews on *This Is Your Life.*"

121. See the photograph of Danny Kaye and Bing Crosby with a boy in braces (at half door with poster). Collection Selechonek.

122. That "ideology" of isolation began to change only in the 1980s, with the advent of a viable disability rights movement and the widespread legitimating of the diagnosis of post-polio syndrome, followed by patient reunions at Warm Springs. See Nancy Baldwin Carter, *Myths and Chicken Feet: A Polio Survivor Looks at Survival* (Omaha:

Nebraska Polio Survivors Association Press, 1992).

123. Acosta, for example, who was actually abandoned, remains at the polio ward so long that she cries when she leaves it: "It is a little like a family." Acosta, *Polio Tragedy of 1941*, 36. Moreover, the doctor's wife says, "Sometimes we think that Virginia Lee is our little girl." Ibid., 68.

124. Lorraine Beim, *Triumph Clear* (New York: Harcourt, Brace, 1946), 5, 48.

125. Allan Moore, *Growing Up with Barnardo's*, ed. Joan Clarke (Sydney: Hale & Iremonger, 1990). The reference is to Dr. Barnardo's homes in the United Kingdom and elsewhere. See June Rose, *For the Sake of the Children: Inside Dr. Barnardo's—120 Years of Caring for Children* (London: Hodder & Stoughton, 1987).

126. On the "submerged" role of polio, see Brad Byrom, "A Pupil and a Patient: Hospital Schools in Progressive America," in *The New Disability History*, ed. Paul K. Longmore and Lauri Umansky (New York: New York Press, 2001), 133 ff.

127. Journals sprang up around this time: the *American Journal of Care for Cripples* (1914–1919) and especially *Crippled Child* (published by the International Society for Crippled Children beginning in 1923 and lasting until 1949, when its name changed to include adults).

128. Alice Sink, *The Grit Behind the Miracle: A True Story of the Determination and Hard Work behind an Emergency Infantile Paralysis Hospital, 1944–1945* (Lanham, Md.: University Press of America, 1998).

129. For pictures of performances by the Poliopolitan Opera, see Tony Gould, *A Summer Plague: Polio and Its Survivors* (New Haven, Conn.: Yale University Press, 1995), insert between 80 and 81.

130. Plagemann, *My Place to Stand*, 120 ff., 212, 213 ff.

131. For the reference to the "pain" in Roosevelt's radio voice, see Acosta, *Polio Tragedy of 1941*, 77.

132. Plagemann, *My Place to Stand*, 215.

133. This particular story line would seem to have been Beim's idea. See Beim, *Triumph Clear*, 154 ff., esp. 162.

134. Acosta met Roosevelt at Saint Luke's in December 1942. Acosta, *Polio Tragedy of 1941*, 22. Beim, *Triumph Clear*, 170, where she writes about her production of Shakespeare's *Othello;* also 196.

135. Marc Shell, *Elizabeth's Glass* (Lincoln: University of Nebraska Press, 1994).

136. Rogers, *Dirt and Disease*, 108; also "Written in Haste," ibid.

137. Schlesinger Library, Harvard University.

138. See John Gliedman and William Roth, *The Unexpected Minority, Handicapped Children in America* (New York: Harcourt, Brace, Jovanovich, 1982), 1–51. See also Philip L. Safford and Elizabeth J. Safford, *A History of Childhood and Disability* (New York: Teachers College Press, 1995), 90–121.

139. *Elizabeth Sings: The Collected Writings of Elizabeth du Preez*, ed. J. J. and E. I. du Preez (Cape Town: Maskew Miller, 1957), 51.

140. Caverly catalogues many minor epidemics that occurred earlier in the eighth century. There is disagreement as to whether earlier reports of an epidemic actually de-

scribe polio; for example, "the pestilence that is called baccach," recorded under the year 708–709 in the Annals of Ulster. William MacArthur, "The Medical Identification of Some Pestilences of the Past," *Transactions of the Royal Society of Tropical Medicine and Hygiene* 53 (1959): 423–439.

141. See Shell, *Stutter.*

142. See Carlos H. Espinel, "Masaccio's Cripple: A Neurological Syndrome: Its Art and Medicine," *Lancet* 346 (1995): 1684–1686.

143. So Claudius appears as a polio in the never-completed movie *I, Claudius* (1937–39) and the great television shows (1976–77) of the same name, and hence Claudius is so depicted. The film, made at the height of the hysteria about the traumatic epidemics of polio, about a partly immobilized emperor with broken bones, is informed, in ways not heretofore recognized, by a culture of poliomyelitic paralysis. It is part of a socio-pathology that at once expresses and represses polio—an important theme of *Polio and Its Aftermath.*

144. Jean de La Fontaine, "Les Dieux voulant instruire un fils de Jupiter" (also known as "Pour Monseigneur le Duc de Maine"), bk. 11, fable 2. V. M. Hillyer, *A Child's History of the World* was originally published in 1924. The edition I had was revised, with new material by Edward G. Huey, with illustrations by Carle Michel Boog and M. S. Wright (New York: Appleton-Century-Crofts, 1951).

145. Jim Marugg, *Beyond Endurance* (London: Rupert Hart-Davis, 1955).

146. Ruth Ben'ary (her name is also spelled Benari, Ben-ari, Ben Ary, and so on), *Prelude to Love* (New York: Arcadia House, 1943). On the novel: Strauss, *In My Heart,* 87. Ruth Ben'ary originally wrote her typing manual at Warm Springs for the benefit of polio patients.

147. Joni Mitchell, *Mingus,* audio CD (Elektra/Asylum, 1979).

148. Kathryn Black, *In the Shadow of Polio: A Personal and Social History* (Reading, Mass.: Addison-Wesley, 1996). Like many who made little progress in rehabilitation, Virginia Black had to reconcile herself to life on a "rocking bed," a device that breathed for a patient who had graduated from the iron lung. She was subjected to the routine cruelty of a staff psychiatrist. "How does it feel," he asked, "to know you'll never hold your children again?" Her daughter vividly imagines the double pain of those who fell short of the ideal "good" handicapped person. "Perhaps the biggest obstacle to acceptance was the much-touted expectation that anyone could, through hard work, be restored to the previous undamaged self. Even the news of Sister Kenny's miracles and the N.F.I.P.'s ballyhooed successes must have undermined those struggling to accept the unchangeable."

149. Plagemann, *My Place to Stand,* 138.

150. Alice Lou Plaistridge was first recruited in 1927 to Warm Springs, where she took over as director of physiotherapy in 1931. Plaistridge's articles for the *Polio Chronicle* (Warm Springs, Ga.: Warm Springs Foundation) include "Late Care of Poliomyelitis: Chronic Stage—After Two Years from Onset," *Polio Chronicle* (Warm Springs Foundation, Ga.) 1, no. 4 (October 1931), and "Corrective Walking," *Polio Chronicle* 1, no. 3 (October 1932).

151. Plagemann, *An American Past: An Early Biography* (New York: William Morrow, 1990), 166.

152. "Alice Lou Plaistridge first treated Roosevelt at Horseneck Beach, Massachusetts, in 1925. They took an instant liking to each other. Due to her efforts, walking with crutches became much easier for Roosevelt. He spoke enthusiastically of his Warm Springs plans during their sessions, and in 1927 Alice was hired." William Warren Rogers, Jr., "The Death of a President, April 12, 1945: An Account from Warm Springs," *Georgia Historical Quarterly* 75, no. 1 (Summer 1991).

153. Kriegel, *Falling into Life*, 21, 89. "The virus had claimed more than my legs with which to feed its hunger. I was a writer whose imagination was literally 'disease-ridden.'" (41). "Until I met with my virus, I was a monotonously average eleven-year-old boy" (42). "But that virus gave me a writer's voice" (85).

154. An example is *Poliomyelitis: A Source Book for High School Students* in Collection Selechonek.

155. Florence M. Taylor and Lucile P. Marsh, *Growing Pains* (Philadelphia: R. R. Donnelley and Sons), 1948. Johanna Spyrie, *Heidi* (New York: Puffin, 1956 [1880]).

156. Dorothy Baruch and Elizabeth Montgomery, *The Girl Next Door*, illustrated by Ruth Steed (Chicago: Scott, Foresman, 1946), 102. In the illustration on 108, the children wave good-bye to the polio as they leave for school. The caption reads: "Which picture shows the better thing to say? Why?"

157. Sigmund Freud, "The Uncanny," in *Standard Edition of the Complete Psychological Works of Sigmund Freud*, ed. and trans. James Strachey (London: Hogarth, 1957–1974), 17:226 (Freud is quoting Ernst Jentsh here), 244. See also Freud, "Wolf-Man," ibid., esp. section 8 in vol. 17.

158. A cripple seeks revenge for an outrage that had been done to his companion Trippetta.

159. Edgar Allan Poe, "The Premature Burial," in *The Works of the Late Edgar Allan Poe*, ed. N. P. Willis, J. R. Lowell, and R. W. Griswold (New York: Redfield, 1850), 1:325–338. Poe's "Premature Burial" was first published in *A Dollar Newspaper*, July 31, 1844. For the use of *trance* in this context ("a tendency to trance"), see *The New Sydenham Society Lexicon of Medicine and the Allied Sciences*, Henry Power and Leonard William Sedgwick, eds. (London: New Sydenham Society, 1899), s.v. "Trance": "Trance, catalepsy; ecstasy—'The hypnotic state: a prolonged abnormal sleep, in which the vital functions are reduced to a very low ebb, and from which the patients cannot ordinarily be aroused.'"

160. David J. Rothman, *Beginnings Count: The Technological Imperative in American Health Care* (New York: Oxford University Press, 1997). The iron lung plays an important role also in *Wealth Well-Given: The Enterprise and Benevolence of Lord Nuffield*, ed. F. J. Minns (Stroud, England: Dover, 1994).

161. Philip Drinker and Louis Agassiz Shaw at the Harvard School of Public Health invented the iron lung in 1928—or so goes one history of the device. Other scientists had invented earlier forms of the machine. See Robert V. Bruce, *Alexander Graham Bell and the Conquest of Solitude* (Ithaca, N.Y.: Cornell University Press, 1990). After Bell's

son Edward died of respiratory problems, Bell designed a metal vacuum jacket to facilitate breathing. The Harvard machine, however, was the first to be widely used. See Louise Joy Short, "Four Pioneers: The Making of the Harvard Program for Industrial Hygiene, 1918–1935," bachelor's honors thesis, Harvard University, 1982; Philip Drinker, "Breathing Machine (Experiments Conducted) 26 September, 1927 to 16 December, 1928, at Harvard University," 1927–1928, comprises original notes on early experiments leading to development of the iron lung; they are found in the manuscript collection at the Francis A. Countway Library of Medicine, Harvard University, Boston. Warren E. Colins of Boston manufactured a second respirator after the Consolidated Gas Company of New York donated money to Harvard University. John Rodman Paul, of the Yale Poliomyelitis Commission (later called the Yale Poliomyelitis Study Unit), says that he, Paul, was the first to use the device for a small infant. Paul, *History of Poliomyelitis*, 327.

162. See Susan Hulme, "Doctors Revamp Iron Lung for Sick Babies," *New Scientist* 125 (March 17, 1990): 35; Theodore H. Stanley, "Iron Lung," Grolier's *Encyclopedia Americana: International* (Danbury, Conn.: Grolier, 1995), 15:466; Helen Eckman Zimmerman, "Ventilation Therapy Flashback!" *RN* 59, no. 12 (1996): 26–31.

163. Regina Woods, *Tales from inside the Iron Lung and How I Got out of It* (Philadelphia: University of Pennsylvania Press, 1994); Richard Chaput, *Not to Doubt* (New York: Pageant, 1964), about a boy and his life in iron lung; Ann Armstrong, *A Breath of Life* (London: British Broadcasting Corporation, 1985), the story of a victim of severe respiratory polio dependent on an iron lung to breathe; Leonard C. Hawkins, *The Man in the Iron Lung* (New York: Doubleday, 1956); Jane Boyle Needham, as told to Rosemary Taylor, *Looking Up* (New York: Putnam's Sons, 1959); Phyll Western, *I Haven't Washed Up for Thirty-Five Years* (n.p.: Desne, 1993); Paul Bates, with John Pellow, *Horizontal Man* (London: Pan, 1966). See also Mark Finley, *2000 and Beyond* (Boise, Idaho: Pacific Press Club, 1996).

164. June Opie, *Over My Dead Body* (London: Methuen, 1957). June Opie, *Over My Dead Body Forty Years On* (Birkenhead, New Zealand: Reed, 1996).

165. Mark O'Brien, *Breathing* (Berkeley, Calif.: Lemonade Factory, 1990); Mark O'Brien and Susan Fernbach, *Love and Baseball: Poems on America's Favorite Pastimes* (Berkeley, Calif.: Lemonade Factory, 1997); Mark O'Brien, *The Man in the Iron Lung* (Berkeley, Calif.: Lemonade Factory, 1997); and Mark O'Brien, *Sonnets and Strikeouts: More Poems on Love and Baseball* (Berkeley, Calif.: Lemonade Factory, 1999).

166. On the "worm's eye view," see Lowe, *Diary of Frida Kahlo*, 263.

167. On claustrophobia, see Farrell, *Lung*, 77; on living deaths, see my earlier remarks concerning the iron lung and *Rear Window*.

4. Paralytic Polio and Moving Pictures

1. See Helen Cathcart, *Lord Snowdon* (London: W. H. Allen, 1968), 71.

2. Francis J. Mott, *Play Therapy and Infantile Paralysis: An Elementary Book for Parents on the Psychosomatic Aspects of Poliomyelitis and Aids to Prevention* (New York: Integration Publishing, 1952), 85.

3. This remark of Archimedes was quoted by Pappus of Alexandria in his "Collection" from ca. 340 CE, *Synagoge*, bk. 8, ed. Friedrich Hultsch (Berlin: n.p., 1878), 1060.

4. V. M. Hillyer, *A Child's History of the World*, revised and expanded edition, ed. Edward G. Huey, illustrated by Carle Michel Boog and M. S. Wright (New York: Appleton-Century-Crofts, 1951). V. M. Hillyer, *A Child's Geography of the World* was first published in 1929. The edition I had had also been revised by Edward G. Huey, illustrated by Mary Sherwood Wright Jones (New York: Appleton-Century-Crofts, 1951).

5. See catalogue for the exhibition *Helen Nestor: Personal and Political*. This exhibition was held at the Oaks Gallery, Oakland Museum, Oakland, California, from June 24 to October 15, 2000.

6. "Rear Window," (also known as "It Had to Be Murder") is collected in William Irish (pseudonym of Cornell Woolrich), *After-Dinner Story* (New York: Lippincott, 1936).

7. See Cathcart, *Lord Snowdon*, 71.

8. Bert Kopperl, *With Two Wheels and a Camera*, foreword by Helen Hayes (Hicksville, N.Y.: Exposition, 1979). See Sally Stein, "Peculiar Grace: Dorothea Lange and the Testimony of the Body," in *Dorothea Lange: A Visual Life*, ed. Elizabeth Partridge (Washington, D.C.: Smithsonian Institution Press, 1994).

9. Allen V. Lee, *My Soul More Bent* (Minneapolis, Minn.: Augsburg, 1948), 82.

10. For one account of this early camera with tripod, which was used for composing pasted-up panoramas, see Eva Antonatos and Marie Mauzy, *Early Photographic Panoramas of Greece*, (Athens: Patomos, 2003).

11. *OED*, s.v. *Double exposure* ("The good pun makes a double exposure on the mind"), led me to Robert Withington, "Verbal Pungencies," *American Speech* 14 (1939): 271.

12. "When the world [of a child] collapses," says Coppola, "it collapses completely."

13. *Elsevier's Dictionary of Photography*, comp. A. S. H. Craeybeckx (Amsterdam: Elsevier, 1965).

14. W. A. Newman Dorland and E. C. L. Miller, *Medical Dictionary*, 18 ed. (Philadelphia: Saunders, 1938) 1272/2.

15. On seeing that the heroine isn't there, the narrator observes, "They use the expression 'delayed action.' I found out then what it meant. For two days a sort of formless uneasiness, a *disembodied* suspicion. I don't know what to call it, had been flitting . . . around in my mind, like an insect looking for a landing place. . . . Now, for some reason, within a split second after he tossed over the empty mattresses, it landed— *zoom!* And the point of contact expanded—or exploded, whatever you care to call it— in a certainty of murder.—In other words, the rational part of my mind was far behind the instinctive, subconscious part. Delayed action. Now the one caught up with the other. The thought-message that sparked from the synchronization was: He's done something to her" (155).

16. Woolrich's story was published in February 1942, Fischer's in May 1939, both in *Dime Detective*.

17. Eadweard Muybridge, *Animal Locomotion* (Philadelphia: University of Pennsylvania and Photogravure Company, 1887). Muybridge did the photographs for *The*

Horse in Motion, with Jacob Davis Babcock Stillman, executed and published under the auspices of Leland Stanford (Boston: James R. Osgood, 1882). Eadweard Muybridge, *The Human Figure in Motion* (New York: Dover, 1955 [1901]).

18. For *creek* meaning "artificial contrivance," see *OED,* s.v. *Creek,* 7.

19. See Lynne Kirby, "The Railroad and the Cinema, 1895–1929: Institutions, Aesthetics, and Gender," Ph.D. diss., University of California, Los Angeles, 1989.

20. *OED,* s.v. *Photography.* The word comes from the Greek *phōs.*

21. "Locked-in syndrome" leaves the patient almost completely paralyzed and mute, but able to receive and understand sensory stimuli.

22. Says American moviemaker Jonas Mekas: "I may not be completely correct, but I ascribe a great deal of Dwoskin's art to his physical incapacities. He has transcended them and made them into a source of energy." See http://www.abm-medien.de/filmbuero/dwoski_e.htm.

23. He also made a movie for a disability series on Channel 4 called *Face of Our Fear.*

24. Martin F. Norden, *The Cinema of Isolation: A History of Physical Disability in the Movies* (New Brunswick, N.J.: Rutgers University Press, 1994), 20–24.

25. See Naomi Rogers, *Dirt and Disease: Polio before FDR* (New Brunswick, N.J.: Rutgers University Press, 1992), 10; Manton M. Carrick, "Preparedness: Our Best Weapon," *Southern Woman's Magazine* (1917): 28.

26. Hillyer, *Child's Geography,* 99.

5. Handi-Capitalism and Cinema Business

1. Charles Mee, *A Nearly Normal Life: A Memoir* (Boston: Little, Brown, 1999), 39.

2. See Pat Barker, *The Eye in the Door* (New York: Dutton, 1994), a fictionalized account of World War I based partly on the work of the British psychiatrist and anthropologist William Rivers with shell-shocked English soldiers.

3. "And one thing I think we can make a pretty good guess about, and that is that here at Warm Springs we are going to have, in the days to come, a great many more men in uniform. After all, infantile paralysis is not a respecter of age; and in the Army, Navy, Marine Corps and Coast Guard, including the WAACs, WAVES and the other girls, we are going to have, out of more than seven million Americans, a good many cases of infantile paralysis, even if we don't have any great epidemic in this country." Extemporaneous remarks by President Roosevelt, Warm Springs, Georgia, April 15, 1943.

4. On their losing money, see Pat Cunningham Devoto, *My Last Days as Roy Rogers* (New York: Time Warner, 1999), 3. Also: During the great epidemic in New York City, people younger than sixteen were barred from the movies.

5. Bing Crosby sang at the end of a typical March of Dimes campaign ad.

6. Devoto, *My Last Days,* 24, 25. In the context of the book the title of the song turns out to be ironic, since, at the end, the polio is quite abandoned by her friend—the feeling of guilt from which abandonment is, in some ways, the explanation for why the author writes the book in the first place (352–353).

7. "You'll Never Walk Alone" has been recorded by dozens of pop, rock, gospel, country western, and opera singers. In the United States in recent years, "You'll Never Walk Alone," long associated with Jerry Lewis's Labor Day muscular dystrophy tele-thons, has also been adopted by such causes as Hurricane Andrew relief and the annual national AIDS Walk campaigns. Marilyn Horne, Joan Baez, and others have sung "You'll Never Walk Alone" at AIDS Walk rallies in New York, Los Angeles, San Francisco, Philadelphia, and Chicago, and in 1992 Patti LaBelle made a new recording of the song for a national AIDS Walk public service announcement. At the 1994 AIDS Walk New York, Shirley Verrett and the cast of the Broadway production of *Carousel* sang "You'll Never Walk Alone" on the Great Lawn in Central Park before a crowd of thirty thousand. See Glynda Gardner, http://www.glyndas.com/story.asp.

8. Eddie Cantor's programs were broadcast on the radio from 1931 until the 1950s. When Franklin D. Roosevelt asked him to help raise money for the NFIP, Cantor came up with the phrase *March of Dimes*. The phrase gained great currency, thanks partly to the popular *The March of Time* newsreels. See the "Eddiecantor.ra" file, in Collection Selechonek.

9. *Miracle at Hickory,* publication no. 53 (New York: National Foundation for Infantile Paralysis, 1944), 5.

10. Alice E. Sink, *The Grit behind the Miracle: A True Story of the Determination and Hard Work behind an Emergency Infantile Paralysis Hospital, 1944–1945* (Lanham, Md.: University Press of America, 1998), begins with an account of a 1994 reunion of former patients, most of whom had not seen each other for some fifty years.

11. See Michael Troyson, *A Rose for Mrs. Miniver: The Life of Greer Garson* (Lexington: University Press of Kentucky, 1998).

12. On this transition, see *See It Now,* ed. Edward R. Murrow and Fred W. Friendly. On *The March of Time* program: *Time* magazine began issuing daily releases throughout the country in 1928 called *NewsCasts*. The following year *Time* supplemented these *NewsCasts* with electrical transcription dramas, five minutes in length, called *NewsActing*. The two were combined into a fifteen-minute show in 1929 under the title *The March of Time*. The show was built around a narrator who led listeners into the dramatized events.

13. Douglas Gomery, "Two Documents: 'Your Priceless Gift' and 'The 1946 Film Daily Yearbook,'" *Historical Journal of Film, Radio, and Television* 15, no. 1 (March 1995).

14. For Schenck, see *Variety* (March 5, 1969); Dore Schary, *Heyday: An Autobiography* (Boston: Little, Brown, 1979) tells what it was like to work for Schenck.

15. See Alfred W. Crosby, *America's Forgotten Pandemic: The Influenza of 1918* (Cambridge: Cambridge University Press, 1989).

16. "And being removed out of sight, quickly also he is out of mind." Thomas à Kempis, *Imitation of Christ,* trans. William Benham (London: Swan Sonnenschein, 1889), bk. 1, chap. 23.

17. Part of *The Crippler* (aka *The Daily Battle*) is included in the PBS movie *A Paralyzing Fear: The Story of Polio in America* (1998), directed by Nina Gilden Seavey.

18. T. S. Eliot, "The Hollow Men" (1925), in T. S. Eliot, *Complete Poems and Plays of T. S. Eliot* (London: Faber, 1969).

19. Robert F. Hall, *Through the Storm: A Polio Story* (St. Cloud, Minn.: North Star Press of St. Cloud, 1990). Other illustrations can be found in Leonard F. Peltier, *Orthopedics: A History and Iconography from Medical History* (London: Wellcome Trust, 1994), 1.

20. The paintings from 1944 of corsets and casts appear in Andrea Kettenmann, *Frida Kahlo, 1907–1954* (Cologne: Benedikt Taschen, 1993), 68. Other Kahlo works directly relevant to polio but not discussed elsewhere in *Polio and Its Aftermath* include the mutually contrasting *Without Hope* (1945) and *Tree of Hope* (1946), in Frida Kahlo, *The Diary of Frida Kahlo: An Intimate Self-Portrait*, introd. Carlos Fuentes, trans. Sarah M. Lowe (New York: Abrams; Mexico: La Vaca Independiente S. A. de C.V., 1995), 233, 263, 274; *"Naturaleza" bien muerta!* [A very still "still life"!]; worm's-eye view painting; *Feet what do I need them for / If I have wings to fly* (1953); and *Footprints*, in Kahlo, *Diary*, 274, 238. See Kahlo's reference to infantile paralysis and Farill, ibid., 251.

21. See Christopher Reeve's autobiography, *Still Me* (New York: Random House, 1998), and official statements of the Christopher Reeve Paralysis Foundation.

22. The Hemlock Society argues for "death with dignity" by means of suicide. See the society's booklet by Derek Humphry, *Final Exit: The Practicalities of Self-Deliverance and Assisted Suicide* (Eugene, Ore.: Hemlock Society, 1991).

23. See the movie-documentary *Flanders and Swann* (BBC, 1994, produced and directed by Kenneth Corden), about Michael Flanders (a polio) and Donald Swann, who became famous between 1956 and 1967. Their partnership ended with their T.V. show on Broadway.

24. *The Poetics of Aristotle*, ed. and trans. Samuel Henry Butcher, annotated 2nd ed. (New York: Macmillan, 1898), sect. 9.

25. Consider the once widespread allegations that HIV was God's way of punishing homosexuals and the promiscuous.

26. *OED*, s.v. *Infantolatrous*—"infant worshipping."

27. Quoted on back dust jacket of David Crosby and David Bender, *Stand and Be Counted: Making Music, Making History. The Dramatic Story of the Artists and Events that Shaped America* (San Francisco: HarperCollins, 2000).

28. Luke 4:23.

29. John C. Hughes, "The Wounded Healer," is reprinted at http://www.positive health.com/permit/Articles/People/wounded.htm by permission of *Journal of Hypnotism*, the National Guild of Hypnotists, Merrimack, N.H. Erickson continued to be troubled with various physical problems throughout his life, and suffered a second attack of paralytic polio at the age of fifty-one—a very rare occurrence, as normally one attack confers immunity. Milton Erickson's physical problems are recounted in a letter dated December 10, 1984, from his wife, Elizabeth Erickson: "About Erickson: His Physical Struggles."

30. On Sarah Bernhardt, whose leg was eventually amputated, see Martin F. Norden, *The Cinema of Isolation: A History of Physical Disability in the Movies* (New Brunswick, N.J.: Rutgers University Press, 1994), 69.

31. An accident having injured his arthritis-affected legs, Barrymore was eventually wheelchair-bound. As such, he played Dr. Gillespie in the fifteen Kildare movies

(1938–1947). "His legs are hopelessly crippled," says a hospital administrator in *The Secret of Dr. Kildare* (1939).

32. John Wells, one of the three producers of *ER,* says: "Laura Enders's character was conceived when I met one of the attendees at a local hospital who was East Indian or Pakistani and who had had polio and used crutches. He worked twelve-hour shifts, and his disability didn't interfere with his job." Interview with Zara Buggs Taylor, "Honest Portrayals of Disabilities Drive Popular Television Show," *Disability Messenger,* http://www.independentliving.org/docs1/taylor.html.

33. See Irving Zola, "Any Distinguishing Features—The Portrayal of Disability in the Crime Mystery Genre," in Stephen C. Hey, Gary Kiger, and Daryl Evans, eds., *The Changing World of Impaired and Disabled People in Society* (Salem, Ore.: Society for Disability Studies and Willamette University, 1989), 144–148.

34. For Oedipus and the riddle, see Marc Shell, *The Economy of Literature* (Baltimore, Md.: Johns Hopkins University Press, 1978), chap. 3.

35. Bruno Fischer's pseudonyms include Russell Gray and Adam Train.

36. Bruno Fischer, "Prey for the Creeping Death," *Dime Mystery* (July 1939). Other stories by Fischer include "The Dead Hand Horrors," *Dime Mystery* (April 1939), and "Flesh for the Monsters," *Dime Detective* (May 1939).

37. According to Robert Jones, the Kane series was "simply too grotesque to last"; see Don Hutchison, *The Great Pulp Heroes* (Buffalo, N.Y.: Mosaic Press, 1996).

38. Enid Foster, *It Can't Happen to Me* (Cape Town: Timmins, 1959), 162.

39. "To love the sinner, hate the sin": Jesus never did say that.

40. Blindness is "by far the most curable of movie disabilities." Norden, *Cinema of Isolation,* 59, 67, 213, 85. *The Miracle Man* (1919, by Paramount/Artcraft), was remade with sound in 1932.

41. See illustrations in Collection Selechonek.

42. Norden, *Cinema of Isolation,* 212.

43. Ibid., 212, 67.

44. See Marion's autobiography, *Off with Their Heads: A Serio-Comic Tale of Hollywood* (New York: Macmillan, 1972).

45. Humphrey was elected state chairperson of the women's division of the National Foundation for Infantile Paralysis and served with Mary Pickford, the screen star.

46. One detects echoes of nineteenth-century scandals involving murder—for example, the scandal of William Burke and William Hare, who murdered in order to supply bodies to the Scottish anatomist Robert Knox. Burke was hanged in 1829 for the murders.

47. *The Ape* (1940, directed by William Nigh, Monogram).

6. The Cast of *Rear Window*

1. J. M. Hayes's collaboration with Hitchcock is the subject of Steven DeRosa, *Writing with Hitchcock: The Collaboration of Alfred Hitchcock and John Michael Hayes* (London: Faber & Faber, 2001).

2. Martin F. Norden, *The Cinema of Isolation: A History of Physical Disability in the Movies* (New Brunswick, N.J.: Rutgers University Press, 1994), 97.

3. Alice Munro, "Open Secrets," in *Open Secrets* (Toronto: McClelland and Stewart, 1994), esp. 133; Catherine Marchant, *House of Men* (London: Corgi Paperback, 1963). In the latter, Rossiter is an embittered victim of polio, subject to fits of temper and depression.

4. Concerning the Marlon Brando movie, compare it with *Born on the Fourth of July* (1989), directed by Oliver Stone, in which Ron Kovic (Tom Cruise) joins up for the Vietnam War. He returns from the war an embittered veteran, paralyzed from the midchest down.

5. Kriegel says that Trumbo's novel is an extreme form of "the cripple novel"—perhaps even outside the genre: Leonard Kriegel, *Falling into Life: Essays* (San Francisco: North Point, 1991), 141.

6. *Johnny cogió su fusilo: Guión cinematográfico de Dalton Trumbo y Luis Buñuel* (Teruel, Spain: Instituto de Estudios Turolenses, Departamento de Cultura y Educación, 1993).

7. Bentz Plagemann, *My Place to Stand* (London: Gollancz, 1950), 122.

8. Paul Bates, with John Pellows, *Horizontal Man* (London: Longmans, Green, 1964); Wendell Phillips, *Qataban and Sheba: Exploring Ancient Kingdoms on the Biblical Spice Road of Arabia* (London: Gollancz, 1955). Phillips embarks on his explorations after his "recovery" from polio.

9. Craik's fictional lame prince did not really have polio: he was crippled, presumably by accident, when his nurse let him fall; yet there are other circumstances to take into account when seeking to understand this lameness, including the role of the wicked uncle. In any case, many readers have recognized Craik's lame prince as an obvious polio survivor; *The Lame Prince* was the main narratological model for tens of children's books written by adults for child-polios, and adult novelists, themselves polios, have also seen Craik's crippled hero as essentially a polio.

10. The first part of J. D. Beresford's trilogy (1911–1915) is *The Early History of Jacob Stahl* (Boston: Little, Brown, 1911). For the ambiguity surrounding the injury, see esp. 19–29.

11. See the recently restored version of *Rear Window*, Collectors Edition DVD (hereafter RW-DVD), March 6, 2001; run time 113 minutes, ASIN-B00003CXC7; here 1.25.50 (hour, minutes, seconds). John Michael Hayes, *Rear Window* (screenplay, Final White Script, December 1, 1953); here scene 345.

12. *Leg art:* exploitation of sex appeal in pictures. Robert Johnston, "Slanguage of Amateur Photographers," *American Speech* 15 (1940): 359.

13. Polios were put into casts to keep the muscles forcibly from doing any work. It was against the doctrine of keeping muscles still by means of heavy casts that Sister Kenny fought.

14. Owing to the polio and its weakening of the muscles, her spine had curved gradually: "scoliosis" as she explained to Martin later. Judith Rossner, *Looking for Mr. Goodbar* (New York: Simon and Schuster, 1975), 43. "She was in the hospital for a year,

her torso encased in a plaster cast both before and after the operation" (16).

15. Owen Dixson, *My Way with Polio: An Autobiography* (London: Merritt & Hatcher, 1960), 99.

16. In *The Affair* (directed by Gilbert Cates), Wood stars as a polio-crippled songwriter, and Robert Wagner (in reality her husband or soon to be) is the man who is her first love. Joan McDonnell, *A Spring in My Step* (Wilton, Ireland: Collins, 2004), 136–154.

17. Sophie uses Polo perfume and sometimes identifies herself as a polio. In apparently "more honest" moments, she admits that her paralysis stems from viral encephalitis. Sophie tells people she had polio because, as she says, more people have heard of polio than viral encephalitis.

18. Polios, like other people, and perhaps even more frequently than others, would break their legs in the normal course of their "after polio" lives. And then they would be put into casts.

19. The polio director Lewin first wrote the script for *Lucky Break* as part of his coming to terms with the real physical effects of his own bout with childhood polio. The woman whom Lewin hired to teach Carideas how to act like a person paralyzed by polio had been Lewin's nurse during his polio treatment.

20. *OED*, s.v. *Akinesia.*

21. RW-DVD, 1.48.18, 1.25.50, 0.58.73.

22. Ibid.; Hayes, *Rear Window*, scenes 208, 209.

23. Christine Brooke-Rose, The *Languages of Love* (London: Secker & Warburg, 1957), 15; quoted in *OED*, s.v. *Jay-walker.*

24. Hayes, *Rear Window*, scene 89.

25. Though this is in the script, we do not see it all recorded in the movie.

26. Hayes, *Rear Window*, scene 474.

27. D. H. Lawrence, *Etruscan Places* (London: Secker, 1932), 127; the book was written in 1927 and published posthumously. *Lady Chatterley's Lover*, in which Sir Clifford Chatterley is the paralyzed veteran, was published in Florence in 1928.

28. Laura Mulvey, "Visual Pleasure and Narrative Cinema," *Screen* 16, no. 3 (1975): 16.

29. *Jack* (1996) concerns a ten-year-old boy who, because he has a medical condition that causes him to age much faster than other children, now inhabits a forty-year-old body. "I think it was Hemingway who said that to be a great artist you have to have an unhappy childhood," said Coppola: "I had polio as a child and was kept from any contact with kids. There was a lot of longing. And I think that was why I empathized with this movie."

30. Hayes, *Rear Window*, scene 1; RW-DVD, 0.03.28.

31. *OED*, s.v. *Cast*, 24.

32. One still picture "freezes" an automobile crash at a race, RW-DVD, 0.03.42. Another, 0.03.45, shows men running from a truck bursting into flame.

33. Ibid., 0.16.02.

34. *OED*, s.v. *Cast*, a. John Lydgate, *The Life of Saint Alban and Saint Amphibal*, ed.

J. E. van der Westhuizen (Leiden, The Netherlands: Brill, 1974 [ca. 1400]), Cij. More on the apparently hidden problem of sibling—and hence incestuous or literally chaste—marriage follows later in this chapter.

35. "Photography's Earliest Days," and "Grace Kelly—Hollywood's Brightest and Busiest Star," *Life,* April 26, 1954.

36. Princess Grace visited—and donated funds to—Saint Edmond's Home for Crippled Children in 1976. Saint Edmond's had been founded in Philadelphia in the 1920s as a home for children crippled by polio. See Anne W. Breidendtein, "Saint Edmond's Home for Crippled Children, Women's Auxiliary," in Jean Barth Toll and Mildred S. Gillam, eds., *Invisible Philadelphia* (New York: Atwater Kent Museum, 1995), 405.

37. RW-DVD, 0.01.53. As it turns out, we see only later (at 0.15.38) that the "wheel-chair" is *perhaps* another kind of moving chair—a rocking chair a little like the one in Hitchcock's movie *Psycho* (1960). Other references to the child and the child's caretakers appear ibid., 1.50.05, 1.23.06, and 0.43.25.

38. Ibid., 0.01.02.

39. In particular, there are the children we see playing in the street, ibid., 0.08.05, 0.16.00, and 0.36.40, and sometimes there follows a water-sprinkler vehicle (0.03.16).

40. Jeff asks about the absence of a doctor for the Thorwalds, ibid., 0.47.30. For the image of Lisa, see 0.03.53. In the opening shot, we see a framed negative of a blonde woman's face; the same photograph, now a positive, of the woman appears on the cover of a large stack of *Life* magazines labeled "Paris Fashions." *OED,* s.v. *Cast:* "A model . . . Sometimes applied to the negative impression taken from the original; more usually to the copy of the original moulded." RW-DVD, 0.03.57, 0.16.02.

41. RW-DVD, 1.49.00.

42. Ibid., 0.10.29, 0.09.03.

43. Garth Drabinsky, *Closer to the Sun: An Autobiography* (Toronto: McClelland and Stewart, 1995), 1. Drabinsky is the author of *Motion Pictures and the Arts in Canada: The Business and the Law* (Toronto: McGraw-Hill Ryerson, 1976). On sprinklers, see RW-DVD, 0.03.16.

44. RW-DVD, 0.10.37, 0.04.24, 0.05.59. In Hayes's script, Editor Gunnison seems to know that Jeff has been in his cast longer than Gunnison says. Hayes, *Rear Window,* scene 2.

45. RW-DVD, 0.26.2, 0.02.38 (and so on), 0.04.44.

46. Hayes, *Rear Window,* scene 42. Compare with RW-DVD, 0.16.02.

47. RW-DVD, 0.01.51.

48. William Irish (pseudonym of Cornell Woolrich), "Rear Window" (also known as "It Had to Be Murder"), in *Six Times Death* (Toronto: Better Publications of Canada, 1948), 181. The short story was first published in book format in William Irish, *After Dinner Story* (New York: Lippincott, 1936). Collection Selechonek.

49. McDonnell, *A Spring in My Step,* 19.

50. Allen V. Lee, *My Soul More Bent* (Minneapolis, Minn.: Augsburg, 1948), 81–82.

51. Elaine Strauss, *In My Heart I'm Still Dancing* (New Rochelle, N.Y.: Strauss, 1979), 25. Strauss provides an example of the error, on 85.

52. Robert Mauro, *Real Crip Sex*, available via the Web; also Richard Bruno, "Sex and Polio Survivors." Robert Mauro, *Sucking Air, Doing Wheelies* (Levittown, N.Y.: People Net, 1999). See also J. G. Farrell, *The Lung* (London: Hutchinson, 1965), 173–177; J. G. Farrell, *A Girl in the Head* (London: Cape, 1967).

53. *Shadows of the Heart* (1990, produced by Jock Blair, directed by Road Hardy, starring Josephine Byrne, Marcus Graham, and Jason Donovan).

54. Dixson, *My Way with Polio*, 72 ff.

55. The film, directed by Bryan Forbes, stars Malcolm McDowell and Nanette Newman. The autobiography is Peter Marshall, *Two Lives* (London: Hutchinson, 1962).

56. The historian Charles Rosenberg writes of the rise of America's hospital system in terms of the care of strangers but does not consider how the family may become strange after hospitalization. Charles Rosenberg, *The Care of Strangers: The Rise of America's Hospital System* (New York: Basic, 1987).

57. Richard Chaput writes convincingly that the ways in which the religious celibate and the totally paralyzed person deal with sexuality are much the same. (The image of an iron lung as a coffin for the living thus resembles the idea of monks and nuns' dying to the world, although they live on after that.) Richard Chaput, *Not to Doubt* (New York: Pageant, 1964). The book details a boy's struggles with polio and an entire life in an iron lung.

58. Bernard F. Stehle, *Incurably Romantic* (Philadelphia: Temple University Press, 1985). Since 1960, the home has also been known as Inglis House.

59. Strauss, *In My Heart*, 183.

60. Michel Eyquem, seigneur de Montaigne, "Of Cripples," in *The Essays* 3.11, trans. Charles Cotton, ed. William Carew Hazlitt (London: Reeves and Turner, 1877 [ca. 1575]). "La philosophie ancienne . . . dict, que les jambes & cuisses des boiteuses, ne recevans à cause de leur imperfection, l'aliment qui leur est deu, il en advient que les parties genitales, qui sont au dessus, sont plus plaines, plus nourries, et vigoureuses. Ou bien que ce défaut empeschant l'exercice, ceux qui en sont entachez, dissipent moins leurs forces, et en viennent plus entiers aux jeux de Venus."

61. The example of detective Oedipus, who has lost the use of his foot but still has too much sex drive, does not convince us otherwise, though his tearing out of his eyes might. Consider the topos of the modern detective (in the defective-detective genre) who is missing a foot or leg and also a testicle. One example is Jerry Allen's detective character, Samuel Clemens Tucker; see Gary Hoppenstand and Ray Brown, eds., *The Defective Detective in the Pulps* (Bowling Green, Ohio: Bowling Green State University Popular Press, 1983), and its sequel, Gary Hoppenstand and Ray Brown eds., *More Tales of the Defective Detective in the Pulps* (Bowling Green, Ohio: Bowling Green State University Popular Press, 1983).

62. Sholem Asch, *East River: A Novel of New York*, trans. A. H. Gross (New York: Putnam's Sons, 1946).

63. Sigmund Freud, "The Aetiology of Hysteria," in *Standard Edition of the Complete Psychological Works of Sigmund Freud*, ed. and trans., James Strachey (London: Hogarth, 1957–1974), 3:191–221. For the reference to paraplegia, see section 3.

64. Sigmund Freud, *Infantile Cerebral Paralysis* [translation of *Infantile Cerebral-*

lähmung], trans. Lester A. Russin (Coral Gables, Fla.: University of Miami Press, 1968). On Freud's "cure" of Bruno Walter's paralysis, see E. Garcia, "Bruno Walter Consults Sigmund Freud: Notes on an Unconventional Therapeutic Cure," *Journal of the Conductor's Guild* 11, nos. 1–2 (Winter–Spring 1990): 24–31. Richard F. Sterba, intrigued by Bruno Walter's 1946 account of his treatment by Freud, interviewed the conductor after the war. Walter said: "I endeavored to adapt my conducting technique to the weakness of my arm without impairing the musical effect. So, by dint of much effort and confidence, by learning and forgetting, I finally succeeded in finding my way back to my profession." In Bruno Walter, *Themes and Variations* (London: Hamish Hamilton, 1947), 167–168. Walter, who was paralyzed around 1904, recalls the ensuing exchange with his analyst: " 'But I can't move my arm.' 'Try anyway.' 'And if I have to stop?' 'You won't!' 'How could I face being responsible for a possible interruption in the performance?' 'I will take that responsibility upon myself.' " (184). See Peter Fonagy, Keynote Address to the Spring Meeting of Division 39 of the American Psychological Association, New York, April 16, 1999.

65. Hugh Gregory Gallagher, *FDR's Splendid Deception* (New York: Dodd, Mead, 1985), 54.

66. For an example of an early thesis linking polio and the brain, see R. L. Bruno, J. Cohn, T. Galski, and N. M. Frick, "The Neuroanatomy of Post-Polio Fatigue," *Archives of Physical Medicine and Rehabilitation* 75 (1994): 498–504.

67. Writes William James: "In the wonderful explorations by Binet, Janet, Breuer, Freud, Mason, Prince and others of the subliminal consciousness of patients with hysteria, we have revealed to us whole systems of underground life, in the shape of memories of a painful sort which lead a parasitic existence, buried outside the primary fields of consciousness, and making irruptions thereunto with hallucinations, pains, convulsions, paralyses of feeling and of motion, and the whole procession of symptoms of hysteric disease of body and of mind." William James, *Varieties of Religious Experience* (New York: Longmans, Green, 1902), 230. See also B. A. van der Kolk and O. van der Hart, "Pierre Janet and the Breakdown of Adaptation in Psychological Trauma," *American Journal of Psychiatry* 146 (1989): 1530–1540.

68. Arthur Miller, *Broken Glass* (New York: Dramatists Play Service, 1994), depicts a woman who has been paralyzed either by the thought of the European Holocaust or by her unsatisfying marriage.

69. Pierre Boileau and Thomas Narcejac, *D'entre les morts,* translated as *Vertigo* [originally titled *The Living and the Dead*] (New York: Dell, 1956).

70. One of Kahlo's painted corsets (1944), an "oil on plaster cast with straps," includes a depiction of Kahlo's broken spinal column; see Andrea Kettenmann, *Frida Kahlo, 1907–1954* (Cologne: Benedikt Taschen, 1993), 68.

71. Franklin D. Roosevelt to Robert W. Lovett, November 13, 1922, Robert W. Lovett Collection of the Francis A. Countway Library of Medicine, Harvard University, Boston; quoted in Richard Thayer Goldberg, *The Making of Franklin D. Roosevelt: Triumph over Disability* (Cambridge, Mass.: Abt, 1981), 52.

72. RW-DVD, 1.31.30.

73. R. C. Emsllie, *The Care of the Invalid and Crippled Children in School* (London: School of Hygiene Publishing Company, 1911), 9. On amputation as treatment for polio, see Gallagher, *Splendid Deception,* 31.

74. See John Belton, *Hitchcock's Rear Window* (Cambridge: Cambridge University Press, 2001), 6.

75. In apoterpnophilia, the amputation is the result of an obsession focused usually on the self. If the patient has not requested surgery, an amputation may be self-induced.

76. In 1998, Richard Bruno said, of people who pretend to be disabled, that many devotees and wannabes suffer from a form of "factitious disorder." Richard Bruno, "Devotees, Pretenders and Wannabes: Two Cases of Factitious Disability Disorder," *Overground: Dedicated to Providing Support for Those of Us Who Are Attracted to Others with Disabilities,* www.overground.be. Another view on wearing prostheses in the absence of any physical need to do so is that it is a form of dysmorphophobia or dysmorphobia. Compare also the condition of apotemnophobia.

77. Hayes, *Rear Window,* scenes 27 (RW-DVD, 0.10.36), 48, 249.

78. Wolfgang E. H. Rudat, "Sexual Dilemmas in *The Sun Also Rises:* Hemingway's Count and the Education of Jacob Barnes," *Hemingway Review* 8 (Spring 1989): 2–13.

79. Gloria (aka Gregory) Hemingway, *Papa: A Personal Memoir,* preface by Norman Mailer (Boston: Houghton Mifflin, 1976).

80. Actor Reeve's hero, Kemp (an architect), is divorced now, and as permanently paralyzed as any quadriplegic could be, but he behaves as if he were not, thanks to computer technology and a black male attendant (corresponding roughly to the camera in Hitchcock's film and the male attendant, Sam in Cornell Woolrich's story).

81. Walter Everaerd, "A Case of Apotemnophilia: A Handicap as Sexual Preference," *American Journal of Psychotherapy* 37, no. 2 (April 1983): 285–293.

82. Dr. John Money coined the term *disability paraphilia* to describe people fascinated by disabilities. Dr. Money termed the attraction to leg braces, wheelchairs and the people who use them abasiophilia. See John Money, "Paraphilia in Females: Fixation on Amputation and Lameness: Two Accounts," *Journal of Psychology and Human Sexuality* 3, no. 2 (1990): 165–172.

83. John Currin, *The Cripple* (1997), Andrea Rosen Gallery, Basel. A famous image by Jeff Koons is one of an attractive girl in leg braces. The model has posed in many of Koons's photo shots. Some call this sort of artwork caliper fetishism.

84. Hayes's script suggests sometimes that Lisa was cold and Jeff was hot so that she is his cast, or casing.

85. The heroine of the novel has dreams in which a person is a sort of statue that can't get out. Judith Rossner, *Looking for Mr. Goodbar* (New York: Simon and Schuster, 1975), 24.

86. Luther Robinson, *We Made Peace with Polio* (Nashville, Tenn.: Broodman, 1960).

87. Farrell, *Lung,* 66.

88. Regarding Lisa's having "stolen the case," see RW-DVD, 1.22.16. Some critics

have pointed out that the movie's protagonist is fixated at an infantile level of sexual development and must grow into "mature sexuality." Robert Stam and Roberta Pearson devote one brief paragraph to this issue in their article "Hitchcock's *Rear Window:* Reflexivity and the Critique of Voyeurism," *Enclitic* 7, no. 1 (Spring 1983): 140. Other critics suggest that Jeff is at the mirror stage of development, a placement that makes him like a cinematic spectator in relation to the screen. Metz speaks of "that other mirror, the cinema screen, in this respect a veritable psychical substitute, a prosthesis for our primally dislocated limbs" (138).

89. RW-DVD, 1.26.40.

90. Consider the following dialogue, ibid., 0.23.30:

> *Jeff:* "Miss Lonelyhearts." Well, at least that's something you'll never have to worry about.
>
> *Lisa:* Oh? You can see my apartment from here, all the way up on 63rd Street?
>
> *Jeff:* No, not exactly . . .

91. Ibid., 0.25.00.

92. Hitchcock comments, "One of the things I was unhappy about in *Rear Window* was the music. It didn't work out the way I wanted it to, and I was quite disappointed." See François Truffaut, *Hitchcock* (New York: Simon and Schuster, 1967), 160; originally published as *Le Cinéma selon Hitchcock* (Paris: Robert Laffont, 1966). See also Elizabeth Weis, *The Silent Scream: Alfred Hitchcock's Soundtrack* (Rutherford, N.J.: Fairleigh Dickinson University Press, 1982).

93. See Joan Zlotnick, "The Medium Is the Message, or Is It? A Study of Nathanael West's Comic Strip Novel," *Journal of Popular Culture* 5, no. 1 (Summer 1971): 236–240.

94. RW-DVD, 0.04.44.

95. Virginia Lee Counterman Acosta, *Polio Tragedy of 1941* (n.p., 1999), 94.

96. Interview with Sharon Term in *Living Longer—Medical Advances Further the Fight against Disease,* first broadcast on Monday, June 21, 1999, at 10 PM. *Living Longer* is produced and directed by Peter Ceresole, narrated by John Forsythe. Transcript in Collection Selechonek.

97. Farrell, *Lung,* 63.

98. See Lynne M. Dunphy, "The Steel Cocoon: Tales of the Nurses and Patients of the Iron Lung," *Nursing History Review* (official journal of the American Association for the History of Nursing, ed. Joan E. Lynaugh) 9 (2001): 3–33.

99. *No Pain,* episode 5, season 5, of *Alfred Hitchcock Presents* (CBS), October 25, 1959, directed by Norman Lloyd and starring Brian Keith in the iron lung.

100. *Cell 227,* episode 34, season 5, ibid., June 6, 1960, directed by Paul Henreid.

101. In Dick Francis, *Forfeit* (London: Pan, 1989), the main character, Tyrone, has a wife who is paralyzed. Tyrone investigates some villains, who try to kidnap his wife and threaten to turn off her ventilator.

102. Ray Turner, *Huston's Laws* (Edmonton, Canada: Commonwealth Publications,

1997). In this Canadian polio memoir-novel a leftover iron lung is integrated into the hospital routine to benefit an emphysema patient. Arthur Hailey, *Overload* (Garden City, N.J.: Doubleday, 1979).

103. Omega Baker, "Iron Lung," *Winchester Star*, April 3, 1995, in the column Slice of Life.

104. *OED*, s.v. *Rear*, n. 3. Another favorite photographic subject was the iron-lung resident's book, whose pages a person or a mechanical device would turn.

105. Colleen Adair Fliedner and G. Maureen Rodgers, *Rancho los Amigos Medical Center: Centennial, 1888–1988* (Downey, Calif.: Rancho Los Amigos Medical Center, 1990), 231.

106. "There was a little girl in the Communicable Disease Unit, and she wanted to see what was happening with the movie. The grips approached the producer and said, 'We promise to be super careful if you'll let us take the second mirror and mount it for this little girl.' So, with masks and gowns, they mounted the mirror and wheeled her iron lung over to the window, and adjusted the mirror so that she could see out. The child started to cry, and they asked what was wrong. 'I never knew I could see so good. Everything is so beautiful,' the little girl explained. With that, the crew went back to the studio, and they robbed the studio blind of everything they needed to make dozens and dozens of these mirrors." Notes attached to a photo, ibid., 231.

107. Farrell, *Lung*, 70.

108. Irish (pseud. of Woolrich), "Rear Window," 181.

109. Ibid., 145; emphasis mine.

110. RW-DVD, 0.43.18. At the end, both Jeff's legs are encased. Hayes, *Rear Window*, 162.

111. *OED*, s.v. *El:* "The initial element of jocular, pseudo-Sp. noun and adj. phrases representing colloq. (and often nonce) alternatives to their Eng. bases (nouns or adjs. freq. in turn suffixed by the Sp. masc. ending *-o*), which convey disparagement, emphasis, or amusement: as *El Cheapo a.* (and *n.*), *el creepo, el foldo, el smoggo*, etc."

112. See, for example, Elise Lemire, "Voyeurism and the Post-War Crisis of Masculinity in *Rear Window*," in Belton, *Hitchcock's "Rear Window*," 82. Lemire seems not to know the Douglas book.

113. Hayes, *Rear Window*, 162. The script has her merely picking up a travel book, not by Douglas, so this would presumably have been a not-in-the-script decision by Hitchcock.

114. Belton, *Hitchcock's "Rear Window,"* 90.

115. Charles H. Andrews, *No Time for Tears* (New York: Doubleday, 1951).

116. William O. Douglas, *Go East Young Man: The Early Years. The Autobiography of William O. Douglas* (New York: Random House, 1974), 34.

117. Ibid.; Bernard Lown, *The Lost Art of Healing* (Boston: Houghton Mifflin, 1997).

118. Douglas, *Go East Young Man*, 31.

119. See Hayes, *Rear Window*, scene 11; RW-DVD, 0.05.10.

120. The use of this term to mean "have sexual intercourse" was already common in the earlier part of the twentieth century. *OED*, s.v. *Way*, n. 1.

121. Hayes, *Rear Window*, scene 147; RW-DVD, 0.44.05.

122. Compare the corset in *Vertigo*. *Corset*, whose etymology represents something like "little body," means "a close-fitting body garment, *esp.* a laced bodice worn as an outside garment by women in the middle ages and still in many countries; also a similar garment formerly worn by men." *OED*, s.v. *Corset*, 1.

123. "Plaster casting is an intermediate stage in the production of a piece of sculpture which is often the last process actually to be carried out by the sculptor himself." Peter and Linda Murray, A *Dictionary of Art and Artists* (London: Penguin, 1959), 248.

124. Rupert Brooke, *Collected Poems* (New York: Lane, 1915), vol.` 2.

7. Polio and the Great Wars

1. Christopher J. Rutty, "Forty Years of Polio Prevention! Canada and the Great Salk Vaccine Trial of 1954–55," *Abilities* 19 (Summer 1994): 26, 28.

2. Elliott Roosevelt, ed., *FDR: His Personal Letters, 1905–1928* (New York: Duell, Sloan, and Pearce, 1950), 566.

3. See Theo Lippman, Jr., *The Squire of Warm Springs: F. D. R. in Georgia, 1924–1945* (Chicago: Playboy, 1977), 39.

4. See Roosevelt's extemporaneous remarks to patients at Warm Springs, Georgia, March 24, 1937.

5. E. Roosevelt, *Personal Letters*, 568.

6. Ibid., 623–624.

7. Roosevelt did not—and for political reasons, perhaps he could not—argue in public for including African-Americans at Warm Springs. See Lippman, *Squire of Warm Springs*, 155. There was limited racial integration at Hickory, however, as can be seen from the second photograph in Chapter 8.

8. *Columbus Ledger* (Columbus, Georgia), November 21, 1938, 1.

9. Lippman, *Squire of Warm Springs*, 53.

10. Kenneth Sydney Davis, *FDR: The New York Years, 1928–1933* (New York: Random House, 1985), 295.

11. In 1957, under the aegis of WHO (World Health Organization), the Sabin vaccine went to large groups of children in Russia and other countries. The NFIP and the U.S. Public Health Service opposed this vaccine for the United States for years more.

12. David Sills, *The Volunteers: Means and Ends in a National Organization. A Report* (Glencoe, Ill.: Free Press, 1957).

13. Elizabeth Cox, *Night Thoughts: A Novel* (Saint Paul, Minn.: Graywolf, 1997).

14. W. F. Carroll, *Whence? Why? Whither?* (San Francisco: Cummings Engraving & Printing, 1948). On the front cover of this book we read: "Communism is a horrible pestilence! More deadly than cancer, more devastating than polio, it warps the minds and souls of men. It plots world revolution and destruction of freedom. Communism must be eradicated! Now and forever!" This book has a strongly Christian religious viewpoint.

15. Richard Carter, "The Polio Triumph," in *The Gentle Legions* (Garden City, N.Y.:

Doubleday, 1961), 91. With regard to public assistance, see Christopher J. Rutty, " 'Do Something! . . . Do Anything!' Poliomyelitis in Canada, 1927–1962," Ph.D. diss., University of Toronto, 1995, 171. Canadian counterparts of the NFIP and the March of Dimes were relatively small.

16. Rutty, " 'Do Something!' " 381.

17. Susan Sontag, *AIDS and Its Metaphors* (New York: Farrar, Straus and Giroux, 1989), 94.

18. At least according to Susan Sontag, *Illness as Metaphor* (New York: Farrar, Straus and Giroux, 1978), 66. Cf. Sontag, *AIDS and Its Metaphors,* 8. In this light also Sontag discusses the "fortress metaphor."

19. See the illustration "The Germ Castle," in Emily Martin, *Flexible Bodies: Tracking Immunity in American Culture from the Days of Polio to the Age of AIDS* (Boston: Beacon, 1994), 34–35.

20. President Roosevelt's informal remarks at Thanksgiving dinner, Warm Springs, Georgia, November 23, 1939.

21. "In other words, I think our attitude toward religion, towards helping one's neighbors has changed an awful lot and we believe that there are certain forces of human endeavor that may be called, very properly, war—war against things that we understand about, things that can be improved, ameliorated, bettered in every way because of human endeavor." Ibid.

22. *King of the Royal Mounted,* series in twelve "chapters" (1940, directed by William Whitney and John English, Republic).

23. Basil O'Connor, *The Conquest of Infantile Paralysis* (New York: National Foundation for Infantile Paralysis, 1940).

24. Alton L. Blakeslee, *Polio Can Be Conquered,* prepared with the cooperation of the National Foundation for Infantile Paralysis and the New York Academy of Medicine (New York: Public Affairs Committee, 1949); Robert Coughlan, *The Coming Victory over Polio* (New York: Simon and Schuster, 1954).

25. Virginia Lee Counterman Acosta, *Polio Tragedy of 1941* (n.p., 1999), 13.

26. Leonard Kriegel, *Falling into Life* (San Francisco: North Point, 1991), 4.

27. Marjorie Lawrence, *Interrupted Melody* (Sydney: Invincible, 1949), 205, 225; the book was made into a movie in 1955. See also, on 178, a description of her interest in singing "Waltzing Matilda."

8. Remembering Roosevelt

1. Doris Kearns Goodwin, *Character above All: Ten Presidents from FDR to George Bush,* ed. Robert A. Wilson (New York: Simon and Schuster, 1995), 18. See also Doris Kearns Goodwin, *No Ordinary Time: Franklin and Eleanor Roosevelt—The Home Front in World War II* (New York: Simon and Schuster, 1994).

2. Doris Kearns Goodwin, *Wait till Next Year: A Memoir* (New York: Simon and Schuster, 1997).

3. Sholem Asch, *East River: A Novel of New York,* trans. A. H. Gross (New York:

Putnam's Sons, 1946). Daniel Kirk, *Breakfast at the Liberty Diner* (New York: DK Publishing, 1997).

    4. Quoted in Goodwin, *No Ordinary Time.*

    5. Frances Perkins, *The Roosevelt I Knew* (New York: Viking, 1946). The quotation is from Richard Thayer Goldberg, *The Making of Franklin D. Roosevelt: Triumph over Disability* (Cambridge, Mass: Abt, 1981), 67.

    6. Perkins, *The Roosevelt I Knew,* 28, 29–30.

    7. John Gunther, *Roosevelt in Retrospect: A Profile in History* (New York: Harper, 1950).

    8. John Gunther, *Death Be Not Proud: A Memoir* (New York: Harper, 1949).

    9. Jim Bishop, *FDR's Last Year: April 1944–April 1945* (New York: William Morrow, 1974); cited in Hugh Gregory Gallagher, *FDR's Splendid Deception* (New York: Dodd, Mead, 1985), 209. See also NBC's TV movie starring Jason Robards, *FDR: The Last Year* (1980).

    10. Goldberg, *Making of Franklin D. Roosevelt.*

    11. Gallagher, *Splendid Deception.*

    12. Geoffrey C. Ward, *Before the Trumpet: Young Franklin Roosevelt, 1882–1905* (New York: Harper & Row, 1985); Geoffrey C. Ward, *First-Class Temperament: The Emergence of Franklin Roosevelt* (New York: Harper & Row, 1989).

    13. Ruth Butts Stevens, *Hi-ya Neighbor: Intimate Glimpses of Franklin D. Roosevelt at Warm Springs, Georgia, 1924–1945* (New York: Tupper and Love, 1947).

    14. Turnley Walker, *Roosevelt and the Warm Springs Story* (New York: A. A. Wyn, 1953).

    15. Goldberg, *Making of Franklin D. Roosevelt,* 167, 68, 135.

    16. Gallagher, *Splendid Deception,* 168.

    17. Goldberg, *Making of Franklin D. Roosevelt,* 172 (1976 interview with Thomas Corcoran).

    18. Ibid. (interview with Alice Roosevelt Longworth in Washington, D.C., on September 9 and 10, 1976), 172–173.

    19. Gallagher, *Splendid Deception,* 209.

    20. Hugh Gallagher, *Black Bird Fly Away: Disabled in an Able-Bodied World* (Arlington, Va.: Vandamere, 1998).

    21. Goldberg, *Making of Franklin D. Roosevelt,* 170; the passage refers to Fred Botts's article, *Polio Chronicle* 2, no. 9 (April 1933): 2.

    22. Franklin D. Roosevelt, first inaugural address, March 4, 1933, Washington, D.C.

    23. Quoted in Susan Sontag, *Illness as Metaphor* (New York: Farrar, Straus and Giroux, 1978), 59. See also Wilhelm Reich, *The Mass Psychology of Fascism,* 3rd ed. (New York: Farrar, Straus and Giroux, 1970).

    24. Cited in Goldberg, *Making of Franklin D. Roosevelt,* 173.

    25. Earle Looker, "Is FDR Physically Fit to Be President?" *Liberty,* July 25, 1931. A reporter once publicly asked Eleanor Roosevelt whether polio had affected her husband's mind. There was a long pause. Then she replied, Yes, that it had affected his mind—it had made him more sensitive to the pain of others. (The polio Mark O'Brien, who re-

tells this story from his iron lung, thinks that the polio affected Roosevelt's mind to the point where he thought he could serve four full terms!) On Earle Looker, see also Gallagher, *Splendid Deception,* 84–85. Gallagher suggests that it was an inside, "put-up" job coming from the Roosevelt side itself.

26. As cited in Theo Lippman, Jr., *The Squire of Warm Springs: F. D. R. in Georgia, 1924–1945* (Chicago: Playboy, 1977), 178.

27. Cited ibid., 178.

28. See James George Frazer, *The Golden Bough: A Study in Comparative Religion* (London: Macmillan, 1890).

29. Jessie Weston, *From Ritual to Romance* (Cambridge: Cambridge University Press, 1920). See especially T. S. Eliot, *The Waste Land* (1922), in *Complete Poems and Plays* (New York: Harcourt, Brace, 1952).

30. See the illustration "Kings-Evil" in Dorothy Sterling and Philip Sterling, *Polio Pioneers: The Story of the Fight against Polio,* photos by Myron Ehrenberg and the National Foundation for Infantile Paralysis (Garden City, N.Y.: Doubleday, 1955).

31. Ronald Reagan, *Where's the Rest of Me?* written with Richard G. Hubler (New York: Duell, Sloan, and Pearce, 1965), 5. Reagan's transformation from actor to politician, his book explains, was the result of a similar shock: his realization that "to remain an actor was to be only 'half a man.' He left the movie 'monastery' (his word suggests both holiness and impotence) to put his ideals into political practice, 'find the rest of me,' and become whole" (57). Eureka College library dedication, September 18, 1967; first inaugural address, January 20, 1981.

32. The play is one of his subjects in Ralph Bellamy, *When the Smoke Hits the Fan* (New York: Doubleday, 1979).

33. Gallagher, *Splendid Deception,* 211.

34. Goldberg, *Making of Franklin D. Roosevelt,* 37.

35. Dore Schary, *Sunrise at Campobello: A Play in Three Acts* (New York: Random House, 1958), 44, 47, 48.

36. Gallagher writes, "Roosevelt had led a fortunate childhood; he had not confronted the feelings of abandonment and helplessness experienced by so many children." Whatever effect polio had on Roosevelt, who had polio in 1921 at the age of forty-nine, it might be expected to be different in quality, if not also quantity, from the effect on young adults like Gallagher (who had polio in 1952 at the age of nineteen) and also from the effect on those "so many children" with whom Gallagher seems to empathize. Yet even mature adult polios such as FDR and—perhaps Gallagher—find themselves suddenly "infantilized" by polio. As Gallagher construes the life of the historical Roosevelt, "here in mid-life . . . FDR found himself helpless, the object of pity." Gallagher, *Splendid Deception,* 121.

37. Lela Stiles, *The Man behind Roosevelt: The Story of Louis McHenry Howe* (Cleveland, Ohio: World Publishing, 1954). See also Alfred Brooks Rollins, *Roosevelt and Howe* (New York: Knopf, 1962).

38. Schary, *Sunrise at Campobello,* 35.

39. Ibid., 25, 79, 75–76.

40. Tom Burke, "On the Rights Track," in Pietro Nivola, ed., *Comparative Disadvantages? Social Regulations and the Global Economy* (Washington, D.C.: Brookings Institution Press, 1997), 247.

41. In Pennsylvania, disabled people, including polios, were officially termed antisocial beings; in Washington, they were said to be "unfitted for companionship with other children"; in Vermont, a "blight on mankind"; in Wisconsin, a "danger to the race." A Utah government report said that a "defect . . . wounds our citizenry a thousand times more than any plague." Martha Russell, "No Nursing Homes on Wheels," *ZNet*, November 5, 2002. United States Supreme Court, views cited in an opinion by Justice Oliver Wendell Holmes upholding the constitutionality of a Virginia law authorizing the involuntary sterilization of disabled persons. Timothy M. Cook, *A Little History Worth Knowing* (Lucky, Ohio: Nth Degree, n.d.).

42. Wilfrid Sheed, *In Love with Daylight: A Memory of a Recovery* (New York: Simon and Schuster, 1995), 29.

43. Larry Kramer, *The Normal Heart*, foreword by Joseph Papp (New York: Dutton, 1985).

44. Thanks to Irving Kenneth Zola, Temple University Press issued *Women with Disabilities: Essays in Psychology, Culture, and Politics,* Michelle Fine and Adrienne Asch, eds. (Philadelphia: Temple University Press, 1988), which made connections between feminism and the study of disability.

45. Enid Foster, *It Can't Happen to Me* (Cape Town: Timmins, 1959), 133.

46. On Edward V. Roberts, see Joseph Shapiro, *No Pity: People with Disabilities— Forging a New Civil Rights Movement* (New York: Times Books, 1994), 41, 56 ff. See also Irving Kenneth Zola, *Missing Pieces: A Chronicle of Living with a Disability* (Philadelphia: Temple University Press, 1982). When, in 1967, I first visited Cowell, a sort of hospital at the University of California, a dozen students there were fighting successfully for various rights or privileges. Governor Jerry Brown appointed Roberts to the Center for Independent Living. Zola explores independent living centers generally in *Missing Pieces.* On Judy Heumann, see Shapiro, *No Pity,* 56–57. Dart organized the first integration club at Houston. Three of five members of this black-white integration group were disabled (109, 111). *Coming to Terms* (directed by Ray Schmit, produced by Frank B. McArdle for Red Earth Productions) is distributed by Cinema Guild, New York.

47. See Joseph F. Sullivan, *The Unheard Cry* (Nashville, Tenn.: Smith & Lamar, 1914); Randolph Bourne, "The Handicapped—By One of Them," *Atlantic,* September 1911. For the journal, see Brad Byrom, "A Pupil and a Patient: Hospital Schools in Progressive America," in *The New Disability History,* ed. Paul K. Longmore and Lauri Umansky (New York: New York Press, 2001), 151; ibid., "A Pupil," 37.

48. See Daniel J. Wilson, "A Crippling Fear: Experiencing Polio in the Era of FDR," *Bulletin of the History of Medicine* 72 (Fall 1998): 464–495. On the league and FDR, see Paul Longmore, "The League of the Physically Handicapped and the Great Depression: A Case Study in the New Disability History," *Journal of American History* (December 2000).

49. A few had cerebral palsy, tuberculosis, or heart conditions.

50. On the League for the Physically Handicapped, see especially Paul Longmore,

"League for the Physically Handicapped," in *Why I Burned My Book and Other Essays on Disability* (Philadelphia: Temple University Press, 2003), and the Web sites he mentions. Paul K. Longmore and David Goldberger, "The League of the Physically Handicapped and the Great Depression: A Case Study in New Disability History," *Journal of American History* 87, no, 3 (December 2000).

51. See Goldberg, *Making of Franklin D. Roosevelt*, 146–151.

52. There were many supposed "causes" for polio, among them "fathers chewing tobacco." See the *Purity and Truth—Self and Sex*, series by Mary Wood-Allen, M.D. (London: Vir Publishing, n.d.), and by William Briggs, Toronto.

53. Hence the importance of such photos showing racial integration in the polio wards as that in *Miracle at Hickory*, publication no. 53 (New York: National Foundation for Infantile Paralysis, 1944). Many of these photos are now part of the Collection Selechonek.

54. A transcription of this speech is in the National Archives, Washington, D.C. For FDR's speeches and remarks at Warm Springs, see listings of the Carl Vinson Institute of Government at the University of Georgia, Athens, at http://www.cviog.uga.edu.

9. What We Can Learn, If We Hurry

1. Franklin Delano Roosevelt, commencement address, Oglethorpe University, 1932.

2. See Nancy Baldwin Carter, *Myths and Chicken Feet: A Polio Survivor Looks at Survival* (Omaha: Nebraska Polio Survivors Association Press, 1992), 9: "Polio is second only to stroke among causes of paralyzing conditions in this country, and yet those in the business of helping people who are handicapped don't even consider it when listing possible existing disability circumstances? Why is this?"

3. It is likely that this figure should be a good deal larger.

4. The National Organization for Rare Diseases (NORD) lists 140 not-for-profit health organizations serving people with rare disorders and disabilities; NORD publishes the newsletter *Orphan Disease Update*. Orphan diseases are illnesses for which, because they do not affect a specified number of people, NIH and similar organizations do not fund research.

5. Why has it taken so long to eradicate the disease? Part of the failure is due to the poor state of international and intranational distribution of the vaccine—as has been the case in India and some African countries. The inadequate distribution may be attributable to lack of will or "economic 'classism.'"

6. The Cutter laboratory scandal has too often been replicated. See Aaron E. Klein, *Trial by Fury: The Polio Vaccine Controversy* (New York: Scribner's, 1972). In Brazil, polio vaccination "unleashed the severest polio epidemic the world had ever known." Hans Ruesch, *Naked Empress or the Great Medical Fraud* (Milan: CIVIS, 1992), 80. Compare, however, João Baptista Risi, Jr., "Poliomyelitis in Brazil," in *Polio*, ed. Thomas M. Daniel and Frederick C. Robbins (Rochester, N.Y.: University of Rochester Press, 1997), 159–181. On comebacks, see Joseph Laurance Marx, *Keep Trying: A Practical Book for the Handicapped by a Polio Victim* (New York: Harper & Row, 1974), 196:

"Allowing a disease that has been effectively eliminated to return is another form of murder."

7. See Bernice E. Eddy, "Persistent Infection of Human Carcinoma and Primary Chick Embryo Cell Cultures with Simian Virus 40," *Proceedings of the Society for Experimental Biology and Medicine* 111 (1962): 718–722. "Before means for detecting the virus were known, SV-40 had been administered to man as a contaminant of poliomyelitis and adenovirus vaccines and as a contaminant of the respiratory syncytial virus tested experimentally in man." See Kamel Khalili and Gerald L. Stoner, eds., *Human Polyomaviruses: Molecular and Clinical Perspectives* (New York: Wiley-Liss, 2001), as well as the controversial claims made in 1973 by J. Clausen at the Institute of Preventative Medicine, University of Odense, Denmark, about the dangers of SV40 virus.

8. The American pathologist Simon Flexner, of the Rockefeller Institute for Medical Research, published a series of influential, interrelated papers in 1909–1913 about growing the polio virus in laboratory animals, especially monkeys, and about related subjects. He directed the institute until 1935.

9. *The Last Word* (1996), produced by Csillag es Adam Film, Budapest, and distributed by Bullfrog Films, won the Prix Leonardo, Italy, in 1997.

10. John La Montagne, deputy director of the National Institutes of Allergies and Infectious Diseases at the National Institutes of Health, as quoted in Rick Weiss, "Scientists Make Polio from Scratch: Replicating Process Is Termed 'Alarming,'" *International Herald Tribune*, Friday, July 12, 2002, 1, 6. Eckard Wimmer (State University of New York at Stony Brook) led the research team, which reported its results in July 2002; the team produced paralysis in mice.

11. Florence Nightingale, *Notes on Nursing for the Labouring Classes* (London: Harrison, 1861), 71: "It is the last straw that breaks the camel's back."

12. See *OED*, s.v. *Trauma*.

13. Anne Kristine Schanke, "Psychological Distress, Social Support and Coping Behaviour among Polio Survivors: A Five-Year Perspective on Sixty-Three Polio Patients," *Disability and Rehabilitation* 19, no.3 (March 1997): 108–116.

14. Enid Foster, in her Rhodesian memoir, refers to her "hallucination experienced by a brain partially paralyzed from polio." Enid Foster, *It Can't Happen to Me* (Cape Town: Timmins, 1959), 10. Past research claiming a link between polio and schizophrenia has already been discredited, but those working on variants of "brain fatigue" are not discouraged.

15. Horace, *Odes* 2.10.5.

16. Arthur C. Clarke, "Painful Memory of a Silent Stalker," *Times Higher Education Supplement*, June 29, 2001, 34.

17. W. Geiger, "Über progrediente postpoliomyelitische Zustandsbilder," *Deutsche Zeitschrift für Nervenheilkunde* 16, no. 84 (1952).

18. On the tendency to ignore clinical findings, see H. V. Wyatt, "Provocation Poliomyelitis: Neglected Clinical Observations from 1914–1950," *Bulletin of the History of Medicine* 55 (1981): 543–557.

19. Bill Phillips, "Témoignage," in Sally Aitken, Pierrette Caron, and Gilles

Fournier, eds., *Histoire vécue de la polio au Québec* (Montreal: Carte Blanche, 2000), 196. "Aussi étrange que cela puisse paraître, j'étais soulagé d'apprendre que je souffrais du syndrome post-polio. 'Mieux vaut un démon connu qu'un inconnu.'"

20. Owen Dixson, *My Way with Polio* (London: Merritt and Hatcher, [1960]), 4, 144.

21. Charles Caverly in *New York Medical Record* 46 (1894): 673. Quoted in W. R. MacAusland, *Poliomyelitis: With Especial Reference to Treatment* (Philadelphia: Lea & Febiger, 1927), 88.

22. On secondary injury, see Eddie Bollenbach, *Polio Biology VII: Holistic Polio,* a Lincolnshire Post-Polio Library Publication, October 17, 1999. He cites W. J. W. Sharrard, "Correlations between the Changes in the Spinal Cord and Muscular Paralysis in Poliomyelitis," *Proceedings of the Royal Society of London* 40 (1953): 346.

23. R. Debré and S. Thieffrey, "Symptomatology and Diagnosis of Poliomyelitis," in *Poliomyelitis* (Geneva: World Health Organization, 1955), 109–136. On the various percentages cited, see W. F. Brown, "Functional Compensation of Human Motor Units in Health and Disease," *Journal of Neurological Science* 20 (1973): 199–209. The facts here were already known, thanks to B. Bodian, "Poliomyelitis: Pathologic Anatomy," in *Poliomyelitis: Papers and Discussions Presented at the First International Poliomyelitis Conference* (Philadelphia: Lippincott, 1949), 62–84.

24. On "overuse" in PPS, see J. Perry, G. Barnes, and J. Key, "The Post-Polio Syndrome: An Overuse Phenomenon," *Clinical Orthopedics* 233 (1988): 145–162.

25. See G. Grimby, E. Stählbeg, A. Sandberg, and K. S. Sunnerhagen, "An Eight-Year Longitudinal Study of Muscle Strength, Muscle Fiber, Size, and Dynamic Electromyelograms in Individuals with Late Polio," *Muscle and Nerve* 21 (1998): 1428–1437.

26. See J. Ramlow, M. Alexander, R. Laporte, C. Jaufmann, and L. Kuller, "Epidemiology of Postpolio Syndrome," *American Journal of Epidemiology* 136 (1992): 769–786. On the failure to diagnose polio in one twin, see L. Ee, J. Dambrosia, E. Bern, R. Eldridge, and M. Alaska, "Post-Polio Syndrome in Twins and Their Siblings: Evidence that Post-Polio Syndrome Can Develop in Patients with Nonparalytic Polio," *Annals of the New York Academy of Science* 753 (1995): 378–380.

27. Tiina Rekand, Bjorn Karlsen, Nina Langeland, and Johann A. Aarli, "Long-Term Follow-up of Patients with Nonparalytic Poliomyelitis," *Archives of Physical Medicine and Rehabilitation* 83 (April 2002). The cases mentioned are those of patients numbers 2 and 3.

28. "Apparently certain white blood cells have polio virus receptors on their surfaces and can shuttle this extremely tiny virus around." Bruno Blondel, Gillian Duncan, Therese Couderc, Francis Delpeyroux, Nicole Pavio, and Florence Colbère-Garapin, "Molecular Aspects of Poliovirus Biology with a Special Focus on the Interactions with Nerve Cells," *Journal of Neurovirology* 4 (1998): 1–26.

29. See, for example, James Hogle, "Poliovirus Cell Entry: Common Structural Themes in Viral Cell Entry Pathways," *Annual Review of Microbiology* 56 (2000): 677–702.

30. Recent reports by Casey D. Morrow in *Nature Biotechnology* (September 2000)

suggest that this is an idea whose time has come: apparently researchers have succeeded in using the altered poliovirus to ferry genes as well as anti-inflammatory agents into and near the relevant neurons in mice. "The research may also lead to treatments for tough neurological illness such at Lou Gehrig's disease and multiple sclerosis." Andrea W. Bledsoe, Cheryl A. Jackson, Sylvia McPherson, and Casey D. Morrow, "Cytokine Production in Motor Neurons by Poliovirus Replicon Vector Gene Delivery," *Nature Biotechnology* 18 (September 2000): 964–969.

31. J. L. Melnick, *American Journal of Public Health* 44, no. 1 (1954): 572. Melnick, who led the team that developed thermostabilized live polio vaccines, demonstrated that the polio virus usually invades the intestines rather than the central nervous system. For more than forty years, Melnick served as director of the Collaborating Center for Virus Reference and Research, World Health Organization.

32. On Coxsackie A9, see M. Gromeier, S. Mueller, D. Solecki, B. Bossert, G. Bernhardt, and E. Wimmer, "Determinants of Poliovirus Neurovirulence," *Journal of Neurovirology* 3 (1997), supp. 1, S35–S38. On enteroviruses 70 and 71, see J. L. Melnick, "Enterovirus Type 71 Infections: A Varied Clinical Pattern Sometimes Mimicking Paralytic Poliomyelitis," *Review of Infectious Diseases* 6 (1984), supp. 2, S387–S390. On Japanese encephalitis virus, see T. R. Solomon, N. M. Kneen, V. C. Dung, T. T. N. Kanh, D. Q. Thuy, N. P. J. Ha, A. Day, D. W. Nisalak, and N. J. Vaughn, "Poliomyelitis-like Illness due to Japanese Encephalitis Virus," *Lancet* 351 (1998): 1094–1097.

33. For the isolations: P. Muir, F. Nicholson, M. K. Sharief, E. J. Thompson, N. J. Cairns, P. Lantos, G. T. Spencer, H. J. Kaminski, and J. E. Banatvala, "Evidence for Persistent Enterovirus Infection of the Central Nervous System in Patients with Previous Paralytic Poliomyelitis," in M. C. Dalakas, H. Bartfeld, and L. T. Kurland, eds., *The Post-Polio Syndrome: Advances in the Pathogenesis and Treatment* (New York: New York Academy of Sciences, 1995), 219–232. On whether this is a common event, see Marcia Falconer and Eddie Bollenbach, *Non-Paralytic Polio and PPS*, A Lincolnshire Post-Polio Library Publication (January 1999).

34. Sven Gard, "Exit Poliomyelitis—What Next?" *Yale Journal of Biological Medicine* 34 (1961–62): 277–288.

35. Richard L. Bruno, "Can a Traumatic Event Trigger Post-Polio Sequelae? . . . Yes and No," *New Mobility Magazine* (May 1997).

36. The role of traumatic injury or accidents in MS has been controversial for many years.

37. On Creutzfeldt-Jakob disease, see D. P. Wientjens, Z. Davanipour, A. Hofman, K. Kondo, et al., "Risk Factors for Creutzfeldt-Jakob Disease," *Neurology* 46, no. 5 (May 1996): 1287–1291. John M. *Eagles*, "Are Polioviruses a Cause of Schizophrenia?" *British Journal of Psychiatry* 160 (May 1992): 598–600, postulates that prenatal infection with polioviruses could contribute to the subsequent development of schizophrenia.

38. This statement is a reworking of Charles Laughton's line in the unfinished movie *I, Claudius* (1936–37). See Marc Shell, *Stutter* (Cambridge, Mass.: Harvard University Press, forthcoming), for a discussion of the Roman emperor himself as Suetonius describes him.

39. "There are growing indications that stutterers have some type of central nervous system deficit." Einer Boberg, "The Winding Trails of Therapy: Convergence at Last?" Presentation at Speak Easy symposium 11, reprinted in *Speak Easy* newsletter (Winter 1992). See also Marty Jezer, *Stuttering: A Life Bound Up in Words* (New York: Basic, 1997), 250–251.

40. Adoniram Brown Judson, *The Influence of Growth on Acquired and Congenital Deformities* (New York: William Wood, 1905), discusses Pott's disease as well as polio. Mary A. Keenan, *Post-Polio Syndrome as a Model for Musculo-Tendinous Overuse Syndromes in Military and Civilian Populations* (Philadelphia: Albert Einstein Medical Center, July 1999), 119.

41. For the misdiagnosis of Lou Gehrig, see the *Baltimore Evening Sun*, June 21, 1939. In 1953 Alexis Shelokov, a polio expert, was called to Chestnut Lodge Hospital on a mission to determine whether an outbreak of something like chronic fatigue syndrome might not have been polio. Consider also the outbreaks of atypical polio—so named in 1934 by A. G. ("Sandy") Gilliam; see "Epidemiological Study of an Epidemic, Diagnosed as Poliomyelitis, Occurring among the Personnel of the Los Angeles County General Hospital during the Summer of 1934," *U.S. Public Health Bulletin* 240 (1938): 1–90. The same condition is sometimes called Iceland Disease and benign myalgic encephalomyelitis. Hillary Johnson, *Inside the Labyrinth of the Chronic Fatigue Syndrome* (New York: Crown, 1996), 200.

42. Alan M. Kraut, *Silent Travellers: Germs, Genes, and the "Immigrant Menace"* (New York: Basic, 1994), esp. 108–113.

43. Geoffrey Marks and William K. Beatty, *Epidemics* (New York: Scribner's, 1976), 271.

44. Susan Sontag, *AIDS and Its Metaphors* (New York: Farrar, Straus and Giroux, 1989), 48.

45. William H. McNeill, in a 1983 book review, cited ibid., 57 n.

46. See, as an example, Edward Hooper's untrustworthy *The River: A Journey to the Source of HIV and AIDS* (Boston: Little, Brown, 1999).

47. Jeff Walsh, "Larry Kramer 'Just Says No' to Being Angry Anymore" (interview with Larry Kramer), www.oasismag.com.

48. Larry Kramer, *The Normal Heart*, foreword by Joseph Papp (New York: Dutton, 1985). According to Ned in the play, American Jews of the 1930s, despite overwhelming evidence, did not take action to resist the Holocaust until it was too late. Ned thinks that the U.S. government might "seclude" homosexuals as dangerous, even as it quarantined American polios and interned Japanese-Americans in concentration camps.

49. Sandra Panem, *AIDS Bureaucracy* (Cambridge, Mass.: Harvard University Press, 1988), 14, cited in Patricia M. Sarchet, "Archaeology of Deadly Meanings: Polio and HIV Photographs," M.A. thesis, May 1998, Anthropology Department, State University of New York at Buffalo, 26.

50. Kramer, *Normal Heart*, scenes 10, 12, 80. Speaking to an AIDS activist at this juncture, Dr. Emma Brookner, a polio survivor, compares polio to AIDS: "Polio is a virus, too. I caught it three months before the Salk vaccine was announced."

51. In Larry Kramer's play (ibid.), the polio Emma has an electric wheelchair in the first act, and a manual wheelchair in the second act.

52. The papers of Linda Jane Laubenstein (1947–1992) are at the Schlesinger Library at Harvard University. They include Baby Book, 1947–48; Photographs, 1949–1992, and "My Life, 1952–1958" (scrapbook with autobiographical essays). Her work includes *AIDS: The Epidemic of Kaposi's Sarcoma and Opportunistic Infections,* ed. Alvin E. Friedman-Kien and Linda J. Laubenstein (New York: Masson, 1984).

53. See Tom Burke, "On the Rights Track," in Pietro Nivola, ed., *Comparative Disadvantages? Social Regulations and the Global Economy* (Washington D.C.: Brookings Institution Press, 1997), 249.

54. On Farill's walking disability, see Andrea Kettenmann, *Kahlo, 1907–1954: Pain and Passion* (Cologne: Benedikt Taschen, 1993), 81. Farill served as president of Rehabilitation International during the period from 1942 to 1948.

55. The story is told in the various gospels: Mark 2.9, 11; John 5.8, 11, 12; Luke 5.24; Matt. 9.6.

56. Robert Mauro, *Landscape of My Disability* (Berkeley, Calif.: Lemonade Factory, 1998), 21.

57. Brother John Sellers sings of the healing of the paralytic in his 1957 blues spiritual "He Came All the Way Down," on an LP titled "Blues and Spirituals by Brother John Sellers," Columbia label SEG 7740.

58. Julie Silver, "When You're Looking for Expert Medical Advice, Start with a Physiatrist," *Polio Connection of America Newsletter* (Howard Beach, N.Y.), January 1999.

59. See Douglas C. McMurtrie, T*he Evolution of National Systems of Vocational Reeducation for Disabled Soldiers and Sailors* (Washington, D.C.: U.S. Government Printing Office, 1918); and John Culbert Faries, *Three Years of Work for Handicapped Men: A Report of the Activities of the Institute for Crippled and Disabled Men* (New York: Institute for Crippled and Disabled Men, 1920).

60. On polios turned missionaries, see Evelyn Bauer, *Through Sunlight and Shadow* (Scottdale, Pa.: Herald, 1959), about a polio who is a Mennonite missionary in India; Viola Pahl, *Gold in Life's Hourglass: The Story of an Ordinary Family with an Extraordinary God* (Surrey, Canada: Maple Lane, 1993); and the Lutheran who called himself the Wheelchair Evangelist, Allen Lee, *My Soul More Bent* (Minneapolis, Minn.: Augsburg, 1948); John Earl Lindell and Ethel Brooks, *Oh God, Help Me! for I Cannot Help Myself: A True Story of Polio in the Life of a Polio Survivor* (n.p., 1988); Keith A. Korstjens, *Not a Sometimes Love* (Waco, Tex.: Word Books, 1981); Dorothy Pape, *Walls Are for Leaping* (Robesonia, Pa.: Overseas Missionary Fellowship, 1983). For a relevant third-person account, see Lloyd C. Douglas's *Green Light* (New York: Grosset & Dunlap, 1935) and Alma Murdock, *Crowned* (San Antonio, Tex: Naylor, 1962), the biography of a six-year-old polio who found Jesus before he died. "But if polio had robbed me physically, it had enriched me in other ways. Sitting, perforce, on the sidelines, one develops a philosophy, a greater tolerance and understanding, that found no place in the previous rushing, hustling, bustling existence . . . Polio, because of its dramatic crippling effects, is a

dread disease, yet out of it can come activity of a new kind—activity of the mind and spirit." Foster, *It Can't Happen*, 175.

61. Dore Schary, *Sunrise at Campobello: A Play in Three Acts* (New York: Random House, 1958), 12.

62. Bentz Plagemann, *My Place to Stand* (London: Gollancz, 1950), 181.

63. M. E. Verheyden-Hilliard, *Scientist and Strategist June Rooks* (Bethesda, Md.: Equity Institute, 1988), a thirty-one-page pamphlet about an African-American who contracted polio as a child, struggled against poverty, earned her degree in physics, and became an operations research analyst with the U.S. Navy.

64. Kathleen Krull, *Wilma Unlimited: How Wilma Rudolph Became the World's Fastest Woman* (New York: Troll, 1996). Wayne Coffey, *Wilma Rudolph: Beating the Odds* (Woodbridge, Conn: Blackbirch, 1993). See also the movie *Wilma* (1977, directed by Bud Greenspan).

65. Conrad Dubé—a sports achiever called *le globe-trotteur*—went around the world by bicycle.

66. Confined to a wheelchair because of a childhood bout with polio, Ewry began exercising his legs to enhance his prospects of recovery. He went on to win ten gold medals between 1900 and 1908 in the standing jump.

67. In July 1951, Barbara Hobelmann, who had overcome polio to become an All-American swimmer, appeared on the cover of *Life*.

68. See Karl Whitezel, *Buster Crabbe: A Self-Portrait* (Lewiston, Ida.: Whitezel, 1997).

69. Matt Christopher, *Catcher with a Glass Arm* (Boston: Little, Brown, 1964); a sports novel for young readers about a polio survivor. C. H. Frick, *Five against the Odds* (New York: Harcourt, Brace, 1955); Matt Christopher, *Shoot for the Hoop* (Boston: Little, Brown, 1995); Bill J. Carol, *Crazylegs Merrill* (Austin, Tex.: Steck-Vaughn, 1969).

70. Simon Åhlstad suffered from polio as a child but became a champion swimmer. In the 1992 Barcelona Paralympics, for example, he won the two-hundred-meter medley and two-hundred-meter breaststroke.

71. See Angela Hughes, *Pierre Fournier: Cellist in a Landscape with Figures* (Aldershot, England: Ashgate, 1998). Pierre Fournier (1906–1986) "overcame" childhood polio to become a world-famous cellist.

72. Doc Pomus was also known as Jerome Felder.

73. Walter Jackson (1938–) was part of the '60s Chicago soul movement. Joni Mitchell, while recovering in a children's hospital, began her performing career by singing to the other patients.

74. Israel Vibrations, well known in reggae music circles, comprises Cecil Spence (Skelly), Albert Craig (Apple), and Lascelle Bulgin (Wiss).

75. See Martica Sawin, *Nell Blaine: Her Art and Life* (New York: Thames and Hudson, 1998).

76. See Jack Davis and Dorothy Ryan, *Samuel L. Schmucker: The Discovery of His Lost Art* (Bozeman, Mont.: Old America Antiques, 2001).

77. Mark Alexander, *Canvases of Courage* (Churt, England: Leader Books, 1991), 77. See especially Paul Driver's *Tower Bridge* (oil, 34 × 44 cm.), ibid., 85; also 20, 79–80.

78. Ibid., 150.

79. J. H. Roesler, *God's Second Door,* illustrated by members of the International Association of Mouth and Foot Painting Artists (London: Painted Postcards, 1960), esp. 99, 23, 15, 7. Roesler's book includes discussion of the Australian artist Athol Thompson. See also *Arnulf Erich Stegmann,* introduction by Richard Hiepe (Munich: Verlag Graphik-Press, 1969).

80. "Painting became everything to me. By it I learned to express myself in many subtle ways. Through it I made articulate all that I was and felt, all that went on inside the mind that was housed within my useless body like a prisoner in a cell looking out on a world that hadn't become a reality to me." Quoted in Alexander, *Canvases,* 11. Brown's book was eventually made into the prizewinning movie *My Left Foot* (1989).

81. Betty Cavanna, *Joyride* (New York: William Morrow, 1974), 109.

82. Earlene W. Luis and Barbara Millar, *Wheels for Ginny's Chariot* (New York: Dodd, Mead, 1966), 173.

83. D. M. Greig, "The Cephalic Features of Sir Walter Scott," *Edinburgh Medical Journal* 39 (August 1932): 497.

84. Watty Piper (pseud.), *The Little Engine That Could,* illustrated by Lois Lenski (New York: Platt and Munk, 1930). Earlier versions of the same story had sometimes been written by others, under these titles: *Thinking One Can, The Pony Engine, The Little Steam Engine,* and *the Royal Engine.* They had been appearing on bookshelves since about 1895. The 78-RPM recording that my parents gave me, during my polio convalescence, featured Burl Ives singing the song by Gerald Marks and Milton Pascal as orchestrated by the Percy Faith Orchestra (Columbia Children's Records MJV-113).

85. "In the common parlance of the country, any one, who counterfeits sickness . . . is said to be 'possuming.'" Timothy Flint, *History and of Geography of the Mississippi Valley,* 2nd ed. (n.p., 1822), 1:67.

86. Nancy Baldwin Carter, "The Little Engine That Shouldn't," *Myths and Chicken Feet: A Polio Survivor Looks at Survival* (Omaha, Neb.: Nebraska Polio Survivors Association Press, 1992), 61–62. Nancy Baldwin Carter is the founder of the Nebraska Polio Survivors Association.

87. Richard Bruno, *The Polio Paradox: What You Need to Know* (New York: Warner, 2002). See also Richard Bruno, *The Polio Paradox: Understanding and Treating "Post Polio Syndrome" and Chronic Fatigue* (New York: Warner, rpr. 2003).

88. See www.ican.com.

89. *OED,* s.v. *Possum,* n. 2. See *Responaut* 13 (Autumn 1976), 2: "My window on the world, apart from my eyes, is 15 inches by 7, the size of the tilting mirror attached to my respirator. Reflected through this I can see my two Possum indicators revealing the 21 electrical devices I am able to control."

90. *OED,* s.v. *Possum.* This usage dates at least as far back as 1822.

91. For a related argument, see N. M. Frick, "The Contribution of Childhood Physical and Emotional Trauma to the Development of the Post-Polio Personality,"

Proceedings of the Ontario March of Dimes Conference on Post-Polio Sequelae (Toronto: Ontario March of Dimes, 1995). See also Al Siebert and Bernie S. Siegel, *The Survivor Personality: Why Some People Are Stronger, Smarter, and More Skillful at Handling Life's Difficulties . . . and How You Can Be, Too* (New York: Penguin, 1996), especially the passages on polio survivors.

92. Irving K. Zola, "Whose Voice Is This Anyway? A Commentary on Recent Collections about the Experiences of Disability," *Medical Humanities Review* 2 (1988): 6–15.

93. Jan Little, *If It Weren't for the Honor—I Would've Rather Walked* (Cambridge, Mass.: Brookline Books, 1996).

94. Roxanne Frigon, "Témoignage," in Aitken, Caron, and Fournier, *Histoire vécue*, 66. "La polio pour moi n'a eu aucun effet positif, bien au contraire. Toute ma vie a été très difficile, remplie d'échecs, d'erreurs, et d'incompréhensions."

95. Charles Conley Ward, "Crippled Thunder: The Autobiography of Charles Conley Ward, the Last Authentic Cripple," 1996. Charles Conley Ward sent the manuscript to me in 1999. Collection Selechonek.

96. Some critics say that Virginia Black's story, as told in Kathryn Black, *In the Shadow of Polio* (Reading, Mass.: Addison-Wesley, 1996), challenges the genre of polio narratives. On returning from the polio ward to Boulder to her young children, Virginia Black had lost the power to touch. Dependent on her parents when her husband decamped, she appears to have lost the will to live.

97. *Cripple's Reward* record album cover (K-Town Records, 1950s), art by Buddy Robertson. Robertson sings "Cripple's Reward," a song about being handicapped and how God is going to give him a mansion someday.

98. Oliver Sacks, *An Anthropologist on Mars: Seven Paradoxical Tales* (New York: Knopf, 1995).

99. Eileen Gagnon, "Témoignage," in Aitken, Caron, and Fournier, *Histoire vécue*, 7: "Si on me disait aujourd'hui qu'on peut me débarrasser de ma polio à la condition de m'enlever aussi tout ce que j'ai appris à travers cette maladie, j'hésiterais."

100. Georgina Bailey, "I'm Glad I Had Polio," *MacLean's Magazine*, October 1, 1950.

Acknowledgments

I am grateful to the John D. and Catherine T. MacArthur Foundation and to the Harvard Medical School for financial support. Work for this project required purchasing hundreds of books, scrapbooks, and unpublished manuscripts available only from private vendors worldwide. Some of the items acquired have been included in a display at the Smithsonian Institution, the exhibition "Whatever Happened to Polio?" at the National Museum of American History (2005). Eventually I will donate the Collection Selechonek to an institution open to the public.

Many organizations generously provided access to books, papers, and works of art: the Association of Mouth and Foot Painting Artists in Liechtenstein, the Center for History in the Media in Washington, the Harvard libraries in Cambridge and Boston, the March of Dimes archives in White Plains, New York, the New York City Ballet, La Salpêtrière in Paris, the Warm Springs Foundation in Georgia, and numerous others.

One great pleasure in writing *Polio and Its Aftermath* was meeting and learning from polio survivors and scholars of polio history. Among these are Diana Barrett, Susan Aiken, Ernie Bollenbach, Timothy Gould, Larry Kramer, Leonard Kriegel, Anne Harpin, Robert Mauro, Charles Mee, Mark O'Brien, David Rubin, Nina Seavey, Bapsi Sidwa, and Daniel Wilson. I am also grateful to many more.

Colleagues in the medical field in the Boston area were especially accommodating. Dorothy Aiello, Laura Diamond, Walter Frontera, Richard

Goldberg, and Sally Johnson helped with the study of poliomyelitic treatment. Among those who guided work in the history of science and disability studies are Adrienne Asch, Arthur Kleinman, and Charles Rosenberg. Julie Silver helped see *Polio and Its Aftermath* through to completion; as director of the Post-Polio Center at Spaulding Rehabilitation Hospital, she provides an authentic model for careful and caring medical practice and research.

Judith Palfrey was chair of Harvard's Children's Initiative while I was chair of the Disability Studies Initiative. Together we worked with Walter Schalick, Evangeline Stefanakis, and Dorothy Weiss to organize a conference in 2000 on the interdisciplinary aspects of disability studies. Some of the ideas raised in *Polio and Its Aftermath* were discussed there. The following year (2001), I delivered a series of lectures entitled "What We Can Learn about Polio If We Hurry" at Spaulding Rehabilitation Hospital. Paralysis and culture in European perspective was the subject of my lectures at the *Zentrum für Literaturforschung* in Berlin and in the Americas.

Graduate and undergraduate students in seminars on paralysis contributed to my thinking about medical history; many seminar participants have now gone on to do further work in the field. In particular, I want to thank Alvan Ikoku, Vaia Sigounas, and Kate Taylor. Casiana Ionita helped brilliantly with myriad issues of writing, permission, and logic.

Susan Shell, Stanley Cavell, and Elaine Scarry read a very long first draft of my study of paralysis. Each of them remarked that the manuscript focused equally on problems of bodily and verbal stasis, and each made the same Solomonic recommendation: divide the manuscript into two parts, devoting the first to the subject of walking and the second to that of talking. Lindsay Waters at Harvard University Press had the same good idea. So *Polio and Its Aftermath* is the firstborn of what was, or were, conjoined twins. *Stutter* will follow in due course, also from Harvard University Press.

Hanna Rose Shell commented on issues of cinematography and the history of science. Jacob Adam Shell assisted with organizing considerable reference material and emphasized the role of urban architecture and planning. This book is dedicated to my uncle Benjamin Cytrynbaum.

TEXT CREDITS

Prologue

George Orwell, *Coming Up for Air* (London: Gollancz, 1939), 184. Copyright © George Orwell 1939, reprinted by permission of Bill Hamilton as the Literary Executor of the Estate of the late Sonia Brownell Orwell and Secker & Warburg, Ltd.; COMING UP FOR AIR, copyright 1950 by the Estate of Sonia Brownell Orwell, reprinted by permission of Harcourt, Inc.

Mark Twain, *Three Thousand Years among the Microbes* (1905), in Mark Twain, *Which Was the Dream? and Other Symbolic Writings of the Late Years,* ed. John Tuckey (Berkeley: University of California Press, 1967).

Larry Kramer, *The Normal Heart,* foreword by Joseph Papp (New York: Dutton, 1985), 40. Used by permission of Larry Kramer.

Emily Dickinson, "Pain—Expands the Time." Reprinted by permission of the publishers and the Trustees of Amherst College from *The Poems of Emily Dickinson,* Thomas H. Johnson, ed. (Cambridge, Mass.: The Belknap Press of Harvard University Press), Copyright © 1951, 1955, 1979, 1983 by the President and Fellows of Harvard College.

1. One Polio Story

Mark O'Brien, "How I Survived Childhood," in Mark O'Brien and Susan Fernbach, *Love and Baseball: Poems on America's Favorite Pastimes* (Berkeley, Calif.: Lemonade Factory, 1997), 1.

Robert Mauro, "My Iron Lung et Cetera," in *Landscape of My Disability* (Berkeley, Calif.: Lemonade Factory, 1998). Used by permission.

Kurt Weill and Bertolt Brecht, "Alabama Song" (1928). Original work, *Mahagonny* by Bertolt Brecht © 1927 by Universal-Edition A. G., renewed in 1955 by Bertolt Brecht. Translation copyright © 1979 by Stefan S. Brecht. Reprinted from *The Rise and Fall of the City of Mahagonny* by Bertolt Brecht, trans. W. H. Auden and Chester Kallman, ed. John Willett and Ralph Manheim, published by Arcade Publishing, New York. Used by permission of Methuen Publishing.

W. J. W. Sharrard, "The Distribution of the Permanent Paralysis in the Lower Limb in Poliomyelitis: A Clinical and Pathological Study," *Journal of Bone and Joint Surgery* 37, no. B.4 (November 1955). Reproduced with permission and copyright © of the British Editorial Society of Bone and Joint Surgery.

2. In the Family

Elizabeth P. Rice, "The Families of Children with Poliomyelitis," in *Poliomyelitis: Papers and Discussions Presented at the First International Poliomyelitis Conference* (Philadelphia: Lippincott, 1949), 308. Used by permission of the March of Dimes and Lippincott, Williams & Wilkins, © 1949.

F. S. Copellman, "Follow-Up of One Hundred Children with Poliomyelitis," *The Family* 25 (1944): 289–297. Reprinted with permission from *Families in Society* (www.families insociety.org), published by the Alliance for Children and Families.

T. S. Eliot, *The Waste Land*, in T. S. Eliot, *Complete Poems and Plays of T. S. Eliot* (New York: Harcourt, 1922).

Emily Dickinson, "Oh give it Motion." Written on the back of printed directions for lighting a lamp. Reprinted by permission of the publishers and the Trustees of Amherst College from *The Poems of Emily Dickinson*, Thomas H. Johnson, ed. (Cambridge, Mass.: The Belknap Press of Harvard University Press), Copyright © 1951, 1955, 1979, 1983 by the President and Fellows of Harvard College.

3. A Polio School

P. Dieppe, "Die Bedeutung des Mittelalters für den Fortschritt der Medizin" (1924), in *Essays on the History of Medicine Presented to Karl Sudhoff on the Occasion of His Seventieth Birthday, November 26, 1923*, ed. Charles Singer and Henry E. Sigerist (London: Oxford University Press, and Zurich: Verlag Seldwyla, 1924), 99–120. Cited by Charles-Edward Amory Winslow, *The Conquest of Epidemic Disease: A Chapter in the History of Ideas* (Princeton, N.J.: Princeton University Press, 1943; rpr. Madison: University of Wisconsin Press, 1980), 88.

Homer, *The Odyssey with an English Translation*, ed. and trans. A. T. Murray, 2 vols. (London: William Heinemann, 1919 [9th–8th century BC]), 8:493–494.

Frank Freidel, *Franklin Delano Roosevelt: The Ordeal* (Boston: Little, Brown, 1954), 113.

Ana Castillo, *Peel My Love Like an Onion* (New York: Doubleday, 1999), 4.

Franklin Delano Roosevelt, letter to Eleanor Roosevelt, December 4, 1938, written from Warm Springs, in *FDR: His Personal Letters*, ed. Elliot Roosevelt, foreword by Eleanor Roosevelt, 4 vols. (New York: Duell, Sloan, and Pearce, 1947).

Edgar Allan Poe, "The Premature Burial" in *The Works of the Late Edgar Allan Poe*, ed. N. P. Willis, J. R. Lowell, and R. W. Griswold (New York: Redfield, 1850), 1:325–338.

II. Stasis and Kinesis

Alexander Bakshy, *The Path of the Modern Russian Stage, and Other Essays* (London: Palmer & Hayward, 1916), 221.

4. Paralytic Polio and Moving Pictures

Dorothea Lange, *The Making of a Documentary Photographer*, an oral history interview conducted in 1960 and 1961 by Suzanne Riess, Regional Oral History Office, Bancroft Library, University of California, Berkeley, 1968, p. 17. Used by permission.

5. Handi-Capitalism and Cinema Business

Charles Dickens, *A Christmas Carol*, introduction by Andrew Lang (London: Chapman and Hall, 1897 [1843]).

The lyric excerpt from "You'll Never Walk Alone," by Richard Rodgers and Oscar Hammerstein II, copyright © 1945 by Williamson Music, copyright renewed, international copyright secured, all rights reserved, is used by permission of Williamson Music, a division of Rodgers and Hammerstein.

6. The Cast of *Rear Window*

J. G. Farrell, *The Lung* (London: Hutchinson, 1965), 47. Copyright © J. G. Farrell, 1965. Reproduced by permission of the Estate of J. G. Farrell, c/o Rogers, Coleridge & White Ltd., 20 Powes Mews, London W11 1JN.

L. B. "Jeff" Jeffries to Editor Gunnison, in Alfred Hitchcock's *Rear Window*, 0.04.17.

Robert Mauro, "White Cocoon," in *Landscape of My Disability* (Berkeley, Calif.: Lemonade Factory, 1998). Used by permission.

7. Polio and the Great Wars

Franklin Delano Roosevelt, informal extemporaneous remarks at the annual Thanksgiving dinner held at Georgia Hall, Warm Springs Foundation, Warm Springs, Georgia, November 28, 1935.

8. Remembering Roosevelt

Turnley Walker, *Roosevelt and the Warm Springs Story* (New York: A. A. Wyn, 1953).

Signs at a civil rights demonstration. Shown in a photograph on the front cover of Richard Bryant Treanor, *We Overcame: The Story of Civil Rights for Disabled People* (Falls Church, Va.: Regal Direct, 1993).

9. What We Can Learn, If We Hurry

Lorraine Beim, *Triumph Clear* (New York: Harcourt, Brace, 1946), 193. Excerpt from page 193 in TRIUMPH CLEAR, copyright 1946 by Lorraine Beim, renewed 1973 by Andrew Beim, reprinted by permission of Harcourt, Inc.

Wallace Stegner, *Crossing to Safety* (New York: Random House, 1987), 273.

Robert Mauro, "On the Rack of Perfection," in *Landscape of My Disability* (Berkeley, Calif.: Lemonade Factory, 1998). Used by permission.

Leonard Kriegel, *Falling into Life: Essays* (San Francisco: North Point, 1991), 19. Used by permission.

Aftermath

Ludwig Wittgenstein, *Culture and Value* [*Vermischte Bemerkungen*], ed. G. H. von Wright and Heikki Nyman, trans. Peter Winch (Oxford: Blackwell, 1980), 17.

ILLUSTRATION CREDITS

Frontispiece: Picking up where he left off. Black and white photograph of the author, by Benjamin Cytrynbaum. © 1951, Collection Selechonek.

Part 1. The face of polio. Linda Gunther, eight (left), and Mary Jo Moss, two, lie in their iron lungs in the Memphis Isolation Hospital, Tennessee. Their parents watch through an observation window. This was often the only way parents could visit their polio-stricken children. The children have rearview mirrors and puppets. Bettmann/CORBIS. All rights reserved.

Part 2. Vaccination day, 1955. Photograph by Ernie Sisto/The New York Times. Used by permission.

Part 3. *Arm und Reich* (Poor and rich), by Arnulf Erich Stegmann. Oil, 75 × 101 cm. Used by friendly permission of the Association of Mouth and Foot Painting Artists Worldwide, headquartered in Schaan, principality of Liechtenstein.

Figures:

1. Military quarantine at Hickory, North Carolina. Armed serviceman ensuring the quarantine at the Emergency Infantile Paralysis Hospital (1940). Used by permission of the March of Dimes.

2. *Self-Portrait in Bed with Polio,* by John Perceval. Reed pen and ink on paper, 20.9 × 30.4 cm. © 1943. © 2004 Artists Rights Society (ARS) New York/ VI$COPY, Australia. Photograph courtesy of the National Gallery of Australia.

3. Polio at the mirrors. Black and white photograph. Used by permission of the March of Dimes. Special thanks to Tim Gould and Nina Seavey.

4. Courage comes in all sizes. Crutches being handed out to children. Prizewinning photograph and poster by Esther Bubley, 1953. Museum of Modern Art and Collection Selechonek.

21. *Christina's World,* by Andrew Wyeth, 1948. Tempera on panel, 32¼ × 47¾ in. Used by permission of the Wyeth Collection. Digital image © The Museum of Modern Art (MOMA)/Licensed by SCALA/Art Resource, New York.

5. Olly's infant. Photograph by Hugo van Lawick, in Jane Goodall, *In the Shadow of Man* (Boston: Houghton Mifflin, 1971). Copyright © 1971 by Hugo and Jane van Lawick-Goodall. Reprinted by permission of Houghton Mifflin Company. All rights reserved.

6. Franklin D. Roosevelt on horseback. Photo courtesy of the Franklin D. Roosevelt Presidential Library and Museum, Hyde Park, New York.

7. Franklin D. Roosevelt at the pool complex in Warm Springs, Georgia, on his first visit, in 1924. Photograph courtesy of FDR's Little White House Historic Site, Warm Springs, Georgia. Used by permission of the Georgia Department of Natural Resources.

8. The shadow of polio in *The Crippler.* Scene from the "documentary" movie *The Crippler* (also known as *The Daily Battle*), put out by the National Foundation for Infantile Paralysis. Used by permission of the March of Dimes.

9. Paralysis victim writing with her teeth, September 12, 1949. After three years in a respirator, Carolyn Sandin, eighteen, of Arlington, Virginia, is shown in an iron lung at the Children's Hospital School, Baltimore, writing: "I am helping the polio epidemic drive. Are you?" Bettmann/CORBIS. All rights reserved.

10. Georges Balanchine with Mourka the cat. Photograph by Martha Swope, in Tanaquil LeClercq, *Mourka: The Autobiography of a Cat* (New York: Stein and Day, 1964), written after LeClercq was paralyzed. Used by permission of Martha Swope.

11. Growing pains. Illustration from an official elementary school textbook used in much of North America. Florence M. Taylor and Lucile Patterson Marsh, *Growing Pains* (Philadelphia: R. R. Donnelly and Sons for Westminster Press), 1948.

12. Double exposures showing the almost totally paralyzed dancer Elizabeth Twistington in a wheelchair, circa 1970. Marc Alexander, *The Dance Goes On: The Life and Art of Elizabeth Twistington Higgins MBE,* foreword by Philip, Duke of Edinburgh, photographs by Graham and Jaquie Sergeant (London: Leader Books, 1980), 141. Courtesy of Widener Library Photographic Services.

13. Serial photographs of crippled boy in motion. Eadweard Muybridge, *The Human Figure in Motion: An Electro-photographic Investigation of Consecutive Phases of Muscular Actions,* a series commenced in 1872 and completed in 1885. Fourth impression

(London: Chapman & Hall, 1913). Courtesy of the Fine Arts Library, Harvard University.

14. "Here lie the broken bones of L. B. Jeffries" (inscription on the plaster cast). *Rear Window* (1954), directed by Alfred Hitchcock, starring Jimmy Stewart (in wheelchair) as Jeff and Grace Kelly as Lisa. Courtesy of the British Film Institute.

15. Grace Kelly on polio campaign, December 1954. Kelly, who played Lisa in Alfred Hitchcock's *Rear Window* (1954), here contributes materials to leaders of the Mothers March on Polio in Philadelphia. Used by permission of the March of Dimes.

16. "Don't Let That Shadow Touch Them." Poster by Lawrence Beall Smith. Offset lithograph, 20 × 14″. 1942. Issued by the U.S. Department of the Treasury. Photo courtesy of New Hampshire State Library, Concord, New Hampshire.

17. Ralph Bellamy as FDR, in a scene from Dore Schary's stage play *Sunrise at Campobello*, 1958. Photograph by Friedman-Abeles. Used by permission of Friedman-Abeles, the Billy Rose Theatre Collection, New York Public Library for the Performing Arts, Astor, Lenox and Tilden Foundations, New York.

18. Integration of the races in the polio wards, 1944: a first for the South. Original photograph from Scrapbook #31, 1947, Collection Selechonek.

19. Polio and AIDS. Scene from Larry Kramer's play *The Normal Heart* (1985), starring Concetta Tomei and Brad Davis. Used by permission of Martha Swope.

20. *Self-Portrait with Portrait of Dr. Farill*, by Frida Kahlo. Oil on Masonite, 16½ × 19¾ in. 1951. © Banco de México Diego Rivera & Frida Kahlo Trust, Av. Cinco de Mayo, No. 2, Co. Centro, Del. Cuauhtémoc 06059, México, D.F. Mexico City) © Instituto Nacional de Bellas Artes y Literatura de México.

List of Boxes

Name Index

Subject Index

Accident: *The Automobile Accident,* 137; in *The Early History of Jacob Stahl,* 152; the fall in *Rear Window,* 155, 156, 157, 161, 166; in *Lucky Break,* 154; versus necessity, 144; in Reeve's *Rear Window,* 168

AIDS, 3; comparison with flu, 212; epidemic not recognized, 212–213; L. Kramer on polio and, 21, 59, 151, 200, 212–213, *214;* and J. Laubenstein, 213; narratives and sexuality, 20; patient's time to write about, 19; as sociological successor to polio, 9, 34, 213; S. Sontag on, 14, 186; terminal and comorbid, 36

Akinesia, 155

ALS, 122, 210; and M. Schwartz, 220; as slow polio, 211

Amputation, 137, 151, 166; and early movies, 139–140; R. Reagan on, 195–196; and *Rear Window,* 166; self-induced, 60, 166–167; and *The Wizard of Oz,* 56. *See also* Apoterpnophilia; Castration

Animals: animal-based therapies, 95–99; bird-people, 55, 105–106, 131–132; chimpanzee polio outbreak, 80–82; cows, 97; experimentation on, 149, 219; as family pets, 75, 96, 97, 253n81, 257n17;

fish-people, 105–107; horse-people, 95, 98, 104–105; as prosthetic devices, 114. *See also* Horses; Prosthesis

Apotemnophilia, 169

Apoterpnophilia, 166, 169

Aristotelian poetics, 136, 139, 144, 239n45

Arthritis, 56, 71, 182, 4, 271n31

Autobiographies: Virginia Lee Counterman Acosta, 52, 64, 97, 118, 119, 172, 189; Charles H. Andrews, 70, 176; Ann Armstrong, 126; Tom Atkins, 33; Earl Bailly, 31, 222; Nancy Carter Baldwin, 37, 224, 264n122, 287n2; Paul Bates, 126, 152; Susan Hyun Sook Beidel, 58; Lorraine Beim, 118, 119, 204; Richard Chaput, 19, 126, 164; Jenny Danielson, 31; Owen Dixson, 31, 75, 103, 153, 163, 208; William O. Douglas, 95, 98; Garth Drabinsky, 30, 42, 45, 161; J. G. Farrell, 10, 71, 104, 150, 163, 169, 173–174; Mia Farrow, 30; Enid Foster, 14, 46, 73, 105, 146, 200, 218; Kenny Fries, 39; Hugh Gregory Gallagher, 193; Amy Gardner, 85; Robert F. Hall, 68, 143; Leonard Hawkins, 126; Peg Kehret, 5, 34; Tony Kemeny, 58, 132; Bert Kopperl, 131; Leonard Kriegel, 10; Edward Le